Researching Corporations and Global Health Governance

Researching Corporations and Global Health Governance

An Interdisciplinary Guide

Edited by
Kelley Lee and Benjamin Hawkins

ROWMAN &
LITTLEFIELD
INTERNATIONAL
London • New York

Published by Rowman & Littlefield International Ltd
Unit A, Whitacre Mews, 26-34 Stannary Street, London SE11 4AB
www.rowmaninternational.com

Rowman & Littlefield International Ltd. is an affiliate of Rowman & Littlefield
4501 Forbes Boulevard, Suite 200, Lanham, Maryland 20706, USA
With additional offices in Boulder, New York, Toronto (Canada), and Plymouth (UK)
www.rowman.com

British Library Cataloguing in Publication Data
A catalogue record for this book is available from the British Library
ISBN: HB 978-1-7834-8359-4
PB 978-1-7834-8360-0

Library of Congress Cataloging-in-Publication Data is Available

ISBN 978-1-78348-359-4 (cloth: alk. paper)
ISBN 978-1-78348-360-0 (pbk: alk. paper)
ISBN 978-1-78348-361-7 (electronic)

∞™ The paper used in this publication meets the minimum requirements of American National Standard for Information Sciences—Permanence of Paper for Printed Library Materials, ANSI/NISO Z39.48-1992.

Printed in the United States of America

Contents

Preface

This book is the product of long-standing and recent collaborations brought together and solidified through two workshops held at the Faculty of Health Sciences, Simon Fraser University, atop Burnaby Mountain (outside Vancouver, Canada). We organised the first workshop in 2012 as part of the Research Programme on Global Health Diplomacy, funded by the Rockefeller Foundation and led by Richard Smith and Kelley Lee at the London School of Hygiene and Tropical Medicine. Having examined the role of governments and civil society organisations in the negotiation of global health governance (GHG) arrangements, we recognised the need to better understand the role of for-profit actors, notably corporations. The first workshop brought together a small group of established scholars who generously shared their findings to date, and ideas for developing an expanded research agenda on corporations and GHG. This meeting was followed by a second workshop in 2013, funded by the Canadian Institutes for Health Research (CIHR Planning Grant No. 126667), which, with the participation of additional scholars, graduate students and postdoctoral fellows, significantly expanded this conversation. Following each workshop, we made extensive efforts to write a single paper setting out a definitive research agenda that would move thinking and practice beyond increasingly polarised debates in public health. However, given the diverse range of disciplines represented, theoretical perspectives and business sectors studied, we found that encapsulating the full breadth of the group into one journal article proved impossible to achieve.

This book project arose from this intellectual impasse. Workshop participants agreed that there was a shared concern about the relationship between corporations and emerging forms of GHG. A loosely structured Corporations and Global Health Research Network (COGHREN) was formed. However, like the parable of the blind men feeling an elephant, with each describing a different part of the same animal, the study of corporations has been approached to date from many different perspectives, generating findings within silos, and thus too often unshared across disciplines, geographies and/or sectors. Moreover, we recognised that more research is urgently needed on GHG per se, from a wider variety of disciplinary perspectives, to make sense of this rapidly shifting global governance sphere.

This book, and the accompanying volume, *Case Studies on Corporations and Global Health Governance: Impacts, Influence and Accountability*, is intended to foster this research need. Our aim is to encourage collaboration and dialogue in three ways. First, we want to bridge disciplinary divides and build greater understanding across discipline-focused and interdisciplinary scholars in such subject areas as anthropology, economics, history, political science, law and sociology, as well as interdisciplinary fields such as business studies, communications, development studies, international relations, public health and policy studies. Our goal is not simply to speak across disciplinary boundaries but to build understanding of how research on corporations is undertaken by, and located within, different disciplines.

Second, we seek to broaden analytical attention beyond the selected geographies and sectors, which have been the principal focus of research in this area to date. Given our understanding of global health as located within, and driven by, patterns of globalisation that have impacts both within and across all societies and populations, this requires a truly global approach to GHG. In doing so, we give due prominence to industrial sectors producing direct harms to human health such as tobacco, alcohol, food, pharmaceuticals and asbestos, which have been the focus of research to date on corporations and global health. Importantly, we also recognise the importance of indirect impacts generated by how corporations operate as particular forms of business organisations. This extends the industries relevant to GHG to such sectors as garment making, agriculture, gambling and the extractive industries (oil and gas, lead). In reality, many industries have the potential to generate both direct and indirect impacts on health, making the challenge of creating effective GHG more complex.

Third, we seek to build intergenerational bridges, between early-career scholars and established scholars, in this subject area. The workshops actively sought participation by graduate students and early-career scholars conducting research on corporations and global health, providing them with the opportunity to engage with 'battle-scarred' senior researchers. We identified the important need for capacity building through training, mentoring, peer reviewing and sharing of methodological approaches and data sources to create and support a new generation of interdisciplinary scholars. Many are currently working in relative isolation, and few, if any, come from the developing world where the health impacts of corporations can be most profound. The ensuing discussions also recognised the need to draw lessons from longer-standing bodies of knowledge, such as analysis of the tobacco industry, for research on other industries given limited attention to date. Opportunities for longitudinal and comparative analyses abound.

Acknowledgements

This book, and the accompanying volume, seeks to globalise the conversations begun at two workshops in Simon Fraser University. The editors would like to acknowledge the participants in these workshops who, while unable to contribute written material, substantively informed the conceptualisation and writing of these books: Doug Blanke, Dana Brown, Susan Erikson, Ann Florini, Lee Johnston, Catherine Jones, Bruce Lanphear, Anne Roemer-Mahler, Stacey Pigg and Richard Smith. For this volume, we would like to thank the additional support of Jappe Eckhardt, Chris Holden, Benoit Gomis, Eleanor Hutchinson, John Calvert, Julia Smith, Ross MacKenzie, Nora J. Kenworthy, Stefanie Ettelt, Thomas Novotny and Heather Wipfli for peer reviewing selected chapters. Chapter 2, 'Political Science', was strengthened by the helpful comments and suggestions of Patrick Fafard. Carol Anderson and Darrelle Markman provided assistance in reviewing the existing literatures for Chapter 7, 'Anthropology'.

The editors wish to gratefully acknowledge funding from the National Cancer Institute, US National Institutes of Health, Rockefeller Foundation and Canadian Institutes for Health Research which supported two workshops, editorial meetings and dedicated research time by the editors and several chapter authors. The editors wish to express their appreciation to Anna Reeve and Dhara Patel at Rowman & Littlefield International for understanding our vision for these books and providing guidance along the way to their completion. And our warm thanks to our colleagues Ela Gohil, Natalia Carrillo Botero and Linda van Vliet for important logistical support in organising the two workshops and their follow-up. Ela and Natalia, in particular, transcribed many hours of recorded sessions to ensure that the rich discussions were formally captured. Finally, the two books would not have been completed spot on time without the remarkably efficient and patient administrative support of Jennifer Fang.

List of Acronyms

ACA	Affordable Care Act
AMA	American Medical Association
ATC	American Tobacco Company
B&W	Brown & Williamson
BAT	British American Tobacco
BATA	British American Tobacco Australasia
CDC	Centers for Disease Control and Prevention
CEDAW	Convention on the Eradication of Discrimination Against Women
CEIL	Centre for International Environmental Law
CSO	civil society organisation
CSR	corporate social responsibility
DMP	data management plan
ECLT	Eliminating Child Labour in Tobacco Growing Foundation
EPA	Environmental Protection Agency
ERB	ethics review board
EU	European Union
FCTC	Framework Convention on Tobacco Control
FEC	Federal Election Commission
FOI	Freedom of Information
FTC	Federal Trade Commission
GAVI	Global Alliance for Vaccines and Immunization
GDP	gross domestic product
GEBN	Global Energy Balance Network
GHG	global health governance
GM	General Motors
HFCS	high-fructose corn syrup
IFICF	International Food Information Council Foundation

IO	international organisation
IP	intellectual property
IPA	Institute of Public Affairs
IPE	international political economy
IR	international relations
IRS	Internal Revenue Service
LMIC	low- and middle-income countries
MDG	Millennium Development Goal
MUP	minimum unit pricing
NCD	non-communicable disease
NGO	non-governmental organisation
OECD	Organisation for Economic Co-operation and Development
PAC	Political Action Committee
PM	Philip Morris
PPP	public–private partnerships
PR	public relations
QA/QC	Quality assurance and quality control
RCT	rational choice theory
SEC	Securities and Exchange Commission
TAC	transnational alcohol company
TEL	Leaded petroleum
TNC	transnational corporation
TPR	transnational private regulation
TTC	transnational tobacco company
UCSF	University of California, San Francisco
UK	United Kingdom
UN	United Nations
US	United States
WB	World Bank
WHO	World Health Organization
WTO	World Trade Organization

List of Illustrations

Chapter 1

Researching Corporations and Global Health Governance

Kelley Lee, Benjamin Hawkins and William H. Wiist

The increased importance of corporations in societies worldwide, since the end of the Second World War, has been widely acknowledged by scholars, policymakers and practitioners across a range of disciplines and fields (Sklair 2001; Fuchs 2007). This attention initially focused on the growing concentration of economic resources in the hands of a small number of increasingly large corporations within key industrial sectors (Gelles 2014). This economic might led to growing concerns about the capacity of corporations to influence political processes at the national level (Wilks 2013). By the late twentieth century, however, the accelerating processes of globalisation, and the consequent growth of transnational corporations (TNCs) whose business interests transcend national frontiers, led to increasing concerns about the exercise of corporate political power beyond and across states (Korten 2001; Bakan 2004; George 2015).

Concerns about the increasing political power of TNCs arise from three key developments. First, corporate activity has shifted into spheres traditionally deemed to be located in the public sector such as health and education (Wiist 2006). Corporations are no longer just economic actors but position themselves as key stakeholders in policy debates and are increasingly involved in the development and implementation of policy measures. Second, corporations are able to exert significant influence on policy at both the national level and global level (Fuchs 2007), including the United Nations through initiatives such as the Global Compact (Fall and Zahran 2010). Third, the proliferation of bilateral and regional trade agreements concluded during the early twenty-first century, potentially extending the legal standing and rights of corporations to challenge public policy making, may embed corporate political power further (Hawkins and Holden 2016). Through these processes, the interests of TNCs come to be institutionally protected and promoted, while the regulatory capacity of public institutions to act in the collective interest is undermined. This volume and the accompanying one (Kenworthy, Mackenzie and Lee 2016) are a response to these concerns, which aim to support a complete understanding of these developments and to inform more effective responses to them.

CORPORATIONS AND GLOBALISATION

While the focus of this book is on the role of corporations in global governance in the early twenty-first century, it is important to acknowledge the historical context of contemporary challenges. Over the course of the twentieth century, corporations became the most powerful form of economic organisation. As they outgrew their domestic markets, they looked beyond their home countries for 'emerging markets' in order to effectively compete in an increasingly globalised world economy. At the same time, high-income countries (particularly in Europe and North America) remain the headquarters of most of the largest TNCs. The resultant structure of the world economy, in many ways, is an extension of a colonial history whereby 'discovered' lands are taken, natural and human 'resources' are usurped and commodified and local societies are fundamentally altered to fit with the acquisitive and profit-seeking rationale of capitalism (Johnson 2013).

Corporate-led economic globalisation, in this form, has impacted all societies worldwide but is layered upon historically embedded inequities. The concepts of 'Global North' and 'Global South' reflect this perpetuation of colonial principles and practices (Stewart-Harawira 2005; George 2015). The former is advantaged by mobility of capital, labour and ideas, which are used to institutionally expand and reinforce privilege. Access to capital, favourable tax regimes, circumscribed regulatory oversight and public subsidies to support certain forms of economic activity are all examples of embedded advantages, which have enabled corporations to expand and extend their global reach (Farnsworth 2004, 2012, 2013).

The starting point for this book is that corporations are social constructs, defined and enabled by particular normative frameworks, and distributions of material power (Polanyi 1957). Direct forms of influence include lobbying, political campaign contributions and public communications. Corporate interests are furthered by networks among themselves, as to elite levels of state and market institutions (Vitali, Glattfelder and Battiston 2011). These networks extend to international organisations, such as the Group of Twenty, Organisation for Economic Co-operation and Development, World Economic Forum, World Trade Organisation, World Bank and International Monetary Fund (IMF), which govern the increasingly globalised world economy. In addition, corporations further their interests through the regulation of capital markets, forms of corporate governance, philanthropy, business associations and alliances, consultative bodies and public–private partnerships. As Polanyi (1957, 44) described, 'No economy prior to our own, even approximately [has been so] controlled and regulated by markets.'

While remarkably efficient at mobilising and generating absolute levels of wealth, corporations have created complex patterns of inequity within and across societies worldwide. The 'losers' from the late twentieth-century economic globalisation suffer undue levels of hardship, in part, from historical disadvantage and, in part, by bearing a disproportionate share of the consequent social and environmental costs. These costs include financial insecurity and instability, environmental degradation, reduced social protections and lack of access to basic needs. These detrimental effects have led to popular resistance worldwide, broadly described as an anti-globalisation movement, embracing indigenous people's protests against extractive industries (Dunbar-Ortiz 2014), Occupy protests against the extreme concentration of the world's wealth in a few hands, popular protests against trade agreements and austerity measures and the rise in support for radical left- and right-wing political parties. In short, corporate-led globalisation has restructured and divided societies at a pace that has raced ahead of the commensurate development of global governance institutions which are needed to, inter alia, regulate the adverse social and environmental impacts of corporate activity, address market failures and achieve a fair distribution of the costs and benefits arising from globalisation. The present weakness of such institutions is contributing to an increasingly unsustainable world order. Research to strengthen global governance, in ways that meet these complex challenges, must thus address the role of the corporation.

EXISTING LITERATURE ON CORPORATIONS AND GLOBAL HEALTH

Corporations have long been on the analytical radar of the health research community (Relman 1980). Debates about the appropriate balance between the public and private sectors in health financing and service provision date from the establishment of public health systems during the nineteenth century (Freeman 2000). The theme of health reform has been ongoing in high-income countries, intensifying during the debt crises of the 1970s and the rise of neoliberalism and intensifying with the global financial crisis since 2008. This period has seen widespread retrenchment of the public sector via policy measures ranging from privatisation to the introduction of market-inspired practices in the public sector (Hoffman 2003). While these processes were first evident in high-income settings, since the 1980s, they have spilled over to low- and middle-income countries. For example, the introduction of Structural Adjustment Programmes, as a conditionality of World Bank and IMF financing, pressured debtor governments to reduce the size of the public sector. The subsequent increase of private sector actors, including corporations, in the provision of key public services and utilities has received substantial research attention (Freeman 2000; Marquand 2004; Brezis and Wiist 2011).

The epidemiological shift, from communicable to non-communicable disease (NCD) burdens, has focused largely on the contribution to these trends of health-harming industries. The focus to date has largely been on documenting the impacts of certain industries, notably tobacco, alcohol and processed food, on health determinants and outcomes (Jahiel 2008; Stuckler et al. 2012; Baum et al. 2016). Not only the strategies that corporations use to produce and market goods and services with adverse health impacts but also their efforts to prevent or weaken regulation of their activities have become a major concern for the public health community (Michaels 2008; Wiist 2010; Freudenberg 2016). These concerns have divided the public health community on the risks and benefits of engaging with corporate actors (Alexander, Yach and Mensah 2011; Gilmore, Savell and Collin 2011).

A further source of health research on corporations has been the study of global health governance (GHG). GHG research that began in the 1990s heavily focused on the institutional arrangements for collective action. The strengths and weaknesses of specific international organisations, notably the World Health Organization (WHO), have been the subject of much pondering (Walt 1993; Forss, Stenson and Sterky 1996; Lee et al. 1996; Vaughan et al. 1996). By the early 2000s, the growing number of public–private partnerships led to scholarly efforts to understand what they do, assess their effectiveness at achieving global health goals and advise on how they might operate more effectively (Buse and Walt 2000; Widdus 2001). By the mid-2000s, an important distinction began to be drawn, between private sector actors as providers of health financing and services, on the one hand, and participants in rule-making (governance), on the other (Ståhl et al. 2006). Buse and Lee (2005), for example, review the diverse roles of the 'commercial sector' in GHG. A rich literature has since emerged, documenting and interrogating how corporate influence is exerted in GHG (Gill and Benatar 2016).

PURPOSE OF THIS BOOK

This book seeks to support an expanded research agenda on corporations and GHG. This is a complex endeavour, both intellectually and practically, requiring multi-disciplinary perspectives, conceptual and theoretical innovation, mixed-method approaches and diverse data sources. The book is an introductory guide to how researchers in different scholarly disciplines approach this subject and how further research could be undertaken to strengthen knowledge and practice. More specifically, as the companion volume to *Case Studies on Corporations and Global Health Governance* (Kenworthy, MacKenzie and Lee 2016), this book seeks to make three distinct contributions.

First, although research on corporations is being undertaken within many fields and disciplines, a detailed study of corporations and GHG is limited. The book aims to strengthen understanding, and support the development, of new research on a critical aspect of global health at a time when policymakers seek to build more effective forms of collective action. Second, much of the existing literature has been polarised and even deadlocked (Hernandez-Aguado and Zaragoza 2016), with advocates for more public–private partnerships (Majestic 2009; Sturchio and Goel 2012; Quelch 2016) lined up against critics of corporate involvement in policy making and implementation (Richter 2001; Benatar, Bill and Bakker 2011; Hastings 2012). This volume and the accompanying one are intended to stimulate the new application of theories and concepts, and to generate empirical evidence, for understanding and regulating the health-related activities of corporations as a core function of GHG. Third, research on corporations and GHG to date has tended to focus on selected and individual industries. The result is fragmentation of research and public policy. There is a clear need to bring together diverse scholarships across time, space, populations and industries (Brownell and Warner 2009; Dorfman et al. 2012), perhaps through the application of complex systems theory (Hill 2011; Haffeld 2012), in order to draw together findings about the corporation as a health-impacting societal institution (Wiist 2006). Ultimately, the books aim to help rebalance the institutional checks and balances required for sustainable human and planetary health.

KEY CONCEPTS AND TERMINOLOGY

Research on corporations and GHG is hindered, to some degree, by conceptual inconsistency and confusion. This is due, in part, to differences across academic disciplines in the ways in which frequently used terms are defined. While acknowledging disciplinary differences, we provide definitions for key concepts and terms used in this book. In some cases, it is challenging and even impossible to fully reconcile different scholarly traditions and values. Moreover, the study and practice of GHG is divided by diverse normative frameworks (McInnes and Lee 2014). The definitions provided are starting points for this book, which, as part of an expanded research agenda, encourages reflexivity by researchers on how the subject is studied.

The term *private sector* is a useful starting point for locating the subject of this book, which can be broadly defined as those parts of a society that are not a direct part of, or under the control of, government. The private sector can, in turn, be divided into organisations that operate as for-profit and not-for-profit. Buse and Lee (2005, 6) define the commercial sector as the former, namely 'organisations that seek to make profits for their owners (e.g. firms increasing shareholder value). Profit, or a return on investment, is the central defining feature of the commercial sector'. This distinction can often be left unclear, and even conflated, in health research. For example, Sturchio and Goel (2012, 3) appear to refer to both for-profit and not-for-profit organisations when they write, 'The central question is not *whether* the private sector has a role to play . . . in many developing countries the majority of health care services are already delivered through the private sector – but *how* to put the particular skills of the private sector to best use.'

The term *corporation* most often evokes images of large companies, like Coca-Cola or Sony, operating and pursuing markets worldwide. However, it is important to define the specific nature of the corporation, as a particular type of business entity, if we are to understand how it has grown so powerful and what regulatory responses are needed to protect global health. The corporation as an economic institution first emerged in the sixteenth century (Nace 2003, 23). There are many ways to structure the ownership of a business: state or private; sole proprietorship, partnership or limited partnership; for-profit or not-for-profit; limited liability; and corporation (and cooperative). As Bakan (2004, 6) describes:

> Unlike the prevailing partnership form, in which relatively small groups of men, bonded together by personal loyalties and mutual trust, pooled their resources to set up businesses they ran as well as owned, the corporation separated ownership from management – one group of people, directors and managers, ran the firm, while another group, shareholders, owned it.

This book is thus primarily concerned with research about large, for-profit corporations whose stock is publicly traded (or privately held) and whose operations transcend national boundaries.

The term *global health* is used to mean health issues that fall within one of four categories:

1. *Transboundary or crossborder problems*, which originate in one state but have ramifications for others (e.g. communicable disease outbreak)
2. *Commons problems*, which concern disputed access and/or use of international commons (e.g. intellectual property rights over DNA sequencing)

3. *Shared problems*, which are widely experienced across many geographical contexts due to the accelerated globalisation of unhealthy lifestyles, urban environments and cultural practices (e.g. NCDs) and
4. *Planetary problems*, which arise from the actions of individuals and populations in many countries. These actions, such as burning fossil fuels, have cumulative effects that are then detrimental to all (i.e. climate change). This category of problem requires collective action to address but, arguably, is also the most difficult on which to achieve policy agreement because of the broad responsibility for causing the problem.

Thus, this book is concerned with not only corporate actors but corporations of sufficient size and reach to affect global health determinants and outcomes. In this respect, we are largely, although not exclusively, interested in corporations frequently designated by the prefix *Big* – as in Big Tobacco, Big Food and Big Pharma. While some dispute the relative importance of major corporations to global health (Alexander, Yach and Mensah 2011), others dismiss them as wholly incompatible with public interests (Stuckler et al. 2012).

Finally, the term *global health governance* lies at the heart of this book. Beyond documenting the impacts of corporations on global health, as defined earlier, this book is about the formal and informal rules, standards, norms and principles governing global health determinants and outcomes (Dodgson et al. 2002; Lee and Kamradt-Scott 2014). Formal governance is concerned with the rules and procedures of treaties, traditionally adopted by international organisations, themselves established by international treaty, having three or more members, and maintaining a permanent secretariat (Colgan and Van de Graaf 2013). Moreover, formal governance can be contained within binding (e.g. International Health Regulations, World Trade Organization Agreement on Trade-Related Intellectual Property Rights and WHO Framework Convention on Tobacco Control) or non-binding (e.g. WHO Global Code of Practice on the International Recruitment of Health Personnel, Pandemic Influenza Preparedness Framework) instruments. Informal governance is 'the systematic influence of unwritten rules, shared expectations or norms within international organizations that substantially modify or substitute for formal treaty provisions. Informal governance prevails when informal influence overrides legal procedures, or when important rules are unwritten' (Stone 2013, 123). While scholars disagree on why informal governance arises, and have largely focused on the role of states in international organisations, there is consensus about the increased, and even greater, importance of informal influence in global governance (Wiist 2011, 207–8). As per this statement, GHG embraces institutions with an explicit health mandate (e.g. WHO, United Nations Programme on HIV/AIDS), with health as part of a broader mandate (e.g. World Bank) and with mandates that impact on health determinants and outcomes (e.g. WTO).

AN EXPANDED RESEARCH AGENDA ON CORPORATIONS AND GHG

This book aims to support research that improves our understanding of the role of corporations in formal and informal GHG. As described earlier, existing public health research has largely focused to date on measuring the health impacts of specific products, processes or sectors. For the purpose of strengthening research, this book supports an expanded agenda that conceptualises the relationship between corporations and GHG in three main ways.

First, there is need for research on *corporations as subjects of GHG*. Building on evidence of the adverse health impacts of corporations worldwide, what global governance is needed to mitigate the adverse health impacts of corporations (e.g. formal treaties, soda taxes, plain packaging)? There is much evidence that regulatory measures at the global level are currently sparse, poorly resourced and weakly implemented. Key questions to address include the following:

- How can corporations operating across jurisdictions, in an increasingly globalised world economy, be effectively regulated to protect and promote public interests?
- What forms of governance are needed to address specific industries, products, impacts and so on?
- How should the capacity of public health actors be strengthened to enable effective regulation of corporations in ways that protect and promote population health (Stuckler and Nestle 2012)?
- How do corporations evade GHG by venue shopping and other strategies?

Second, there is need for research on *corporations as participants in GHG*. The study of public policy, including health policy, is traditionally focused on state actors and intergovernmental organisations (Strange 1996). These approaches are out of step with the rise in importance in recent decades of non-state actors, including corporations (George 2015). Influence of GHG may be exerted through a variety of means – financial contributions, public–private partnerships, political lobbying of governments and knowledge generation – which serve private interests. This raises the following research questions:

- How have corporations formally and informally shaped the agendas of public and private institutions involved in GHG in ways that serve corporate interests (Dorfman et al. 2012; Shiffman 2014)?

- When and how, if at all, should corporate actors engage with GHG? Can and, if so, when, might corporate and public interests coincide?
- To what extent should public institutions, or those ostensibly seeking to serve the public interest (e.g. non-governmental organisations), accept funding and endorse the corporate social responsibility activities of, or even directly partner with, corporations (Quelch 2016)?
- How do we ensure good governance (transparency, accountability, democratic principles) in a world in which powerful corporations seek to influence public policy making?
- What checks and balances are needed to prevent undue influence by corporations seeking to further their private interests? What protections are needed against conflicts of interest in priority setting?

Third, there is need for research on *corporations as GHG* or the shift of corporations from being rule-takers to rule-makers. Corporations have traditionally been given limited formal authority in intergovernmental organisations. However, their arms-length relationship with GHG may be steadily changing in some regulatory areas. One trend is towards growing corporate involvement to transnational private regulation (TPR) defined as ‘regimes that regulate the conduct of private actors across jurisdictional boundaries primarily through standards, which are voluntary, at least as a matter of formal law’ (Cafaggi 2014, 8). TPR may emerge when international regulatory cooperation fails (e.g. Marine Stewardship Council), when markets are characterised by fast-paced change and highly technical content (e.g. Internet Corporation for Assigned Names and Numbers) or when expertise is needed from private actors (e.g. Basel Committee on Banking Supervision). As May (2015, 2) writes, ‘The global corporation itself has a significant governance role within its own international structures, and we can usefully consider this as a form of global governance in itself.’ Moreover, corporations may be gaining new standing as legal ‘persons’ with the right to challenge public policies, under a growing number of bilateral and regional trade and investment agreements, deemed harmful to their interests. The potential chilling effect on governments, seeking to strengthen public policies to protect human health, in effect gives corporations a new degree of regulatory power. These developments raise the following research questions:

- How are corporations exercising authority in GHG on specific regulatory issues?
- To what extent is a shift in authority, from public to private actors, occurring in GHG?
- What distribution of authority in GHG is appropriate to protect public interests?

STRUCTURE OF THE BOOK

The chapters in this book are organised into two parts. Part I comprises chapters on ten subject areas or disciplines relevant to research on corporations: political science; international political economy; social policy; history; criminology; anthropology; public health; and media, communication and business studies. While this selection of subject areas aims to include those with the potential to offer key insights, the list is not comprehensive. Other fields, such as sociology, geography and psychology, would undoubtedly offer further insights. The aim of Part I is to demonstrate the opportunity, and indeed need, for multidisciplinary research on an increasingly dominant form of social organisation in contemporary society. Given that the book is aimed at non-specialists in the disciplines covered, the chapters begin by identifying key debates in each discipline, before examining how corporations are conceptualised within them. The chapters then discuss key research questions on corporations arising within each discipline, with particular attention paid to how they might contribute to a critical research agenda. This includes key frameworks, concepts and theories offered. Examples of empirical research undertaken within the discipline are discussed to illustrate its contribution to research on corporations and GHG, along with ideas for further research.

The chapters in Part II are intended to provide practical information on specific methods, data sources and research needs when undertaking analysis of corporations and GHG. Four chapters provide the use of methods – key informant interviewing, ethnography, oral history and participant observation. The next six chapters cover sources of data, which researchers can draw on to better understand the role of corporations in GHG – data on corporate influence of democratic processes, internal company documents, social media, business and financial data, freedom of information requests and grey literature. The final two chapters deal with legal and ethical issues when conducting research on corporations, and how to develop an effective data management and security plan. Practical examples are provided in each chapter, along with three further readings for readers seeking deeper understanding.

With these two volumes, the editors and authors hope to stimulate an expanded research agenda focused on corporations as subjects of GHG, corporations as participants in GHG and corporations as GHG. The two books seek to achieve this much-needed task by bringing together scholars with multidisciplinary backgrounds and wide-ranging expertise on different industries. In doing so, we are encouraging readers to venture from their familiar intellectual terrains and meet this important challenge by drawing upon diverse perspectives, analytical methods and data sources. This creates opportunities, not only to deepen our understanding through shared learning but also to bring our knowledge together in a common task. This task is ultimately to support effective GHG in a world dominated by the remarkable growth of large TNCs.

REFERENCES

Alexander, Eleanore, Derek Yach and George A. Mensah. 2011. 'Major Multinational Food and Beverage Companies and Informal Sector Contributions to Global Food Consumption: Implications for Nutrition Policy'. *Globalization and Health* 7: 26.

Bakan, Joel. 2004. *The Corporation.* London: Penguin Books.

Baum Frances, David Sanders, Matt Fisher, Julia Anaf, Nicholas Freudenberg, Sharon Friel, Ronald Labonté, Leslie London, Carlos Monteiro, Alex Scott-Samuel and Amit Sen. 2016. 'Assessing the Health Impact of Transnational Corporations: Its Importance and a Framework'. *Globalization and Health* 12: 27.

Benatar, Solomon, Stephen Gill and Isabella Bakker. 2011. 'Global Health and the Global Economic Crisis'. *American Journal of Public Health* 101(4): 646–53.

Brezis, Mayer and William H. Wiist. 2011. 'Vulnerability of Health to Market Forces'. *Medical Care* 49(3): 232–39.

Brownell, Kelly and Kenneth Warner. 2009. 'The Perils of Ignoring History: Big Tobacco Played Dirty and Millions Died. How Similar Is Big Food?' *Milbank Quarterly* 87(1): 259–94.

Buse, Kent and Kelley Lee. 2005. *Business and Global Health Governance*. London: Centre on Global Change and Health, London School of Hygiene and Tropical Medicine.

Buse, Kent and Gill Walt. 2000. 'Global Public–Private Partnerships: Part I – A New Development in Health?' *Bulletin of the World Health Organization* 78(4): 549–61.

Cafaggi, Fabrizio. 2014. 'A Comparative Analysis of Transnational Private Regulation: Legitimacy, Quality, Effectiveness and Enforcement'. European University Institute. http://papers.ssrn.com/sol3/papers.cfm?abstract_id=2449223.

Colgan, Jeff and Thijs Van de Graaf. 2015. 'Mechanisms of Informal Governance: Evidence from the IEA'. *Journal of International Relations and Development* 18(4): 455–81.

Dodgson, Richard, Kelley Lee & Nick Drager. 2002. '*Global health governance: A conceptual review.*' Department for Health in Sustainable Development, World Health Organization, Geneva.

Dorfman, Lori, Andrew Cheyne, Lissy C. Friedman, Asiya Wadud and Mark Gottlieb. 2012. 'Soda and Tobacco Industry Corporate Social Responsibility Campaigns: How Do They Compare?' *PLoS Medicine* 9(6): e1001241.

Dunbar-Ortiz, Roxanne. 2014. *An Indigenous Peoples' History of the United States.* Boston, MA: Beacon Press.

Fall, Papa Louis and Mohamed Mounir Zahran. 2010. *United Nations Corporate Partnerships: The Role and Functioning of the Global Compact.* Geneva: UN Joint Inspection Unit.

Farnsworth, Kevin. 2004. *Corporate Power and Social Policy in a Global Economy.* Bristol, UK: Policy Press.

Farnsworth, Kevin. 2012. *Social versus Corporate Welfare: Competing Needs and Interests within the Welfare State*. New York: Palgrave Macmillan.

Farnsworth, Kevin. 2013. 'Bringing Corporate Welfare In'. *Journal of Social Policy* 42(1): 1–22.

Forss, K., Bo Stenson and Goran Sterky. 1996. 'The Future of Global Health Cooperation: Designing a New World Health Organization'. *Current Issues in Public Health* 2(3): 138–42.

Freeman, Richard. 2000. *The Politics of Health in Europe*. Manchester, UK: Manchester University Press.

Freudenberg, Nicholas. 2016. *Lethal but Legal: Corporations, Consumption and Protecting Public Health*. Oxford, UK: Oxford University Press.

Fuchs, Doris. 2007. *Business Power in Global Governance*. Boulder, CO: Lynne Rienner Publishers.

Gelles, David. 2014. 'Mega-Mergers Popular Again on Wall Street'. *New York Times*, 17 November. http://dealbook.nytimes.com/2014/11/17/mega-mergers-popular-again-on-wall-street/?emc=edit_th_20141118&nl=todaysheadlines&nlid=68658563&_r=0.

George, Susan. 2015. *Shadow Sovereigns: How Global Corporations Are Seizing Power*. Cambridge, UK: Polity Press.

Gill, Stephen and Solomon Benatar. 2016. 'Global Health Governance and Global Power: A Critical Commentary on the Lancet-University of Oslo Commission Report'. *International Journal of Health Services* 46(2): 346–65.

Gilmore, Anna, Emily Savell and Jeff Collin. 2011. 'Public Health, Corporations and the New Responsibility Deal: Promoting Partnerships with Vectors of Disease?' *Journal of Public Health* 33(1): 2–4.

Haffeld, Just. 2012. 'Facilitative Governance: Transforming Global Health through Complexity Theory'. *Global Public Health* 7(5): 452–64.

Hastings, Gerard. 2012. 'Why Corporate Power Is a Public Health Priority'. *BMJ* 345: e5124.

Hawkins, Benjamin and Christopher Holden. 2016. 'A Corporate Veto on Health Policy? Global Constitutionalism and Investor–State Dispute Settlement'. *Journal of Health Politics, Policy and* Law (epub). doi:10.1215/03616878-3632203.

Hernandez-Aguado, Ildefonso and G.A. Zaragoza. 2016. 'Support of Public–Private Partnerships in Health Promotion and Conflicts of Interest'. *BMJ Open* 6(4): e009342. doi:10.1136/bmjopen-2015-009342.

Hill, Peter. 2011. 'Understanding Global Health Governance as a Complex Adaptive System'. *Global Public Health* 6(6): 593–605.

Hoffman, Beatrix. 2003. 'Health Care Reform and Social Movements in the United States'. *American Journal of Public Health* 93(1): 75–85.

Jahiel, Rene. 2008. 'Corporation-Induced Diseases, Upstream Epidemiologic Surveillance, and Urban Health'. *Journal of Urban Health* 85(4): 517–31.

Johnson, Walter. 2013. *River of Dark Dreams: Slavery and Empire in the Cotton Kingdom*. Cambridge, MA: Belknap Press of Harvard University Press.

Kenworthy, Nora, Ross MacKenzie and Kelley Lee, eds. 2016. *Case Studies on Corporations and Global Health Governance*. London: Rowman and Littlefield International.

Korten, David. 2001. *When Corporations Rule the World*, 2nd edition. Bloomfield, CT: Kumarian Press.

Lee, Kelley, Susan Collinson, Gill Walt and Lucy Gilson. 1996. 'Who Should Be Doing What in International Health: A Confusion of Mandates in the United Nations?' *BMJ* 312 (7026): 302–7.

Lee, Kelley and Adam Kamradt-Scott. 2014. 'The Multiple Meanings of Global Health Governance: A Call for Conceptual Clarity'. *Globalization and Health* 10(28). doi:10.1186/1744-8603-10-28.

Majestic, Elizabeth. 2009. 'Public Health's Inconvenient Truth: The Need to Create Partnerships with the Business Sector'. *Preventing Chronic Disease* 6(2): A39.

Marquand, David. 2004. *Decline of the Public*. Cambridge, UK: Policy Press.

May, Christopher. 2015. 'Who's in Charge? Corporations as Institutions of Global Governance'. *Palgrave Communications* 1: 15042. doi:10.1057/palcomms.2015.42.

McInnes, Colin and Kelley Lee, eds. 2014. *Framing Global Health Governance*. London: Routledge.

Michaels, David. 2008. *Doubt Is Their Product: How Industry's Assault on Science Threatens Your Health*. New York: Oxford University Press.

Nace, Ted. 2003. *Gangs of America: The Rise of Corporate Power and the Disabling of Democracy*. San Francisco, CA: Berrett-Koehler.

Polanyi, Karl. 1957. *The Great Transformation*. Boston, MA: Beacon Press.

Quelch, John, ed. 2016. *Consumers, Corporations, and Public Health*. Oxford, UK: Oxford University Press.

Relman, Arnold. 1980. 'The New Medical-Industrial Complex'. *New England Journal of Medicine* 303(17): 963–70.

Richter, Judith. 2001. *Holding Corporations Accountable*. London: Zed Books.

Shiffman, Jeremy. 2014. 'Knowledge, moral claims, and the exercise of power in global health.' International Journal of Health Policy and Management 3(6): 297–9.

Sklair, Leslie. 2001. *The Transnational Capitalist Class*. Malden, MA: Blackwell Publishing.

Ståhl, Timo, Matthias Wismar, Eeva Ollila, Eero Lahtinen and Kimmo Leppo, eds. 2006. *Health in All Policies: Prospects and Potentials*. Helsinki, Finland: Ministry of Social Affairs and Health.

Stewart-Harawira, Makere. 2005. *The New Imperial Order: Indigenous Responses to Globalization*. London: Zed Books.

Stone, Randall. 2013. 'Informal Governance in International Organizations: Introduction to the Special Issue'. *Review of International Organizations* 8(2): 121–36.

Strange, Susan. 1996. *The Retreat of the State: The Diffusion of Power in the World Economy*. Cambridge, UK: Cambridge University Press.

Stuckler, David, Martin McKee, Shah Ebrahim and Sanjay Basu. 2012. 'Manufacturing Epidemics: The Role of Global Producers in Increased Consumption of

Unhealthy Commodities Including Processed Foods, Alcohol, and Tobacco'. *PLoS Medicine* 9(6): e1001235.

Stuckler, David and Marion Nestle. 2012. 'Big Food, Food Systems, and Global Health'. *PLoS Medicine* 9(6): e1001242.

Sturchio, Jeffrey and Akash Goel. 2012. *The Private-Sector Role in Public Health, Reflections on the New Global Architecture in Health.* Washington, DC: Center for Strategic and International Studies.

Vaughan, J. Patrick, Sigrun Mogedal, Stein-Erik Kruse, Kelley Lee, Gill Walt and K. de Wilde. 1996. 'Financing the World Health Organization: Global Importance of Extrabudgetary Funds'. *Health Policy* 35(3): 229–45.

Vitali, Stefania, James Glattfelder and Stefano Battiston. 2011. 'The Network of Global Corporate Control'. *PLoS ONE* 6(10): e25995. doi:10.1371/journal.pone.0025995.

Walt, Gill. 1993. 'WHO under Stress: Implications for Health Policy'. *Health Policy* 24(2): 125–44.

Widdus, Roy. 2001. 'Public–Private Partnerships for Health: Their Main Targets, Their Diversity, and Their Future Directions'. *Bulletin of the World Health Organization* 79(8): 713–20.

Wiist, William H. 2006. 'Public Health and the Anticorporate Movement: Rationale and Recommendations'. *American Journal of Public Health* 96(8): 1370–75.

Wiist, William H. 2010. *The Bottom Line or Public Health: Tactics Corporations Use to Influence Health and Health Policy, and What We Can Do to Counter Them.* New York: Oxford University Press.

Wiist, William H. 2011. 'The Corporate Play Book, Health and Democracy: The Snack Food and Beverage Industry's Tactics in Context'. In *Sick Societies: Responding to the Global Challenge of Chronic Disease*, edited by David Stuckler and Karen Siegel, 204–16. New York: Oxford University Press.

Wilks, Stephen. 2013. *The Political Power of the Business Corporation.* Cheltenham, UK: Edward Elgar.

Part I

DISCIPLINARY APPROACHES TO ANALYSING CORPORATIONS

Chapter 2

Political Science

Benjamin Hawkins

Political science is the branch of the social sciences which focuses on systems of governance and the conduct of politics. While the term *political science* is common in the United States, and much of the rest of the world, in the United Kingdom, the subject is often referred to as *political studies* or simply *politics*. For the purpose of this chapter, we shall treat these terms as synonyms. Political scientists are interested in a range of themes and issues related to the conduct of politics, systems of government and the behaviour of political actors including political parties, trade unions, civil society actors (e.g. charities and non-governmental organisations [NGOs]) and voters. Many study public opinion and voting trends, public administration (sometimes referred to as *government*), while others focus on the structure of political systems from a comparative perspective (comparative politics). The allocation, distribution and exercise of power, within political communities, is the key concept of study for political scientists.

Political scientists focus on politics not only at the national level but also at the subnational and supranational levels (i.e. above the national level). For example, scholars working on subnational politics may focus on political processes at the state or provincial level within federal systems (e.g. Germany, Canada and the United States), within autonomous regions in devolved polities (e.g. Spain) and within even municipalities and local levels of government (e.g. local councils). The conduct of politics at the supranational level is the focus of the sub-discipline of international relations (IR). While some scholars seek to differentiate IR from political science, underlining the multidisciplinary nature of the former, political science and IR share a common concern with governance processes and the exercise of power. As the name suggests, IR focuses principally on the conduct of politics *between* national governments, including how these relationships are mediated by regional and international organisations such as the United Nations (UN) system, and World Trade Organization (WTO) and the African Union. Increasingly, IR has taken account of other non-state actors, active in the supranational context, including international charities, NGOs and expert networks. Chapter 3 in this volume examines the contribution of international political economy (IPE), a specific area of focus for IR scholars, to the study of corporations and global health in more detail. Consequently, this chapter focuses on the analysis of politics at the national level and below, and examines the interaction between national and global politics. The interrelationship between different levels of decision making has led scholars to characterise current policy making arrangements as a system of multi-level governance.

A further sub-discipline of political science, policy studies, focuses on the development and implementation of public policy in a range of areas (e.g. health, transportation, town planning). Chapter 4 discusses the contribution of one specific area of policy studies, social policy, to the study of corporations and health, and should be read in conjunction with this chapter. This chapter highlights other examples of public policy that have been studied by political scientists and are relevant to the study of corporations and/or health. This chapter also addresses attempts by political scientists to theorise the impact of corporations on politics and provide frameworks for the analysis of specific policy debates.

A wide range of approaches are available to the study of politics, which reflect different research foci and different assumptions about the factors shaping politics. For example, institutionalists study how political institutions and the organs of the state are structured and function, and how these structures, and the wider political and constitutional systems in which they are located, shape the political process (Schmidt 2008; Peters 2012). Another influential approach is rational choice theory (RCT), which seeks to explain politics as the result of the individual-level preferences and interests of policy actors and voters (see Dowding 2005). In the field of public administration, public choice theorists have used the principles of RCT in an attempt to explain the functioning of government, and other public bodies, including the civil service and the National Health Service in the United Kingdom (Dunleavy 2013). More recently, scholars have attempted to combine the insights of institutionalism and RCT through the development of rational-choice institutionalism, which recognises both the intentional behaviour and motivation of actors and the constraints placed on their behaviour by the institutional contexts in which they are located.

Political scientists may also make different assumptions about the nature of the political world (ontology) and our access to knowledge about that world (epistemology). The differences among these approaches are reflected in their understanding of the scientific process. On the one hand, what we may term positivist approaches assume the objective of political science, which is analogous to that of the natural sciences – to uncover universal laws about the political world which can explain events over time and space, and predict similar future events with a high degree of accuracy. These approaches undertake empirical observation of events and practices to corroborate or disprove hypotheses and refine theoretical models. On the other hand, post-positivists emphasise the fundamentally different nature of the social and natural worlds, and the impossibility of applying the naturalism paradigm to the world on intelligent reflexive human actors (Fischer 2003). The aim is not to uncover putative laws of the social world but to seek to understand the meaningful practices in which policy actors and citizens are engaged in the conduct of politics. They seek to render these practices comprehensible and, in so doing, explain them in terms of the meanings they have to the actors involved. Political science does not seek to ape the natural sciences but more closely resembles sociological or anthropological research (see Chapter 7).

Political scientists employ a range of qualitative and quantitative methods common to other social science disciplines. These include structured and semi-structured interviews, focus groups, surveys, historical or archival research, document analysis, discourse and narrative analysis, (participant) observation and statistical analysis of both primary and secondary data sets (see Bryman 2001; Johnson and Reynolds 2007, 2012). The choice of methods used is closely related to the researcher's ontological-epistemological position and thus the type of research question(s) to be answered. Researchers working from a post-positive perspective, concerned with the meaning of specific practices, are inclined to use semi-structured interviews and other qualitative data sources to understand self-interpretations of policy actors. Positivist approaches are often associated with quantitative methodologies and macro-level statistical analysis. However, it is possible to conduct research from diverse perspectives, with different methods applied in ways keeping with the underlying assumptions of the researcher. Many of the methods, and potential data sources, used by political scientists are examined in greater detail in Part II of this volume.

POLITICAL SCIENCE AND GLOBAL HEALTH

Bernier and Clavier (2011) have called for a greater engagement by public health researchers with the concepts and approaches of political science. Their aim is to facilitate a move away from traditional concerns with the effectiveness of and supporting evidence for a given policy measure to a more nuanced, political understanding of how health policies are made and implemented. Thus, scholars of public policy, often housed within political science departments, have undertaken extensive analyses of health policy in different contexts. However, the contribution of political science to *global* health may be less obvious than its contribution to understanding health and health policy *within* nation-states. This section thus focuses on the interaction between the national and supranational levels as a key determinant of global health policy. National health policies and health systems, as well as the wider political and institutional contexts in which these are situated, are vital in understanding the dynamics of current debates in global health, and the effectiveness and feasibility of global health programmes.

A good example is how national political factors are of vital importance in understanding the commitment to overseas aid and development spending in donor states, a key factor affecting global health financing. The analytical lens of political science can be used to understand the wider orientation of national governments to development issues and the global health objectives they pursue. For example, in the industrialised world, what factors determine the ongoing commitment of countries to the Global Alliance for Vaccines and Immunization – a global health partnership that funds vaccination programmes for children in the world's poorest countries – during times of austerity and cutbacks across government? How can we explain the failure of certain governments to honour aid spending commitments made to the Millennium Development Goals (MDGs), while others comply? What explains shifts in government commitment between the MDGs and the Sustainable Development Goals which superseded them? In low- and middle-income countries (LMICs), meanwhile, what explains some countries' prioritising health needs and health systems development, while others do not? Political scientists aim to answer these questions by examining the institutional and political contexts in which these policy decisions are made.

National governments also play a key role in shaping global health policy through international organisations. For example, France as a member state of the European Union (EU), World Health Organization (WHO) and WTO (as well as a permanent member of the UN Security Council which plays a role in health crises) is a key actor shaping the policy outputs of these bodies, along with other countries. The insights of political scientists, on the domestic political contexts of key member states, can be vital in understanding the positions they adopt in these international forums and thus how they shape global health. The relationship between national politics and the position adopted by member states within international forums was perhaps most clearly theorised by the liberal-intergovernmentalist analyses of the EU (Moravcsik 1993), although a similar approach is applicable to decision making in other international forums (e.g. WHO). For liberal-intergovernmentalists, the vector of European integration is explained by the policy preferences of (the most powerful) EU member states. However, to understand the positions adopted by member-state governments, it is necessary to look at the preferences of key policy actors in the domestic arena.

While national governments are key actors in shaping policy at the global level, the converse is also true; politics at the national and subnational levels is in turn shaped and constrained by agreements made at higher levels of governance. Countries (and subnational entities) play a key role in implementing regional and global health policies. As a consequence of the interconnected processes of globalisation, including the development of international organisations, national governments are now embedded in a complex and asymmetric system of multi-level governance in which the decisions taken and the political considerations pertinent at one level of authority both shape and are shaped by processes occurring at other levels of government.

For example, in Germany, key health policy decisions, such as smoking bans in bars and restaurants, are taken at the state (*Länder*) level, while decisions about statutory health insurance, standards and quality of health care, as well as smoking bans in places under federal control (e.g. train stations), are taken at the national (federal level). In addition, the EU has competence in health policy issues and passes laws in other policy areas, such as the single market, which affect health (e.g. mandatory warning labels on cigarette packets), and must be implemented by member states (Greer 2009). International organisations like the WHO, WTO, International Monetary Fund (IMF) and World Bank are further sources of rules and agreements, which impact significantly on domestic health policies. This is evident with the structural adjustment programmes put in place by the IMF and World Bank during the 1970s–1990s, which impacted dramatically the provision of health services in LMICs, and are now being replicated in Europe (Greer 2014). Chapter 11 in the accompanying volume to this discusses multi-level governance further (Holden and Hawkins 2016).

POLITICAL SCIENCE AND CORPORATE ACTORS

The political and economic power of large corporations is now widely acknowledged, but the degree of attention they have received from political scientists is out of keeping with the extent of their political and economic influence. As Wilks (2013, 2) writes:

> Until very recently there has been little systematic analysis of the impact of the business corporation on contemporary society. In particular political scientists have been myopic on the subject to the point that instead of mountains of scholarly achievements we have a few oases in an arid landscape.

In the study of global governance, Doris Fuchs (2007) has identified a similar lack of engagement by scholars with the political power of business. She has sought to address this gap in the literature by mapping the different ways in which businesses engage with governance processes since the 1970s. Her analyses reveal that business has become a key actor in global governance. This increased attention to corporations, as political actors, is in keeping with scholars, such as Robert Cox (1981) and Susan Strange (2000), who have examined the role of corporations as part of a wider shift, within IR, to emphasise the role of non-state actors within global governance (see Nye and Keohane 1971).

Despite relatively limited engagement by political scientists, the study of corporations has spawned a number of theoretical perspectives for understanding the influence of corporations on political, and especially governmental, institutions and processes. For example, pluralism sees corporations as one type of interest group among many, attempting to influence the content of government policy, whose success in shaping the policy terrain varies over time (see Vogel 1989). From this perspective, the main tool of the corporation seeking influence is political lobbying (Wilks 2013). For pluralists such as Vogel (1989), the influence of corporations over government is often overstated. Likewise, Grant (1993) argues that the success of business in influencing policy is often limited by a firm's inability to define its interests clearly, and to collaborate with similar market actors to articulate their positioning to government collectively. Moreover, not all businesses are equal, with some (large, strategically important) firms enjoying greater access to decision makers and influence over policy debates than others (Coen 2009).

Others working from an elitist or structuralist perspective have argued that corporations, because of the nature of the specific tasks they perform within the capitalist system, are uniquely influential political actors to which governments and policymakers grant privileged attention (Lindblom 1977; see also Hay 1999). As Lindblom (1977, 175) states:

> Any government official who understands the requirements of his position and the responsibilities that market-oriented systems throw on businessmen will therefore grant them a privileged position. He does not need to be bribed, duped or pressed to do so . . . he simply understands . . . that public affairs in market-oriented systems are in the hands of two groups of leaders, government and business.

From this perspective, the influence of corporations emanates, not from their influencing strategies (i.e. lobbying) but from the structural position they occupy in the economy and the core systemic tasks they perform. The structuralist perspective implies a necessity or inevitability for corporate influence, which is underplayed by pluralist accounts and which poses fundamental challenges to those seeking to rebalance political relationships within the overall framework of the market economy.

One response to this can be found in the 'varieties of capitalism' literature which recognises the way in which corporate influences vary across contexts and seeks to highlight the different functions performed, and positions occupied, by corporate actors within different forms of (capitalist) political economy (Hall and Soskice 2001). Similarly, Hacker and Pierson (2002) argue that decentralised federal systems augment structural power, and several scholars have noted that globalisation increases the structural power of businesses because it facilitates their ability to relocate investment (Farnsworth and Holden 2006). Stopford and Strange (1991) suggest that, in the global context, corporations should be seen as political actors whose powers are comparable to those of countries. As such, it is essential to examine corporate political influence in its spatial and temporal contexts. A more detailed analysis of the engagement by IPE scholars with the corporation and global health is provided in Chapter 3.

In order to understand and evaluate the influence of corporate actors, it is essential to engage with the concept of power. According to Steven Lukes (1974), power comes in three forms: coercion, agenda setting and co-option. The latter form of power is subtle and often hidden and involves the redefinition of individuals' or groups' interests so they become synonymous with those of the corporate sector. Power thus results not simply from the ability to influence political processes but from the ability to set the policy agenda. Thus, analyses of power must focus not just on the structure of political contestation, and whose interests policies serve, but also on those issues which remain unproblematised and, thus, never emerge as policy issues. Suppressing potential policy conflicts, and keeping these issues off the agenda, is a key component of the exercise of power, but it is very difficult for political scientists to observe. The ways in which corporations seek to influence policy agendas thus offer themselves as key research questions for political scientists and students of public policy.

Farnsworth (2004) has developed the concepts of structural and agency power to analyse corporate political influence (see Chapter 4; see also Hacker and Pierson 2002). In many cases, the political power of corporations is derived from the key structural position corporations have within the economy. For example, Johal, Moran and Williams (2013) have examined the political power of the financial services sector in the city of London, in the light of the unbalanced structure of the UK economy and the reliance on financial services as a source of economic growth and employment. At other times, corporations act purposively to shape the direction of government, through lobbying or campaign financing. However, corporations are highly pragmatic political actors, adapting their strategies to the political terrain with which they are confronted. A study of UK alcohol found that corporations attempted to build long-term relationships with political actors to embed their interests in the political process (Hawkins and Holden 2014). However, when these relationships were unable to secure favourable outcomes, they resorted to highly confrontational methods, including legal changes to the government (Holden and Hawkins 2013).

Corporations, and their trade association and front organisations, have also been identified as important policy actors, not just in terms of their structural position in the global economy and the influence they are able to exert through policy-influencing strategies, but because of their increasing role in the development and implementation of policy measures. In this sense, corporations cease being just an interest group, attempting to shape policy debates, and become something much harder to pin down. Wilks (2013) argues that the corporation in many current contexts has become what he terms a *governing institution*. Corporations are engaged in not just the formulation but the delivery of policy responses. The provisions of information to government by corporations have been described as a 'legislative subsidy' (Hall and Deardorff 2006), which is highly valued by resource-stretched policymakers. Bouwen (2002), meanwhile, employs the term *access goods* to describe the information, expertise and capacity possessed by businesses, and desired by government, which guarantee corporate actors access to policymakers. The ability, not just to provide information but to implement policy outcomes through self- and co-regulatory regimes, is an example of this type of 'goods', which facilitate corporations' access to, and potentially influence over, key decision makers. In the United Kingdom, for example, alcohol corporations now perform key policy tasks such as the provision of public information (via *Drinkaware*), the implementation of measures to tackle the sale of alcohol to minors and the regulation of alcohol marketing via the *Portman Group* code of practice (see Hawkins, Holden and McCambridge 2012).

Allowing corporations to take on tasks such as these is intuitively appealing. It relieves government of the responsibility to intervene directly, freeing up resources to focus on other issues. However, it also affords businesses enormous scope to shape policies in ways favourable to their interests and to shift debates towards (potentially less effective) measures in which such partnership-based approaches are feasible. The changing role of corporations creates the idea, in the mind of both policymakers and the public, that corporations are not economic actors in need of regulation but key stakeholders in the policy process which should be involved in addressing key policy problems.

CONCLUSION

The theories and concepts of political science offer important avenues for better understanding corporations and global health governance. There is a close connection between political science and related disciplines, such as social policy and IPE, yet the specific contribution of political science – for instance about the nature of (corporate) political power and the interconnectedness between different levels of political authority – can complement and expand on existing research agendas in these areas. It is vital to understand the domestic political factors shaping health policy decisions within countries, and the engagement of states in international forums and the wider global health agenda. Similarly, the ability of corporations to influence governments will depend on precisely the political-institutional variables studied by political scientists. Finally, the research methodologies used by political scientists, and the theories and concepts they employ, can now be more extensively exploited to expand our knowledge of corporations and global health, especially in policy areas and political contexts which have been under-researched to date. This is especially true in the context of LMICs, in which the impact of corporations over policy and government at the national and subnational levels remains under-researched.

FURTHER READING

Cairney, Paul, Donley Studlar and Hadii Mamudu. 2012. *Global Tobacco Control: Power, Policy, Governance and Transfer*. Basingstoke, UK: Palgrave-Macmillan.

Hay, Colin. 2002. *Political Analysis: A Critical Introduction*. Basingstoke, UK: Palgrave-Macmillan.

Wilks, Stephen. 2013. *The Political Power of the Business Corporation*. Cheltenham, UK: Edward Elgar.

REFERENCES

Bernier, Nicole and Carole Clavier. 2011. 'Public Health Policy Research: Making the Case for a Political Science Approach'. *Health Promotion International* 26(1): 109–16.

Bouwen, Pieter. 2002. 'Corporate Lobbying in the European Union: The Logic of Access'. *Journal of European Public Policy* 9(3): 365–90.

Bryman, Alan. 2001. *Social Research Methods*. Oxford, UK: Oxford University Press.

Coen, David. 2009. 'Business Lobbying in the European Union'. In *Lobbying in the European Union: Institutions, Actors and Issues*, edited by David Coen and Jeremy Richardson, 145–68. Oxford, UK: Oxford University Press.

Cox, Robert W. 1981. 'Social Forces, States and World Orders: Beyond International Relations Theory'. *Millennium: Journal of International Studies* 10(2): 126–55.

Dowding, Keith. 2005. 'Is It Rational to Vote? Five Types of Answer and a Suggestion'. *British Journal of Politics & International Relations* 7(3): 442–59.

Dunleavy, Patrick. 2013. *Democracy, Bureaucracy and Public Choice: Economic Approaches in Political Science*. Oxford: Routledge.

Farnsworth, Kevin. 2004. *Corporate Power and Social Policy in Global Context: British Welfare under the Influence?* Bristol, UK: The Policy Press.

Farnsworth, Kevin and Chris Holden. 2006. 'The Business–Social Policy Nexus: Corporate Power and Corporate Inputs into Social Policy'. *Journal of Social Policy* 35(3): 473–94.

Fischer, Frank. 2003. 'Beyond Empiricism: Policy Analysis as Deliberative Practice'. In *Deliberative Policy Analysis: Understanding Governance in a Network Society*, edited by Maarten Hajer and Hendrik Wagenaar, 209–27. Cambridge, UK: Cambridge University Press.

Fuchs, Doris. 2007. *Business Power in Global Governance*. Boulder, CO: Lynne Rienner.

Grant, Wyn. 1993. *Business and Politics in Britain*, 2nd edition. Houndmills, UK: Palgrave Macmillan.

Greer, Scott. 2009. *The Politics of European Union Health Policies*. Berkshire, UK: Open University Press.

Greer, Scott. 2014. 'Structural Adjustment Comes to Europe: Lessons for the Eurozone from the Conditionality Debates'. *Global Social Policy* 14(1): 51–71.

Hacker, Jacob S. and Paul Pierson. 2002. 'Business Power and Social Policy: Employers and the Formation of the American Welfare State'. *Politics and Society* 30: 277–325.

Hall, Peter and David Soskice. 2001. 'An Introduction to Varieties of Capitalism'. In *Varieties of Capitalism: The Institutional Foundations of Comparative Advantage*, edited by Peter Hall and David Soskice, 1–68. Oxford, UK: Oxford University Press.

Hall, Richard and Alan V. Deardorff. 2006. 'Lobbying as Legislative Subsidy'. *American Political Science Review* 100(1): 69–84.

Hawkins, Benjamin and Christopher Holden. 2014. '"Water Dripping on Stone"? Industry Lobbying and UK Alcohol Policy'. *Policy and Politics* 42(1): 55–70.

Hawkins, Benjamin, Christopher Holden and Jeff McCambridge. 2012. 'Alcohol Industry Influence on UK Alcohol Policy: A New Research Agenda for Public Health'. *Critical Public Health* 22(3): 297–305.

Hay, Colin. 1999. *The Political Economy of New Labour*. Manchester, UK: Manchester University Press.

Holden, Christopher and Benjamin Hawkins. 2013. '"Whisky Gloss": The Alcohol Industry Devolution and Policy Communities'. *Public Policy and Administration* 28(3): 253–73.

Holden, Christopher and Benjamin Hawkins. 2016. 'Health Policy, Corporate Influence and Multi-Level Governance: The Case of Alcohol Policy in the European Union'. In *Case Studies on Corporations and Global Health Governance*, edited by

Nora J. Kenworthy, Ross McKenzie and Kelley Lee, 145–58. London: Rowman & Littlefield International.

Johal, Sukhdev, Michael Moran and Karel Williams. 2013. 'Power, Politics and the City of London: Before and after the Great Crisis'. Sheffield Political Economy Research Institute Working Paper 3. http://speri.dept.shef.ac.uk/wp-content/uploads/2013/01/SPERI-Paper-No.3-Power-Politics-the-City-of-London-Before-After-the-Great-Crisis.pdf.

Johnson, Janet B. and H.T. Reynolds. 2012. *Political Science Research Methods*, 7th edition. London: Sage.

Joseph S. Nye and Robert O. Keohane. 1971. 'Transnational Relations and World Politics: An Introduction.' International Organization 25(3): 329-49.

Lindblom, Charles. 1977. *Politics and Markets: The World's Political-Economic Systems*. New York: Basic Books.

Lukes, Steven. 1974. *Power: A Radical View*. London: MacMillan.

Moravcsik, Andrew. 1993. 'Preferences and Power in the European Community: A Liberal Intergovernmentalist Approach'. *Journal of Common Market Studies* 31(4): 473–524.

Peters, Guy. 2012. *Institutional Theory in Political Science*, 2nd edition. London: Continuum International.

Schmidt, Vivien. 2008. 'Discursive Institutionalism: The Explanatory Power of Ideas and Discourse'. *Annual Review of Political Science* 11: 303–26.

Stopford, John and Susan Strange. 1991. *Rival States, Rival Firms: Competition for World Market Shares*. Cambridge, UK: Cambridge University Press.

Strange, Susan. 2000. 'States, Firms and Diplomacy'. In *International Political Economy: Perspectives on Global Power and Wealth*, edited by Jeffry Frieden and David Lake, 60–68. London: Routledge.

Vogel, David. 1989. *Fluctuating Fortunes: The Political Power of Business in America*. New York: Basic Books.

Wilks, Stephen. 2013. *The Political Power of the Business Corporation*. Cheltenham, UK: Edward Elgar.

Chapter 3

International Political Economy

Jappe Eckhardt

International political economy (IPE) is concerned with the interaction between economics and politics in the global arena. Simply put, the economy can be defined as the system by which the production, consumption and distribution of goods and services and the supply of money are organised. Politics concerns the total set of institutions and rules that govern our social and economic interactions. IPE scholars take as a starting point that, in order to understand the world around us, the economic and political domains cannot be separated in any meaningful way.

In daily life, the notion of a close connection between economics and politics makes perfect sense, as almost all economic behaviour is directly or indirectly regulated by government. Important aspects of our economy are also influenced by economic logic, in particular the forces of supply and demand in the marketplace. A clear example is that whenever resources are scarce, demand exceeds supply and prices are driven up. Oil, for example, is an essential, yet scarce, resource with no cost-effective alternatives available for many of its principal uses. If the global supply of oil decreases (e.g. due to war), while demand remains the same or increases, consumers cannot (easily) switch to another product to keep their vehicles running, so oil prices rise.

At the same time, 'governments can act, consciously or inadvertently, to alter patterns of consumption, supply, demand, prices, and virtually all other economic variables' (Frieden and Lake 2002, 2). For this purpose, a national government has *domestic* economic and regulatory tools at its disposal. Most important, in this regard, are monetary and fiscal policies. Monetary policy enables a government – usually through the central bank – to regulate the size and rate of increase (or decrease) of the money supply in a country, which, in turn, impacts interest rates. In general, when the money supply increases, there is more money in the economy and hence – following the law of supply – the price of it (i.e. the interest rate) decreases and vice versa. Fiscal policy permits a government to adjust public spending levels and tax rates (e.g. income tax and sales taxes levied on many of the products and services we buy) in order to monitor and influence the domestic economy. Governments can also use regulatory tools such as introducing a minimum legal drinking age for alcohol to influence consumer behaviour. *Foreign* economic policies are equally important in determining the price of goods and services. For instance, governments may impose tariffs or other trade barriers on imports or alter the exchange rate between the domestic and foreign currencies. Both measures can have a significant impact on domestic and global prices, production and consumption patterns.

The study of political economy dates from the eighteenth and nineteenth centuries; Adam Smith, John Stuart Mill and Karl Marx, among others, stressed that politics and economics do not operate in separate realms but are closely interrelated. From the beginning of the twentieth century, however, the study of economics and politics started to become more disconnected, developing into two separate scholarly fields, each with its own language and distinct focus (Frieden and Lake 2002). By the 1970s, IPE (re)emerged as a distinct and important object of study within international relations.

Much like their predecessors in the eighteenth and nineteenth centuries, modern IPE scholars analyse and explain the interaction between actors in both the political and the economic domains. Contemporary IPE seeks to answer two broad and interrelated questions (Oatley 2016, 5–6). First, how does politics shape societal decisions regarding the allocation of resources? For instance, how does a society decide whether to use its available land, labour and capital for agriculture or the production of cars? A country's foreign economic policies play a key role in this process as it affects, to a significant extent, the allocation of resources. A government's decision to impose an import tariff on cars, for example, will protect domestic car manufacturers from foreign competition and, as a result, will encourage domestic businesses to invest and workers to seek employment in the car industry. In other words, the introduction of a tariff is likely to lead to an increase of capital and labour in the protected sector. Correspondingly, lowering a tariff has the opposite effect. A decision to impose or remove a tariff, like other economic policy decisions, is, in turn, the result of a political battle between the winners and losers of global economic exchange. These may be either domestic or foreign actors given that both domestic and foreign interests are impacted by such decisions.

A second central question of IPE concerns the *consequences* of societal choices about resource allocation, which are of two types: welfare and distributional. The study of *welfare* consequences examines the extent allocative decisions increase or decrease the overall economic well-being of a country. Returning to the example of import tariffs, if a country imposes a tariff to protect an inefficient or unprofitable sector from foreign competition, capital and labour may flow away from more efficient/profitable sectors. This may mean society expends 'too many of its resources in activities that it does less well and too few resources in activities that it does better' (Oatley 2016, 6). This, in turn, may make a country less well off as a whole than it otherwise could be. *Distributional* consequences refer to the effects of resource allocation on income distribution within a state or among countries in the global system. Students of IPE seek to identify who are the winners and losers from a policy change. If a country introduces a tariff on agriculture imports, for instance, domestic food prices will rise and income is redistributed from consumers to farmers. At the same time, because the tariff makes it harder for foreign farmers to export their products to the protected market, it also leads to a redistribution of income from foreign to domestic farmers.

To answer these two questions, IPE scholars look at the role of, and/or interplay among, interests, institutions and ideas. *Interests* are defined as the goals or policy objectives of the key economic and political actors in a given domain. These can be individuals, firms, non-governmental organisations (NGOs), business federations, professional organisations and governments. In general, actors favour policies that increase their income over those that decrease income and, in order to defend their interest, they will try to influence the policy-making process. The extent actors can influence policy depends to a significant extent on political *institutions*, that is the organisations, rules and norms that organise the policy-making process. The institutional environment in which foreign economic policy making takes place partly determines which actors are likely to have influence. Although the domestic institutional architecture is important in this regard, IPE scholars are particularly interested in the connection between domestic and international institutions. Traditional political science approaches have tended to separate local, domestic, regional and international (inter-state) politics (see Chapter 2). However, as the economies of the market system have become increasingly transnationalised, and thus operate increasingly beyond the direct control of individual states, 'what were once essentially matters of domestic politics have now spilled over and become contentious in relations among states and other actors in the international system' (Underhill 2000, 5). Finally, *ideas* define the range of economic policy options that governments consider or constitute the perception societal actors have of their interests and identities, which may not always be solely determined by material interests.

THE CONTRIBUTION OF IPE TO THE STUDY OF GLOBAL HEALTH

During the twentieth century, the bulk of IPE scholarship focused on what are usually considered to be the key issue areas in the global economy – the international trading system, the international monetary system, the role of multinational corporations and economic development (see Ravenhill 2014; Oatley 2016). Global health issues were not on the radar of most IPE scholars until the beginning of the twenty-first century. Moreover, public health research rarely incorporated insights from IPE.

The prior separation of IPE and public health research was understandable. Health policy was largely a domestic concern of national governments (i.e. low politics). Globalisation, and the transboundary flows of goods, services and people, meant that health determinants and outcomes also began to transcend national borders. Many aspects of health policy, as a result, are now seen as circumventing, undermining or being oblivious to the territorial boundaries of states. Health policy has thus gone 'beyond the capacity of states to address effectively through state institutions alone' (Lee, Buse and Fustukian 2002, 5). This process gave rise to a new research agenda on global health governance (GHG), and health scholars began to draw insights from IPE. At the same time, IPE scholars became increasingly interested in global health issues (McInnes and Lee 2012).

A series of discussion papers published by the London School of Hygiene & Tropical Medicine and the World Health Organization (WHO) on GHG were instrumental in setting out this new research agenda (see, in particular, Dodgson, Lee and Drager 2002). The themes in these papers have been fleshed out in subsequent publications (Lee, Buse and Fustukian 2002; Lee 2003; Kawachi and Wamala 2006; Kay and Williams 2009; MacLean, Brown and Fourie 2009; Hanefeld 2015). Although their precise focus and aims differ, they all deal in one way or the other with the effect of globalisation on health, and how health policy making takes places in a globalised world. While the focus of this body of work is not limited to IPE, and in fact IPE is not always mentioned explicitly, all touch on three interrelated issues at the core of IPE.

First, this literature emphasises the growing importance of crossborder economic activities, such as increased international trade and investment flows, on health issues, as well as processes of commodification and liberalisation in global health. A key question is how economic globalisation changes the way health is, or should be governed, at the global level. Many authors are critical of the current state of GHG (for a review, see Fidler 2007; MacLean, Brown and Fourie 2009). Kay and Williams (2009, 2), for instance, argue 'that there is a wider political economy of global health that is increasingly market driven, and that only by understanding the structuring role of this political economy can we adequately explain the disjuncture between global health needs and contemporary governance'.

Second, the GHG literature recognises that there are increasing linkages between health policy and typical IPE policy areas such as trade and finance. As a result of these linkages, the institutional environment in which health policy is conducted is changing and, therefore, GHG scholars recognise the need 'to define and address the determinants of health from a multi-sectoral perspective' (Dodgson, Lee and Drager 2002, 18) using IPE in their work. Particularly noteworthy is research on the growing role of international economic organisations like the World Bank, International Monetary Fund, World Trade Organization (WTO) in GHG, as well as the increasing importance of economic agreements on health policy (Lee, Buse and Fustukian 2002; Kawachi and Wamala 2006; Hanefeld 2015).

Third, GHG scholarship increasingly acknowledges the importance of non-state actors like NGOs and firms in shaping health policy. This is discussed in detail in relation to research on corporations and GHG.

THE CONTRIBUTION OF IPE TO RESEARCH ON CORPORATIONS

The role of firms in policy making is central to IPE research. There is a long history of IPE scholarship on this topic, especially within the context of traditional IPE fields such as trade policy (Milner 1988; Dür 2008) and monetary and financial affairs (Frieden 1991; Underhill and Zhang 2008). Increasingly, IPE perspectives on corporate actors are also finding their way into the study of GHG.

There is an obvious relationship between government and corporate actors in the field of public health. Some corporations develop, produce and sell health-harming products, like tobacco and alcohol, and governments seek to regulate these markets. Other corporations produce health-enhancing goods and services such as medicines, therapeutic and diagnostic equipment, as well as health care services. Finally, firms actively try to shape, formulate and implement health policies, as the consequences of regulation/legislation can negatively affect their competitiveness.

As a result of globalisation, the role of corporate actors in GHG has become even more important. As Buse and Lee (2005, 6) explain:

> The advent of globalisation has amplified the impact of the commercial sector on health by extending the reach and scale of global firms and industries, by increasing the concentration of ownership in specific industries, by changing how goods

> and services are produced, marketed, traded and sold, and in some situations by altering the balance of power between public and commercial sectors and hence the regulatory framework which governs commercial activities and their impact on health.

In the light of these changes, IPE provides a useful set of tools and concepts to explain the interaction between political and economic actors in GHG. This research focuses on the three core IPE themes set out earlier: interests, institutions and ideas.

Research focused on *interests* analyses the political tactics and impacts of firms on GHG. Particularly noteworthy is research on transnational tobacco companies (TTCs) enabled by the public release of internal industry documents. Initially, research focused on the negative public health implications of the political and economic role of TTCs (e.g. Ling and Glantz 2002; Bero 2003). However, to further understanding of TTC political strategies and influence, scholars have increasingly approached the topic using an IPE lens (for recent literature reviews, see Bump and Reich 2013; Lee, Eckhardt and Holden 2016). As a result, we now have a detailed picture of the many ways TTCs have tried to wield influence over economic policy and legislation.

Research has also shown that, given their historically high degree of access to policymakers and officials at the national and the international levels, TTCs' efforts to influence foreign economic policy outcomes have been successful. For instance, in their analysis of lobbying efforts in Latin America in the 1990s, Holden and Lee (2011) show how British American Tobacco was able to convince policymakers within the Central American Common Market to protect the company's dominant position in the region, by maintaining high tariff rates for cigarette imports by competitors while reducing tariffs for key inputs. Others have shown that, as TTCs have become political pariahs in many countries (Brandt 2012), they have looked for 'creative' ways to reclaim lost legitimacy and access decision makers such as participating in corporate social responsibility (CSR) initiatives (Fooks et al. 2013). While the tobacco sector has received the bulk of the scholarly attention of this kind, due to the availability of internal documents, interesting work has been done on pharmaceutical companies (Abraham 2002; Grover et al. 2012) and the alcohol industry (Hawkins, Holden and McCambridge 2012; Jernigan 2012).

Scholars have also looked at the link between *institutions*, corporate actors and GHG. This research focuses, in particular, on how business–government relations are affected by the transnationalisation of firms, and the institutional complexity of contemporary GHG (Fidler 2010). As stated earlier, there are growing linkages between health and other policy areas like trade and investment. At the same time, decision making and regulation no longer take place only nationally but also at the regional (e.g. the European Union), bilateral and the multilateral levels (e.g. WHO, WTO and International Labour Organization). This increasing 'regime complexity' provides internationally operating firms with ample opportunities to engage in 'forum shopping' and, as such, target institutions more favourably disposed towards their policy preferences. Examples from GHG include TTCs' use of the WTO Dispute Settlement System (Eckhardt, Holden and Callard 2015) and Investor-State Dispute Settlement Mechanisms within bilateral investment treaties to challenge domestic policies (Hawkins and Holden 2016).

A related strand of the institutional literature focuses on the increasingly active and direct role that firms play in regulating public health (see also Chapter 2). First, self-regulation 'concerns efforts by private companies to set and enforce their own rules and policies for operating within a specific domain' (Buse and Lee 2005, 17). Examples include CSR initiatives (Fooks et al. 2013) and voluntary codes of conduct (Grover et al. 2012). Second, co-regulation is when public and private actors (i.e. firms and other non-state actors) agree on a set of sectoral or cross-sectoral policy or regulatory objectives. These objectives will then be implemented by the sector(s) in question (Buse and Lee 2005). One way international organisations can co-regulate, for instance, is through 'orchestration' by which third parties are brought 'into the governance arrangement to act as intermediaries between itself and the targets, rather than trying to govern the targets directly' (Abbott et al. 2015, 3; for an application to global health, see Hanrieder 2015). A good example is transnational public–private partnerships (PPPs) in which 'non-state actors are directly involved in political steering, and co-govern along with state actors' (Schäferhoff, Campe and Kaan 2009, 451). Research shows that PPPs are on the rise in all key policy fields, including GHG (Reich 2002).

Finally, 'ideational' (or constructivist) theories are beginning to attract attention from global health policy scholars. As Harmer (2011, 704) puts it, ideas-based approaches have the 'potential to illustrate how ideational factors construct global health policy, or how the identities and interests of public and private actors might be reconstructed through partnership'. Global health policies are not only determined by material factors but socially constructed and mediated through ideas and discourses. Policy outcomes are shaped by the hard power of well-endowed actors (e.g. transnational corporations), but also by the soft power of actors. Williams and Rushton (2009, 15), for example, describe 'the global biomedical epistemic community' which wields influence in GHG by persuasion and justification of particular (scientific) approaches and solutions. GHG may also offer less materially affluent non-state actors platforms to shape policy decisions through ideational power (Buse and Harmer 2004; Harmer 2011).

CONCLUSION

IPE, as a field of study, offers important contributions to the study of corporations and GHG. IPE takes, as its starting point, that the political and economic domains cannot be separated in any meaningful way. Insights from IPE were originally used to study business–government relations in policy fields such as trade, investment and finance. Since 2000, IPE has expanded to the study of global health, in general, and the role of corporations in GHG, in particular. This emerging body of research has stressed the growing links between health policy and other policy fields, and has analysed how this process has changed the political environment in which GHG is conducted. A key finding is that non-state actors, like NGOs and firms, play increasingly important roles in health policy making. Scholars have looked, in particular, at the interests and political power of corporations, how (changing) institutions shape business–government relations and the role of ideas in GHG.

The IPE and GHG research agenda, however, remains in its infancy, with plenty of avenues for future research. First, we know surprisingly little about how the globalisation of production influences business–government relations and policy outcomes in the field of GHG. Scholars could use insights from recent IPE research on trade policy – which has shown how the emergence of global value chains as a key characteristic of the contemporary world economy has major implications for firms' policy preferences, lobby behaviour and, ultimately, decision making (Eckhardt 2015) – to further develop this research theme. Second, while scholarly attention to regime complexity in GHG is increasing (Fidler 2010), more can be learned about the exact implications for the political role and influence of corporations. The key question is, as Alter and Meunier (2009, 13) put it, whether and how international regime complexity impacts 'decision-making and political strategies, as well as empower some actors and interest groups'. Third, there is ample scope for more comparative research. Comparative analysis could examine business–government relations and health policy making in different countries by drawing on the rich tradition of the 'varieties of capitalism' literature (Hall and Soskice 2003). An IPE approach could also be used to compare, and explain differences in, interactions and outcomes among policymakers and firms in different global health-harming industries (see e.g. Hawkins et al. 2016). Ultimately, such research would provide vital lessons for strengthening the protection and promotion of health through effective GHG.

FURTHER READING

Dodgson, Richard, Kelley Lee and Nick Drager. 2002. *Global Health Governance: A Conceptual Review*, Discussion Paper No. 1. London: London School of Hygiene & Tropical Medicine.

Holden, Chris and Kelley Lee. 2011. '"A Major Lobbying Effort to Change and Unify the Excise Structure in Six Central American Countries": How British American Tobacco Influenced Tax and Tariff Rates in the Central American Common Market'. *Global Health* 7(1): 15.

Oatley, Thomas. 2016. *International Political Economy*, 5th edition. London: Routledge.

REFERENCES

Abbott, Kenneth W., Philipp Genschel, Duncan Snidal and Bernhard Zangl, eds. 2015. *International Organizations as Orchestrators*. Cambridge, UK: Cambridge University Press.

Abraham, John. 2002. 'The Pharmaceutical Industry as a Political player'. *Lancet* 360(9344): 1498–502.

Alter, Karen J. and Sophie Meunier. 2009. 'The Politics of International Regime Complexity'. *Perspectives on Politics* 7(1): 13–24.

Bero, Lisa. 2003. 'Implications of the Tobacco Industry Documents for Public Health and Policy'. *Annual Review of Public Health* 24: 267–88.

Brandt, Allan. 2012. 'Inventing Conflicts of Interest: A History of Tobacco Industry Tactics'. *American Journal of Public Health* 102(1): 63–71.

Bump, Jesse and Michael Reich. 2013. 'Political Economy Analysis for Tobacco Control in Low-and Middle-Income Countries'. *Health Policy and Planning* 28(2): 123–33.

Buse, Ken and Andrew Harmer. 2004. 'Power to the Partners?: The Politics of Public–Private Health Partnerships'. *Development* 47(2): 49–56.

Buse, Kent and Kelley Lee. 2005. *Business and Global Health Governance*. London: London School of Hygiene & Tropical Medicine.

Dodgson, Richard, Kelley Lee and Nick Drager. 2002. *Global Health Governance: A Conceptual Review*. London: London School of Hygiene & Tropical Medicine.

Dür, Andreas. 2008. 'Bringing Economic Interests Back into the Study of EU Trade Policy-Making'. *British Journal of Politics & International Relations* 10(1): 27–45.

Eckhardt, Jappe. 2015. *Business Lobbying and Trade Governance: The Case of EU-China Relations*. London: Palgrave Macmillan.

Eckhardt, Jappe, Chris Holden and Cynthia Callard. 2015. 'Tobacco Control and the World Trade Organization: Mapping Member States' Positions after the Framework Convention on Tobacco Control'. *Tobacco Control*. doi:10.1136/tobaccocontrol-2015-052486.

Fidler, David P. 2007. 'Architecture amidst Anarchy: Global Health's Quest for Governance'. *Global Health Governance* 1: 17.

Fidler, David P. 2010. *The Challenges of Global Health Governance*. New York: Council on Foreign Relations.

Fooks, Gary, Anna Gilmore, Jeff Collin, Chris Holden and Kelley Lee. 2013. 'The Limits of Corporate Social Responsibility: Techniques of Neutralization, Stakeholder Management and Political CSR'. *Journal of Business Ethics* 112(2): 283–99.

Frieden, Jeffry. 1991. 'Invested Interests: The Politics of National Economic Policies in a World of Global Finance'. *International Organization* 45(4): 425–51.

Frieden, Jeffry and David Lake. 2002. *International Political Economy: Perspectives on Global Power and Wealth*, 2nd edition. London: Routledge.

Grover, Anand, Brian Citro, Mihir Mankad and Fiona Lander. 2012. 'Pharmaceutical Companies and Global Lack of Access to Medicines: Strengthening Accountability under the Right to Health'. *Journal of Law, Medicine & Ethics* 40(2): 234–50.

Hall, Peter and David Soskice. 2003. *Varieties of Capitalism: The Institutional Foundations of Comparative Advantage*. Oxford, UK: Oxford University Press.

Hanefeld, Johanna, ed. 2015. *Globalisation and Health*, 2nd edition. Maidenhead, UK: Open University Press.

Hanrieder, Tine. 2015. 'WHO Orchestrates? Coping with Competitors in Global Health'. In *International Organizations as Orchestrators*, edited by Kenneth W. Abbott, Philipp Genschel, Duncan Snidal and Bernhard Zangl, 191–213. Cambridge, UK: Cambridge University Press.

Harmer, Andrew. 2011. 'Understanding Change in Global Health Policy: Ideas, Discourse and Networks'. *Global Public Health* 6(7): 703–18.

Hawkins, Benjamin and Chris Holden. 2016. 'A Corporate Veto on Health Policy? Global Constitutionalism and Investor-State Dispute Settlement'. *Journal of Health Politics, Policy and Law* 41(5): 969–95.

Hawkins, Benjamin, Chris Holden, Jappe Eckhardt and Kelley Lee. 2016. 'Reassessing Policy Paradigms: A Comparison of the Global Tobacco and Alcohol Industries'. *Global Public Health*.

Hawkins, Benjamin, Chris Holden and Jim McCambridge. 2012. 'Alcohol Industry Influence on UK Alcohol Policy: A New Research Agenda for Public Health'. *Critical Public Health* 22(3): 297–305.

Holden, Chris and Kelley Lee. 2011. ' "A Major Lobbying Effort to Change and Unify the Excise Structure in Six Central American Countries": How British American Tobacco Influenced Tax and Tariff Rates in the Central American Common Market'. *Global Health* 7(1): 15.

Jernigan, David J. 2012. 'Global Alcohol Producers, Science and Policy: The Case of the International Center for Alcohol Policy'. *American Journal of Public Health* 102: 80–89.

Kawachi, Ichiro and Sarah Wamala, eds. 2006. *Globalization and Health*. Oxford, UK: Oxford University Press.

Kay, Adrian and Owain Williams, eds. 2009. *Global Health Governance: Crisis, Institutions and Political Economy*. Houndmills, UK: Palgrave Macmillan.

Lee, Kelley, ed. 2003. *Health Impacts of Globalization: Towards Global Governance*. London: Palgrave Macmillan.

Lee, Kelley, Kent Buse and Suzanne Fustukian, eds. 2002. *Health Policy in a Globalising World.* Cambridge, UK: Cambridge University Press.

Lee, Kelley, Jappe Eckhardt and Chris Holden. 2016. 'Tobacco Industry Globalization and Global Health Governance: Towards an Interdisciplinary Research Agenda'. *Palgrave Communications* 2: 16037. doi:10.1057/palcomms.2016.37.

Ling, Pamela M. and Stanton Glantz. 2002. 'Why and How the Tobacco Industry Sells Cigarettes to Young Adults: Evidence from Industry Documents'. *American Journal of Public Health* 92(6): 908–16.

MacLean, Sandra J., Sheri A. Brown and Pieter Fourie. 2009. *Health for Some: The Political Economy of Global Health Governance.* London: Palgrave Macmillan.

McInnes Colin and Kelley Lee. 2012. *Global Health and International Relations.* London: Polity Press.

Milner, Helen V. 1988. *Resisting Protectionism: Global Industries and the Politics of International Trade.* Princeton, NJ: Princeton University Press.

Oatley, Thomas. 2016. *International Political Economy*, 5th edition. London: Routledge.

Ravenhill, John, ed. 2014. *Global Political Economy.* Oxford, UK: Oxford University Press.

Reich, Michael R. 2002. *Public–Private Partnerships for Public Health.* Cambridge, MA: Harvard Center for Population and Development Studies.

Schäferhoff, Marco, Sabine Campe and Christopher Kaan. 2009. 'Transnational Public–Private Partnerships in International Relations: Making Sense of Concepts, Research Frameworks, and Results'. *International Studies Review* 11(3): 451–74.

Underhill, Geoffrey R.D. 2000. 'Conceptualizing the Changing Global Order'. In *Political Economy and the Changing Global Order*, edited by Richard Stubbs and Geoffrey Underhill, 3–24. Don Mills, ON: Oxford University Press.

Underhill, Geoffrey R.D and Xiaoke Zhang. 2008. 'Setting the Rules: Private Power, Political Underpinnings, and Legitimacy in Global Monetary and Financial Governance'. *International Affairs* 84(3): 535–54.

Williams, Owain and Simon Rushton. 2009. 'Global Health Governance as a Contested Space: Competing Discourses, Interests and Actors'. 50th International Studies Association Annual Convention in New York.

Chapter 4

Social Policy

Chris Holden and Kevin Farnsworth

Social policy, as an academic field, is centrally concerned with the study of human well-being; the political, economic and social structures and processes that influence it; and the policies that can protect and enhance it. Social policy analysis has often been focused on the making of government policy and the provision of public welfare services, including health services. A key focus of enquiry for social policy scholars has been the development and operation of welfare states in high-income countries. Social policy analysts often direct their attention to the most socially and economically disadvantaged groups, and to issues of social justice and equity. Historically, social policy as an academic subject paid very little attention to low- and middle-income countries (LMICs), especially where these were lacking state-institutionalised forms of welfare provision. The analysis of key players within processes of welfare reform has also sometimes been quite narrow.

However, social policy is an evolving subject. In recent years, a number of scholars within the field have increasingly turned their attention to a wider array of actors, institutions and processes that may impact on human well-being. There have been new analyses of welfare arrangements in low-income countries and of emerging welfare states in middle-income countries (Surender and Walker 2013). As discussed in more depth later, the focus of analysis has also grown to incorporate not simply analyses of national social policies and comparisons across welfare states but also the social policies of international organisations and the global and transnational processes that affect human well-being, which cut across national boundaries. This includes expanding analysis to private corporations.

Social policy is an interdisciplinary academic subject, which draws on a number of social science disciplines, especially political science and economics. It is allied to the sub-discipline of policy studies, or public policy, within the field of political science (see Chapter 2), with scholars attempting to understand how policy is made and why certain policy approaches lead to particular outcomes (Hill 2012). Particularly relevant to this book is a strong tradition of political economy that runs through social policy analysis (Pierson 2006). As discussed in Chapter 3, this builds on the fundamental insight that political and economic power cannot be separated but are rooted in the same social structures (Holden 2005a).

A number of authors, including O'Connor (1973), Gough (1979) and Offe (1984), sought to explain the contradictory place of welfare states within modern capitalism and the fiscal pressures that economic crises were already placing on them by the 1970s. Esping-Andersen (1990) used the concept of 'decommodification' in his influential comparative analysis of different types of 'welfare regimes' (liberal, conservative and social democratic), to explain how welfare states limited market forces by allowing workers to survive independently of the market in certain situations. Similarly (and relatedly), the 'varieties of capitalism' approach, which draws a distinction between 'liberal' and 'coordinated' market economies, has been used by various authors to understand differences between welfare states and the ways that they intersect with the wider political economy (Ebbinghaus and Manow 2001; Hall and Soskice 2001).

The political economy tradition that runs through much social policy scholarship reminds us that the determinants of health are often fundamentally social and may have their roots in economic structures and relationships. Policy change in areas relating to income, wealth and the economy more broadly may be just as important to ensuring good health as the provision of health services. Furthermore, the social determinants of health may not be confined to the national level but may be global in scope, with processes such as trade liberalisation having a potentially profound impact on health outcomes (McNamara 2015). The wages that transnational corporations (TNCs) pay their workers, the conditions they ask them to work in and the impacts they have on the environment can all be important determinants of health, even where the core activities of the corporations concerned appear to have little to do with health.

Three linked social trends, which developed simultaneously from the 1980s onwards, were highly influential to the further elaboration of political economy approaches in social policy (Holden 2005a). First, the intensifying globalisation of the world economy was seen to place new pressures and constraints on welfare states. Second, governments began to explicitly couple economic and social policies, with social policies being progressively subordinated to economic policies. To this end, social policies were designed to serve the needs of national competitiveness within the world economy, in what Cerny (1997) describes as the substitution of the welfare state by the 'competition state'. Third, there has been an increasing preference by governments for the privatisation and contracting out of core welfare provision to private for-profit companies. The significance of these trends is discussed further later.

Social policy scholars employ the full range of social research methods, including both quantitative and qualitative approaches. Quantitative analysis has been particularly prevalent in comparative welfare state research, with Esping-Andersen's (1990) analysis of the 'three worlds of welfare capitalism' as an important point of departure for many scholars (Powell and Barrientos 2011; Hudson 2015), although qualitative and 'fuzzy set' approaches have also been used in comparative research (Hudson and Kühner 2013). Qualitative approaches have often been used in studies of how policy is made, including at the international level. For example, Bob Deacon's (2013) study of how the Social Protection Floors Recommendation was generated, developed and adopted within the International Labour Organization drew on a combination of qualitative interviews, document analysis and first-hand observation.

In the remainder of this chapter, we discuss the contributions that academic social policy analyses have made to our understanding of global health governance (GHG) and to the impact of corporate actors on human well-being. First, we discuss the development of global social policy analyses and their concern with global governance processes. This is followed by an examination of social policy analyses of corporate actors. We conclude by considering how these analyses can be built upon to enhance our understanding of the effects of corporate activity on GHG.

GLOBAL SOCIAL POLICY AND GLOBAL HEALTH

In keeping with the traditional focus of social policy on national welfare states, social policy analyses relating to health have often been focused on the delivery of health services and the subsequent effects on health inequalities and outcomes. From the 1990s onwards, however, an increasing awareness of economic globalisation and its potential implications for social policy began to transform the subject. These changes sparked a vibrant debate about the extent to which global economic processes undermined established welfare states, or placed constraints on them such that governments were compelled to follow essentially neoliberal or pro-market policies regardless of their political preferences (Yeates and Holden 2009, 269). Mishra (1999, 15), for example, argued that the 'logic' of economic globalisation undermines the ability of national governments to pursue Keynesian welfare policies and high levels of government expenditure, exerts 'a downward pressure on systems of social protection' and 'virtually excludes left-of-centre approaches'.

Such claims have been vigorously challenged by Hay (2005) and Swank (2005), among others, who sought to show that national governments retain significant policy space and that high levels of social protection are not necessarily inconsistent with an open and competitive world economy. Indeed, some have argued that globalisation has increased the importance of robust social policies, as a bulwark against the worst effects of the world market on growing inequalities, unemployment, poverty and poor health (Holden 2014). Others, however, have found that social protection is often inaccessible to those most vulnerable to the effects of liberalisation processes, such as workers laid off by small enterprises and those with informal labour contracts (McNamara 2015).

Most relevant to GHG is a subsequent turn towards the analysis of the global aspects of social policy, or 'global social policy'. These analyses focused not simply on the implications of globalisation processes for welfare states in high-income countries but on the full range of determinants of human well-being in high-, middle- and low-income countries. In doing so, social policy scholars have reached out to forge alliances and collaborations with scholars of development studies, international political economy, global health and a range of other disciplines and fields. Research has focused on the roles of international organisations in social policy, transnational processes that impact on human well-being and the range of non-state actors that operate across borders, including TNCs (Yeates 2014). Analyses of international organisations by Deacon and others have demonstrated how such organisations play a significant role in the social policies (including health policies) adopted and implemented at the country level, particularly in LMICs that rely on funding from the World Bank, International Monetary Fund and foreign donors (Deacon, Stubbs and Hulse 1997; Deacon 2007). Scholars of global social policy have also turned their attention to the full array of global health issues and their governance that scholars in public health and other fields are concerned with (Koivusalo and Ollila 2014).

One important strand of such research has been a concern with the ways in which processes of international trade interact with and impact on health. Holden, for example, has analysed how an increasing trend towards the greater involvement of for-profit providers in the delivery of health services has combined with the liberalisation of global trade and investment to create partially globalised health services markets (2003, 2005b), with a number of implications for social policy goals concerned with equity, efficiency, quality and choice (2009). As health care markets develop and become more global in scope, their effective regulation in the pursuit of these goals becomes ever more complex. Furthermore, a number of World Trade Organization (WTO) and other trade and investment agreements have substantial implications for health systems and the broader health policies pursued by governments. The WTO's General Agreement on Trade in Services, for example, may 'lock in' privatisation policies, effectively making them irreversible, and may constrain the ways that governments choose to regulate their health systems (Holden 2014). Furthermore, the increasing development of global health markets has involved the growth of health-related TNCs, both in the direct delivery of health services and in related sectors such as the pharmaceutical industry (Holden 2005c). Importantly, as the following section discusses, such corporations are not merely economic actors but political actors seeking to influence the policy process in various ways (Holden 2009).

SOCIAL POLICY AND CORPORATE ACTORS

As global analyses of social policy have developed, there has been an increasing return to political economy approaches among some scholars. A particular concern has been to analyse the ways in which corporate actors can enhance or undermine human well-being, including their increasing roles in the provision of welfare services, their influence on the making of social policy and their roles in producing social goods and harms. Of note has been Farnsworth's (2004, 2005, 2014) work to understand corporate power at various levels of national and global governance, including both structural and agency power, and its impact on social policy making and delivery.

Structural power relates to businesses' control over investment and the unequal dependency relationship between capital, labour and the state (Farnsworth 2004). Governments and workers depend on businesses to invest but have no control over private investment decisions. Private sector investment can result in jobs and tax revenues, while a lack of investment can lead to unemployment and fiscal crisis. To encourage investment, governments and workers seek ways of inducing corporations to invest by socialising their risks and reducing their costs. *Agency power* concerns the political mobilisation of business interests, through lobbying activities and the funding of sympathetic political parties or pro-business and anti-trade union groups. For example, one area in which the interests of businesses and health can collide is regulations. Regulations to protect health and welfare, in the workplace or beyond, may bring significant health benefits but may also impose costs on corporations as employers, producers and retailers. Where public policies impose costs on corporations, governments are likely to be subject to various forms of agency power employed to counter such measures.

Of course, structural and agency powers are interrelated (Farnsworth 2004). The power and ability of businesses to shape and influence policy direction is highly variable, temporally (over time), geographically (between nations and regions) and according to strategic importance and size. Furthermore, how business interests try to exercise agency power also varies according to the relative strength of structural power within different spaces. For example, the power of financial capital has generally been higher than industrial capital because the former is far more mobile than the latter and is thus able to use the threat of an 'investment strike' more easily. Similarly, auto manufacturers have tended to wield a great deal of power because they are large employers and, while less mobile than financial companies, are more mobile than oil companies, whose activities are tied to the ability to exploit natural resources in particular locations. Part of the explanation for the power of corporations, therefore, lies in the government's perceptions of their strategic importance within an economy. Thus, the power that individual corporations wield can vary extensively over time. This is especially true where the strategic importance of corporations to a national economy changes or is ambiguous.

Just as businesses' interests and power vary, so too do their political preferences. As with other sectors, business preferences in the health sphere are shaped by a firm's own assessment of its particular interests and the extent to which the firm is involved in political networks with other businesses (Martin 1995; see also Mares 2001). Within this, however, the extent to which businesses choose to act really is a question of the weighing up of the consequences of not acting (see Hacker and Pierson 2002). Thus, certain aspects of health policy may be important for individual companies, but sustained business lobbying is more likely to occur in those more limited cases where interests are common across a number of businesses, and preferences can be pressed by collective organisations, or where particularly large firms can 'go it alone'.

Farnsworth and Holden (2006) set out a comprehensive analytical framework to study different types of corporate inputs into social policy, which takes account not only of structural and agency power but also of the range of roles that corporations can play in the provision and production of welfare services and goods (see also Holden 2005c). Corporate actors are of great significance to the provision of health and other welfare services. To begin with, some corporations directly provide key health services and, therefore, have a keen interest in health policies. Indeed, the significance of private health care providers has increased in recent years as governments have moved to marketise services and/or outsource their delivery to private providers. Businesses may also produce goods (e.g. pharmaceuticals) that are necessary for health; supply various services to direct providers of health services; provide health insurance; invest in facilities such as hospitals; or run occupational welfare schemes for their own employees, such as pensions or health insurance schemes.

Occupational health insurance schemes can be particularly important in countries that lack comprehensive public health care systems. In the United States, for instance, General Motors was the largest provider of occupational health insurance in the mid-2000s, spending US$5.6 billion on it in 2006 alone (Webster 2006). Employers in countries with comprehensive public health care systems, by contrast, can gain substantially from the socialisation of costs provided by such systems, since workers' health is a key factor in determining productivity and, ultimately, profits. This fact is captured well by the World Economic Forum – more often associated with big business than big government – in its 2012 *Global Competitiveness Report*: 'Workers who are ill cannot function to their potential and will be less productive. Poor health leads to significant costs to business, as sick workers are often absent or operate at lower levels of efficiency. Investment in the provision of health services is thus critical for clear economic, as well as moral, considerations' (WEF 2012, 6). Seen in this way, public health systems provide not only essential services to citizens but also indirect financial benefits to private corporations.

The ideas discussed in this section have been applied to the field of global health by Holden and Lee (2009), who analyse the structural and agency power of transnational tobacco companies (TTCs). The structural power of TTCs is found to be higher where countries rely heavily on employment as a result of cigarette manufacturing or tobacco leaf growing and the income taxes or export earnings that flow from this. However, few countries are highly reliant on tobacco-related employment or export earnings. As Jacobs et al. (2000) argue, reductions in tobacco use are likely to be gradual, so that most countries' economies would not be negatively affected by reduced demand. The consumption of tobacco also imposes high economic and social costs as a result of high levels of morbidity and mortality. Many countries have thus been able to introduce effective tobacco control regulations. TTCs have responded by extensive use of agency power, employing a range of political tactics and strategies to attempt to change or weaken governments' policies. These have included both direct and indirect forms of influence, which have been extensively documented by public health researchers (Holden and Lee 2009). Direct efforts at policy influence have included lobbying of policymakers, both directly and via contract lobbyists, political campaign contributions and the use of front groups (Givel and Glantz 2001). Indirect attempts to influence policy have taken the form of efforts to undermine the scientific evidence base relating to tobacco and health (Bero 2003), and diverting of attention to non-tobacco policy issues (Muggli et al. 2008; Petticrew and Lee 2011). TTCs' use of agency power has been extensive and has operated at a range of political levels, from the local through the national to the global. Effective tobacco control has thus necessitated a global approach in the form of the World Health Organization's Framework Convention on Tobacco Control.

CONCLUSION

While social policy as an academic subject has often focused on the national policies and services of advanced welfare states, a number of scholars have increasingly turned their attention to issues of well-being in LMICs, to questions of global governance and to the effects of corporate behaviour on health and well-being. Farnsworth and Holden's (2006) work has provided a useful analytical framework for understanding the roles of different types of corporate actors and corporate behaviours in influencing social and health outcomes. Furthermore, Holden and Lee (2009) have demonstrated how this framework can be applied not only to providers of health services, producers of health-related goods (e.g. pharmaceuticals) and so on, but also to health-harming industries such as tobacco. This kind of framework could be applied to a number of different sectors relevant to global health, such as the alcohol and food industries, in order to develop a greater understanding of the impacts of TNCs on GHG and on health outcomes.

FURTHER READING

Farnsworth, Kevin and Chris Holden. 2006. 'The Business-Social Policy Nexus: Corporate Power and Corporate Inputs into Social Policy'. *Journal of Social Policy* 35(3): 473–94.

Yeates, Nicola, ed. 2014. *Understanding Global Social Policy*, 2nd edition. Bristol, UK: Policy Press.

Yeates, Nicola and Chris Holden, eds. 2009. *The Global Social Policy Reader*. Bristol, UK: Policy Press.

REFERENCES

Bero, Lisa. 2003. 'Implications of the Tobacco Industry Documents for Public Health and Policy'. *Annual Review of Public Health* 24: 267–88.

Cerny, Philip G. 1997. 'Paradoxes of the Competition State: The Dynamics of Political Globalization'. *Government and Opposition* 32(2): 251–74.

Deacon, Bob. 2007. *Global Social Policy and Governance*. London: Sage.

Deacon, Bob. 2013. *Global Social Policy in the Making: The Foundations of the Social Protection Floor*. Bristol, UK: Policy Press.

Deacon, Bob, with Paul Stubbs and Michelle Hulse. 1997. *Global Social Policy: International Organisations and the Future of Welfare*. London: Sage.

Ebbinghaus, Bernhard and Philip Manow, eds. 2001. *Comparing Welfare Capitalism: Social Policy and Political Economy in Europe, Japan and the USA*. London: Routledge.

Esping-Andersen, Gøsta. 1990. *The Three Worlds of Welfare Capitalism*. Cambridge, UK: Polity Press.

Farnsworth, Kevin. 2004. *Corporate Power and Social Policy in a Global Economy*. Bristol, UK: Policy Press.

Farnsworth, Kevin. 2005. 'International Class Conflict and Social Policy'. *Social Policy and Society* 4(2): 217–26.

Farnsworth, Kevin. 2014. 'Business and Global Social Policy'. In *Understanding Global Social Policy*, edited by Nicola Yeates, 77–104. Bristol, UK: Policy Press.

Farnsworth, Kevin and Chris Holden. 2006. 'The Business-Social Policy Nexus: Corporate Power and Corporate Inputs into Social Policy'. *Journal of Social Policy* 35(3): 473–94.

Givel, Michael S. and Stan A. Glantz. 2001. 'Tobacco Lobby Political Influence on US State Legislatures in the 1990s'. *Tobacco Control* 10: 124–34.

Gough, Ian. 1979. *The Political Economy of the Welfare State*. London: Macmillan.

Hacker, Jacob S. and Paul Pierson. 2002. 'Business Power and Social Policy: Employers and the Formation of the American Welfare State'. *Politics and Society* 30(2): 277–325.

Hall, Peter A. and David Soskice, eds. 2001. *Varieties of Capitalism: The Institutional Foundations of Comparative Advantage*. Oxford, UK: Oxford University Press.

Hay, Colin. 2005. 'Too Important to Leave to the Economists? The Political Economy of Welfare Retrenchment'. *Social Policy and Society* 4(2): 197–205.

Hill, Michael. 2012. *The Public Policy Process*. London: Routledge.

Holden, Chris. 2003. 'Actors and Motives in the Internationalization of Health Businesses'. *Business and Politics* 5(3): 287–301.

Holden, Chris. 2005a. 'Social Policy and Political Economy: A Tale of (at least) Two Disciplines'. *Social Policy and Society* 4(2): 173–81.

Holden, Chris. 2005b. 'Privatization and Trade in Health Services: A Review of the Evidence'. *International Journal of Health Services* 35(4): 675–89.

Holden, Chris. 2005c. 'The Internationalization of Corporate Healthcare: Extent and Emerging Trends'. *Competition & Change* 9(2): 185–203.

Holden, Chris. 2009. 'Regulation, Accountability and Trade in Health Services'. In *Ethics and Health in the Global Village: Bioethics, Globalization and Human Rights*, edited by Emilio Mordini, 95–121. Rome: CIC Edizioni Internazionali.

Holden, Chris. 2014. 'International Trade and Welfare'. In *Understanding Global Social Policy*, 2nd edition, edited by Nicola Yeates, 105–28. Bristol, UK: Policy Press.

Holden, Chris and Kelley Lee. 2009. 'Corporate Power and Social Policy: The Political Economy of the Transnational Tobacco Companies'. *Global Social Policy* 9(3): 328–54.

Hudson, John. 2015. 'Twenty-Five Years after *The Three Worlds of Welfare Capitalism*: A Retrospective'. In *Social Policy Review 27*, edited by Zoë Irving, Menno Fenger and John Hudson, 5–10. Bristol, UK: Policy Press.

Hudson, John and Stefan Kühner. 2013. 'Qualitative Comparative Analysis and Applied Public Policy Analysis: New Applications of Innovative Methods'. *Policy and Society* 32(4): 279–87.

Jacobs, Rowena, H. Frederick Gale, Thomas C. Capehart, Ping Zhang and Prabhat Jha. 2000. 'The Supply-Side Effects of Tobacco-Control Policies'. In *Tobacco Control in Developing Countries*, edited by Prabhat Jha and Frank Chaloupka, 311–41. Washington, DC: World Bank.

Koivusalo, Meri and Eeva Ollila. 2014. 'Global Health Policies'. In *Understanding Global Social Policy*, 2nd edition, edited by Nicola Yeates, 159–86. Bristol, UK: Policy Press.

Mares, Isabela. 2001. 'Firms and the Welfare State'. In *Varieties of Capitalism: The Institutional Foundations of Comparative Advantage*, edited by Peter A. Hall and David Soskice, 184–212. Oxford, UK: Oxford University Press.

Martin, Cathie J. 1995. 'Nature or Nurture? Sources of Firm Preference for National Health Reform'. *American Political Science Review* 89(4): 898–913.

McNamara, Courtney. 2015. 'Trade Liberalisation, Social Policies and Health: An Empirical Case Study'. *Globalization and Health* 11: 42.

Mishra, Ramesh. 1999. *Globalization and the Welfare State*. Cheltenham, UK: Edward Elgar.

Muggli, Monique E., Kelley Lee, Quan Gan, Jon O. Ebbert and Richard D. Hurt. 2008. ' "Efforts to Reprioritise the Agenda" in China: British American Tobacco's Efforts to Influence Public Policy on Secondhand Smoke in China'. *PLoS Medicine* 5(12): 1729–36.

O'Connor, James. 1973. *The Fiscal Crisis of the State*. New York: St Martin's Press.

Offe, Claus. 1984. *Contradictions of the Welfare State*. London: Hutchinson.

Petticrew, Mark and Kelley Lee. 2011. 'The "Father of Stress" Meets "Big Tobacco": Hans Selye and the Tobacco Industry'. *American Journal of Public Health* 101(3): 411–18.

Pierson, Christopher. 2006. *Beyond the Welfare State: The New Political Economy of Welfare*. Cambridge, UK: Polity Press.

Powell, Martin and Armando Barrientos. 2011. 'An Audit of the Welfare Modelling Business'. *Social Policy & Administration* 45(1): 69–84.

Surender, Rebecca and Robert Walker, eds. 2013. *Social Policy in a Developing World*. Cheltenham, UK: Edward Elgar.

Swank, Duane. 2005. 'Globalization, Domestic Politics, and Welfare State Retrenchment in Capitalist Democracies'. *Social Policy and Society* 4(2): 183–95.

Webster, Philip. 2006. 'US Big Businesses Struggle to Cope with Healthcare Costs'. *Lancet* 367(9505): 101–2.

WEF. 2012. *Global Competitiveness Report*. Davos, Switzerland: World Economic Forum.

Yeates, Nicola. 2014. 'The Idea of Global Social Policy'. In *Understanding Global Social Policy*, 2nd edition, edited by Nicola Yeates, 1–18. Bristol, UK: Policy Press.

Yeates, Nicola and Chris Holden, eds. 2009. *The Global Social Policy Reader*. Bristol, UK: Policy Press.

Chapter 5

Historical Analysis

Ross MacKenzie

History is the study of the past. However, this simple definition belies the richness of the discipline in terms of subject matter, approaches and purpose. Narrowly focused until the mid-twentieth century on major political and military events, and the 'great men' involved in those events, history today incorporates analysis of society, culture, gender, labour relations and medicine, among other subjects. Within this context, this chapter discusses the particular contributions of history to the study of corporations. It begins with an overview of how the discipline has evolved, in terms of subject matter deemed significant, methods and sources of data. It then reviews the engagement of historical analysis with global health governance (GHG) and corporations, and concludes with a discussion of how historical methods and approaches can expand our understanding of corporations.

HISTORY AS AN EVOLVING DISCIPLINE

Historical scholarship was broadly founded on the assumption that a true account of the past could be revealed through rigorous analysis of primary sources conducted by trained scholars who, by and large, emphasised the progress of Western countries (Iggers 2005). This approach was personified by the Cambridge historian Geoffrey Elton (1967, 44), who described historical analysis as the 'rational reconstruction of the past'. The most notable challenges to this perception of history came from the *Annales* School, Marxist historical materialism, social history and cultural history. Rather than contextualising an event within a linear temporal progression, *Annales* scholars focused on human agency and culture, considering a specific period on its own terms, and sought to understand the whole history of, for instance, a region by examining its economic, political, religious and demographic characteristics (Iggers 2005). Historical materialism emerged after the Second World War as a refinement of Marx's assumption that society is defined by its material conditions, that is the way in which individuals acquire the means to live within society. Key to this analysis is the concept of *history from below*, which analyses the situation of 'the majority of people', as opposed to political and economic leaders (Cohen 2001). This process effectively changed the criteria for what is considered to be historically significant (Southgate 2001).

Social history emerged in the 1960s as an academic reflection of post-war democratisation, and the social and cultural upheavals of the decade. Aspects of *Annaliste* and materialist theory were combined, with greater methodological reliance on quantifiable evidence (Lewis 2013). Researchers focused explicitly on social structures, class and demographics, and their work encompassed analysis of workers' social and political lives, urban and rural populations, women and ethnic minorities.

The ascendance of social history was, in turn, challenged by the rise of cultural history during the 1970s. Influenced by post-modernist philosophers and literary critics, cultural historians questioned the fundamental assumption that history followed an intelligible evolution, arguing instead that there is no coherent, progressive historical narrative. Post-modernists argued that historians do not so much interpret the past as invent it, by imposing their own beliefs that history is coherent and has meaning (White 1973). From the post-modernist perspective, academic history is an inherently conservative undertaking that perpetuates the social status quo by defining the parameters of acceptable visions of the past (Southgate 2001). Cultural historians study the daily lives of ordinary people using anthropological methods and semiotics (the study of the meaning in language) (Burke 2008).

Several key points emerge from these disciplinary debates. First, most historical studies are still presented as narrative, the most viable means of bringing the past 'under control for intelligible, meaningful comprehension' (Partner 2013). Second, history is recognised as being inherently ideological (Schneider and Woolf 2015), and the concept of an objective historical narrative carries little weight today. Finally, approaches to history and topics of study commonly reflect social and cultural contexts. The dramatic social and cultural upheavals in the 1960s, for example, predicated the rise of social history, while women's history reflected the impact of feminism in the West during the 1970s. By the late twentieth century, interest shifted towards the global and transnational, largely in response to economic globalisation (Hopkins 2006), including the rise of corporations to become the 'dominant governance institutions on the planet' (Korten 2001, 60).

HISTORY AND THE STUDY OF GHG

To understand and respond to the complexities of GHG, Loughlin and Berridge (2002) argue that a 'stronger sense of the complex history of this field' is needed but caution that much of the required historical research has not been done. The term *global health* and its predecessor *international health* are often used interchangeably but to historians describe evolving conceptions of health over time. International health broadly refers to cross-border health risks, notably infectious disease outbreaks, which require cooperation across governments (Brown, Cueto and Fee 2006). It also describes the concern with health in low- and middle-income countries, particularly tropical diseases, sanitation and malnutrition, which arose through colonial ties (Koplan et al. 2009). Global health 'refers to the scope of problems, not their location' (Koplan et al. 2009), again a reflection of the closer integration of human societies from the late twentieth century.

The nature of collective action has correspondingly changed over time to address actual and perceived needs. Much of the historical analysis undertaken, according to Birn and Hochman (2008), has been 'aimed at documenting a parade of progress in the name of justifying particular programs and organizations'. One example is the near-consensus that existed among historians that the international sanitary conferences of the nineteenth century represented steady, if slow, progress in forging cooperative responses to infectious disease epidemics. This, according to Birn (2009), overlooks the limited enforcement of agreements, political rivalry among leading European powers that delayed negotiations and British reluctance to commit to anything that threatened its trade routes.

There is much scope for critical analysis of the role of key actors, and strategies to use 'health' in support of economic and political goals. This shift has potentially significant implications for contemporary GHG. Birn (2009) argues that many funders and policymakers 'use historical episodes or precedents . . . to push forward particular agendas based on (mis)perceived successes of the past'. References to smallpox eradication, during discussions by the Gates Foundation of its approach to malaria control, are an example of allusion to previous GHG success stories (Birn 2009). Thus, historians of GHG have two roles: to assess events in the past using rigorous historical methods and to reveal how the selectivity and subjectivity of historical analysis can relate to particular agendas and ideologies.

HISTORY AND THE STUDY OF CORPORATIONS

Corporate histories are 'interpreted account[s] of the historical trajectory and development of an organisation representing an attempt in the present to explain, celebrate, justify, or otherwise make sense of changes over time' (Burghausen and Balmer 2014, 392). It is imperative, however, to distinguish between two broad categories of such research: internal corporate histories and external academic studies. Corporate histories are accounts written in-house, or by a commissioned historian, within clear parameters established by the sponsoring corporation. Such narratives serve corporate strategies to project an image of asocial, ahistorical, forward-looking, modern entities that provide moral and social legitimacy (Rajak 2014). Their value extends to public relations, reinforcement of corporate identity, marketing and communications and strengthening bonds with clients and employees (Corporate History 2007). Such 'corporate eulogies' (Burghausen and Balmer 2014) disregard 'continuity and overlooks the ways in which transnational corporations are themselves territorialized, rooted in place and *history* in ways that cannot simply be transcended or effaced' (Rajak 2014, emphasis in original).

Academic histories of corporations, in contrast, are independent analyses. Business history developed outside of the broader academic discipline of history, first appearing around the turn of the twentieth century. Informed by the German historical school of economics, these studies sought to analyse factors that contributed to economic growth overlooked by traditional economic theory (Berghoff 2015). In the United States, the field emerged in 1927 when the Harvard Business School funded a chair in business history in an effort to rehabilitate a sector that had faced extensive criticism for its treatment of workers; production safety standards, particularly in the food industry; and the enormous power and influence of industry trusts such as Standard Oil (McGerr 2003). From the 1930s, analysis in the United States focused on executive leadership, entrepreneurialism and how forms of business – petty, mercantile and industrial, for example – influenced economic development in different eras. The field was enhanced in the 1950s by the work of Alfred Chandler, widely acknowledged as the founder of modern business history, on the role of organisation building and professional management.

While business history remained a specialised field, it was influenced by theoretical and methodological developments in social and cultural history. Approaches adopted from social history informed analyses of wage differentiation and work incentives, primarily among white-collar employees and middle managers. Cultural history's focus on meaning and reception of language and symbols had clear implications for studies of public relations, marketing and advertising (Fridenson 2009). By the early twenty-first century, academic business history had incorporated critical examination of an expanding range of topics, including organisational and management structures, financial systems, marketing history and the regulatory role of the state.

Research on the corporation reflects much of this evolution, and directions in research have included corporate governance, corporations as political actors, firms as a venue of social interaction (Fridenson 2009; Berghoff 2015) and, notably, the role played by corporations in globalisation. Large corporations 'were at the heart' of the globalisation process (Jones 2009, 141), and historians have assessed ways in which they create, and respond to, global markets; develop integrated supply chains; manage dispersed operations; exploit natural resources; adapt to local culture and practice; and interact with national governments (Jones 2009).

Historical analysis of corporations employs an increasingly sophisticated range of methods and approaches. In the United States, for example, the field is notable for its extensive use of oral history (see Chapter 13). Fridenson (2009) credits Nivens's publication of the life stories of 150 Ford Motor Company managers and employees between 1954 and 1963 with establishing the credibility of this approach. Another approach is to study the connections between the history of corporations and that of technology through the material culture, products, artefacts, machinery, infrastructure and buildings of corporations (Fridenson 2009).

Textual resources are also central data sources and include in the form of annual reports, investor prospectuses and media releases, and corporate submissions to public consultations, trade directories, industry journals, trade catalogues and, in some cases, records of government inquiries. Business organisations, from small companies to transnational corporations (TNCs), keep records of their operations, and these represent a particularly valuable resource for historians (see Chapter 16). Access to corporate documents, however, is a long-standing challenge. In 1943, the American historian Stanley Pargellis (1944) was told by companies he approached that they could not 'trust the average historian to render a just judgement', an experience shared by numerous researchers.

Provenance and comprehensiveness of collections, given corporate concerns about confidentiality, also impact the ability of historians to fully study a corporation (Lewis and Newtown 1981; Rowlinson 2004). Many corporations, such as Coca-Cola (Booker 2011), IBM (2016) and Siemens (2016), have selectively made corporate documents publicly available through company-operated depositories or public archives. While such collections undergo filtering by the company and legal reviewers before release, they can still yield important information. Document collections can also be located in government archives and university holdings, and many, such as the National Archives in London (2016), have online catalogues and guides to their collections. The Directory of Corporate Archives in the United States and Canada (Society of American Archivists 2016) provides extensive listings of holdings in those countries. Published guides to industry records, such as those of the banking (Orbell and Turton 2001), pharmaceutical (Richmond, Stevenson and Turton 2003), brewing (Richmond and Turton 1990) and shipbuilding industries (Ritchie 1992) in the United Kingdom, offer further historical corporate collections. Finally, internal documents made available via court order are generally subject to a lesser degree of filtration. Important examples, including documents of the tobacco, lead, and pharmaceutical industries, are discussed in Chapter 16.

CONTRIBUTIONS OF HISTORICAL RESEARCH ON CORPORATIONS AND GHG

Historians have contributed important studies of corporations and their impact on global health. In *Merchants of Doubt* (2012), historians Naomi Oreskes and Eric Conway analyse the campaigns waged by right-wing think tanks and foundations, and scientists financed by tobacco and fossil fuel industries, to discredit independent environmental science. *Lead Wars: The Politics of Science and the Fate of America's Children* (2013) and *Deceit and Denial: The Deadly Politics of Industrial Pollution* (2002) by historians Gerald Markowitz and David Rosner examine the deleterious health impacts caused by lead content in paint and other everyday products. Their analysis of documents made available through US litigation reveals the commercial, political and scientific factors that enabled the widespread use of lead despite known health risks. Their revelations of corporate misconduct are valuable to policymakers and the general public who can be misled by corporate strategies. As Markowitz and Rosner (2002, 3) argue, 'It is a tenet of democracy that citizens should have full access to information so they can make informed decisions about policies that affect their lives.' Historical analysis has been especially important in this respect:

> What emerges is a history of deceit that is strikingly similar to that of the asbestos and tobacco industries. As with tobacco and asbestos, the lead and vinyl industries knew of dangers from their products but chose to ignore or conceal them. In fact, they actively deceived the public about the safety of their products. (Markowitz and Rosner 2002, 300)

Historians have yet to engage directly with the relationship between corporations and GHG, but there is a significant related literature that suggests potential contributions. Three historical studies of tobacco corporations neatly summarise key distinctions in approach, interpretation and sources between corporate history and historical analysis of corporations. Howard Cox's *The Global Cigarette, Origins and Evolution of British American Tobacco, 1880–1945* (2000), is a chronological narrative of British American Tobacco's (BAT) first half century of operation. A professor of business history at the University of Worcester, Cox notes that BAT was a multinational corporation from its formation in 1902, created by US and UK tobacco companies to control the world cigarette market. BAT prospered by establishing subsidiaries throughout the British Commonwealth, China and other key markets through innovative manufacturing and aggressive marketing. The company markedly expanded its overseas operations in the interwar years, despite increasing competition, with operations in 50 markets by the 1930s. The company's ability to prosper, amid the political and economic uncertainty of the twentieth century, is attributed to strategies such as working in partnership with allied countries on advertising and marketing strategies and establishing relationships with the British government and successive Chinese administrations. Cox was granted access to BAT's archives based on his previous research on the company, which came to the attention of former chairman Duncan Oppenheim who interceded on his behalf to secure company support for his project. Cox describes this as an 'extraordinary act of faith' by a leading figure in an industry that had become 'instinctively suspicious and defensive' (Cox 2000, x). That BAT harboured no such suspicions about Cox's analysis is suggested by the company chairman's foreword to the book, and its dedication to the former editor of BAT NEWS and the company's marketing information officer (Proctor 2011).

However, Proctor (2011, 468) argues that such reliance by an individual historian on unpublished "corporate histories" prepared by BAT's legal department, to which others do not have access, raises questions about whether the account can be meaningfully evaluated. While acknowledging its inherent scholarship, he describes *The Global Cigarette* as 'a celebration of one of the worlds' largest tobacco transnationals' and an example of company-sanctioned corporate histories, which 'typically treats the rise of a particular firm in the form of a business history' (Proctor 2011, 468).

Cox's relationship with BAT stands in marked contrast to the obstacles created for academic researchers seeking access to the Guildford Depository, a collection of company documents made public, with those of other tobacco companies, by a 1998 US legal settlement (Muggli, LeGresley and Hurt 2004). These documents have contributed to histories of the tobacco industry by Allan Brandt and Robert Proctor that provide narratives considerably different to that written by Cox. In *The Cigarette Century: The Rise, Fall and Deadly Persistence of the Product that Defined America* (Brandt 2007),

Brandt, a professor of the history of medicine at Harvard Medical School, analysed secondary sources and internal industry documents to reveal strategies by US tobacco companies to avoid meaningful regulation, promote spurious 'harm reduction' modifications and reframe the debate around smoking and health to incorporate concerns around commercial freedom. The documents also disclose a history of the industry keeping its decades-long knowledge of the health risks of smoking secret, and creating extensive campaigns, not only to deny links to cancer and other diseases but also to discredit the findings of independent scientists.

Proctor, a professor of the history of science at Stanford University, describes his book *Golden Holocaust: Origins of the Cigarette Catastrophe and the Case for Abolition* as 'the history of cigarette design, cigarette rhetoric, and cigarette science', aimed at treating 'the cigarette as part of the ordinary history of technology – and a deeply political (and fraudulent) artefact' (Proctor 2011, 4). His approach to the history of the cigarette as artefact would be familiar to social and cultural historians. Based on industry documents, Proctor concludes that tobacco corporations are 'notorious masters of deception', who 'know how to manufacture ignorance and rewrite history', most notably in their ability to create a narrative of smoking as a solved problem (Proctor 2011, 3).

CONCLUSION

Public concern about the impact of corporations is increasingly focused on the health implications of their products and operations (Wiist 2010; Freudenberg 2014; Kenworthy, MacKenzie and Lee 2016). While confronting corporate power and influence remains a daunting task, historical analysis offers important approaches, data sources and methods to help locate corporations within particular social and cultural contexts over time. Academic histories challenge the notion that corporations are the inevitable product of immutable market forces and that their activities simply arise from the pursuit of economic efficiency and profit. Rather, the global rise of the corporation is the consequence of human agency, played out within certain social and culture settings, with resultant harms and benefits to different interests. Baum and Anaf (2015) suggest four research directions for future historical analysis of corporations: assessing the health and equity impacts of TNCs, evaluating the effectiveness of government regulation to mitigate health and equity impacts, studying civil society strategies that highlight adverse TNC impacts and identifying ways to restrain transnational capitalism. The work of historians, as discussed in this chapter, is well placed to contribute to a deeper understanding of corporate influence on GHG.

FURTHER READING

Markowitz, Gerald and David Rosner. 2013. *Lead Wars: The Politics of Science and the Fate of America's Children*. Berkeley: University of California Press.

Oreskes, Naomi and Eric Conway. 2012. *Merchants of Doubt: How a Handful of Scientists Obscured the Truth on Issues from Tobacco Smoke to Global Warming*. New York: Bloomsbury Press.

Proctor, Robert. 2011. *Golden Holocaust: Origins of the Cigarette Catastrophe and the Case for Abolition*. Berkeley: University of California Press.

REFERENCES

Baum, Fran and Julia Anaf. 2015. 'Transnational Corporations and Health: A Research Agenda'. *International Journal of Health Services* 45(2): 353–62.

Berghoff, Hartmut. 2015. 'Business History'. In *International Encyclopedia of the Social and Behavioral Sciences*, 2nd edition, volume 3, edited by James D. Wright, 21–26. Oxford, UK: Elsevier.

Birn, Anne-Emanuelle. 2009. 'The Stages of International (Global) Health: Histories of Success or Successes of History?' *Global Public Health* 4(1): 50–68.

Birn, Anne-Emanuelle and Gilberto Hochman. 2008. 'Communication, Control, and Co-operation: (Latin) American Interchanges in the History of International Health'. *Canadian Bulletin of Medical History* 25(1): 7–16.

Booker, Jamal. 2011. 'A Virtual Walk through the Coke Archives!!'. Accessed 12 March. http://www.coca-colacompany.com/stories/2011/04/a-virtual-walk-through-the-coke-archives/.

Brandt, Allan. 2007. *The Cigarette Century: The Rise, Fall and Deadly Persistence of the Product That Defined America*. New York: Basic Books.

Brown, Theodore M., Marcos Cueto and Elizabeth Fee. 2006. 'The World Health Organization and the Transition from "International" to "Global" Public Health'. *American Journal of Public Health* 96(1): 62–72.

Burghausen, Mario and John M.T. Balmer. 2014. 'Repertoires of the Corporate Past: Explanation and Framework: Introducing an Integrated and Dynamic perspective'. *Corporate Communications: An International Journal* 19(4): 384–402.

Burke, Peter. 2008. *What Is Cultural History?* 2nd edition. Malden, MA: Polity Press.

Cohen, Gerald. 2001. *Karl Marx's Theory of History: A Defence*, 2nd edition. Princeton, NJ: Princeton University Press.

'Corporate History; Past Rites'. 2007. *The Economist*, 6 September 6. Accessed 19 January 2016. http://www.economist.com/node/9767599.

Cox, Howard. 2000. *The Global Cigarette: Origins and Evolution of British American Tobacco, 1880–1945*. Oxford, UK: Oxford University Press.

Elton, Geoffrey R. 1967. *The Practice of History*. London: Metheun.

Fridenson, Patrick. 2009. 'Business History and History'. In *The Oxford Handbook of Business History*, edited by Geoffrey Jones and Jonathan Zeitlin, 9–36. Oxford, UK: Oxford University Press.

Freudenberg, Nicholas. 2014. *Legal but Lethal: Corporations, Consumption and Protecting Public Health*. Oxford, UK: Oxford University Press.

Hopkins, Anthony. 2006. *Global History: Interactions between the Universal and the Local*. Basingstoke, UK: Palgrave Macmillan.

IBM. 2016. 'Using the Archives Site'. Accessed 11 April 2016. http://www-03.ibm.com/ibm/history/using/index.html.

Iggers, Georg. 2005. *Historiography in the Twentieth Century: From Scientific Objectivity to the Postmodern Challenge*. Hanover, NH: Wesleyan University Press.

Jones, Geoffrey. 2009. 'Globalization'. In *The Oxford Handbook of Business History*, edited by Geoffrey Jones and Jonathan Zeitlin, 141–68. Oxford, UK: Oxford University Press.

Kenworthy, Nora, Ross MacKenzie and Kelley Lee, eds. 2016. *Case Studies on Corporations and Global Health Governance: Impacts, Influence and Accountability*. London: Rowman & Littlefield International.

Koplan, Jeffrey, Christopher Bond, Michael Merson, Srinath Reddy, Mario Henry Rodriguez, Nelson Sewankambo, Judith Wasserheit for the Consortium of Universities for Global Health Executive Board. 2009. 'Towards a Common Definition of Global Health'. *Lancet* 373: 1993–95.

Korten, David. 2001. *When Corporations Rule the World*, 2nd edition. Bloomfield, CT: Kumarian Press.

Lewis, Brian. 2013. 'The Newest Social History: Crisis and Renewal'. In *The SAGE Handbook of Historical Theory*, edited by Nancy Partner and Sarah Foot, 225–37. London: Sage.

Lewis, W. David and Wesley Newtown. 1981. 'The Writing of Corporate History'. *Public Historian* 3(3): 62–74.

Loughlin, Kelly and Virginia Berridge. 2002. *Global Health Governance: Historical Dimensions of Global Governance*. London: London School of Hygiene & Tropical Medicine.

Markowitz, Gerald and David Rosner. 2002. *Deceit and Denial: The Deadly Politics of Industrial Pollution*. Berkeley: University of California Press.

Markowitz, Gerald and David Rosner. 2013. *Lead Wars: The Politics of Science and the Fate of America's Children*. Berkeley: University of California Press.

McGerr, Michael E. 2003. *A Fierce Discontent: The Rise and Fall of the Progressive Movement in America, 1870–1920*. New York: Free Press/Simon & Schuster.

Muggli, Monique, Eric LeGresley and Richard Hurt. 2004. 'Big Tobacco Is Watching: British American Tobacco's Surveillance and Information Concealment at the Guildford Depository'. *Lancet* 363: 1812–19.

National Archives, United Kingdom. 2016. 'Businesses'. Accessed 5 March. http://www.nationalarchives.gov.uk/help-with-your-research/research-guides/businesses/.

Orbell, John and Alison Turton. 2001. *British Banking: A Guide to Historical Records*. Aldershot, UK: Ashgate.

Oreskes, Naomi and Eric Conway. 2012. *Merchants of Doubt: How a Handful of Scientists Obscured the Truth on Issues from Tobacco Smoke to Global Warming*. New York: Bloomsbury Press.

Pargellis, Stanley. 1944. 'The Corporation and the Historian'. *Journal of Economic History* 4: 29–37.

Partner, Nancy. 2013. 'Foundations: Theoretical Frameworks for Knowledge of the Past'. In *The SAGE Handbook of Historical Theory*, edited by Nancy Partner and Sarah Foot, 1–8. London: Sage.

Proctor, Robert. 2011. *Golden Holocaust: Origins of the Cigarette Catastrophe and the Case for Abolition*. Berkeley: University of California Press.

Rajak, Dinah. 2014. 'Corporate Memory: Historical Revisionism, Legitimation and the Invention of Tradition in a Multinational Mining Company'. *Political and Legal Anthropology Review* 37(2): 259–80.

Richmond, Lesley, Julie Stevenson and Alison Turton. 2003. *The Pharmaceutical Industry: A Guide to Historical Records*. Aldershot, UK: Ashgate.

Richmond, Lesley and Alison Turton. 1990. *The Brewing Industry: A Guide to Historical Records*. Manchester, UK: Manchester University Press.

Ritchie, L.A. 1992. *The Shipbuilding Industry: A Guide to Historical Records*. Manchester, UK: Manchester University Press.

Rowlinson, Michael. 2004. 'Historical Analysis of Company Documents'. In *Essential Guide to Qualitative Methods in Organizational Research*, edited by Catherine Cassell and Gillian Symon, 301–11. London: Sage.

Schneider, Axel and Daniel Woolf. 2015. 'Introduction'. In *The Oxford History of Historical Writing Volume 5: Historical Writing since 1945*, edited by Axel Schneider and Daniel Woolf, 1–12. Oxford, UK: Oxford University Press.

Siemens. 2016. 'Corporate Archives'. Accessed 12 March. https://www.siemens.com/history/en/siemens_historical_institute/corporate_archives/.

Society of American Archivists. 2016. 'Directory of Corporate Archives in the United States and Canada'. Accessed 12 April 2016. http://www2.archivists.org/groups/business-archives-section/directory-of-corporate-archives-in-the-united-states-and-canada-introduction.

Southgate, Beverley. 2001. *History, What and Why?* 2nd edition. London: Routledge.

White, Hayden. 1973. *Metahistory: The Historical Imagination in Nineteenth-Century Europe*. Baltimore, MD: Johns Hopkins University.

Wiist, William, ed. 2010. *The Bottom Line or Public Health: Tactics Corporations Use to Influence Health and Health Policy, and What We Can Do to Counter Them*. Oxford, UK: Oxford University Press.

Chapter 6

Criminology

Raymond Michalowski

Criminology is most often understood as the study of why people commit crimes, with particular emphasis on the psychological and social background of criminals; how to more effectively police, prosecute and punish criminal offenders; and how to reintegrate convicted offenders back into society. This *orthodox* approach is devoted to explaining the 'ordinary' crimes that consume most of the time, money and energy of justice systems worldwide, and serve as routine fodder for newspaper headlines, detective novels, films and television dramas. Because of this focus on lawbreakers as *individual* agents of crime, orthodox criminology offers few insights into how structured *social organisations*, such as corporations, can threaten human and planetary well-being. In contrast to orthodox approaches, *critical criminology* is explicitly grounded in analyses of the relationship between power and law. This branch of criminology provides a starting point for studying the crimes of the powerful, including power centres such as corporations.

This chapter explores the relationship between corporations and global health governance from a criminological perspective. It focuses on the study of 'state-corporate crime' as it has evolved in the sub-discipline of critical criminology. The chapter first examines the tensions within criminology between studying common 'street crimes' by relatively powerless individuals versus crimes and social harms emanating from corporate and political power centres. It argues that it is essential to study corporate and political power if we hope to understand the forces driving many of the gravest threats to human health worldwide. It then examines the concept of *state-corporate* crime and social harms resulting from systemic relationships between business and government. Finally, it examines the potential of the state-corporate crime model for analysing the relationship between global health and the threats that emerge from their intersection with corporations and governments.

THEORISING CRIME

As a topic, rather than a discipline, criminology has relied primarily on theories and methods developed within core social science disciplines to create mid-range theories about the making, breaking and enforcement of law. For example, criminological theories concerning the deterrent effect of law and punishment are grounded in economic theories of rational choice (Zimring and Hawkins 1973). Criminological theories about how people begin and persist in deviant or criminal acts draw on psychological theories about social learning (Bandura and Walters 1963), sociological theories of routine socialisation (Sutherland 1939) and social psychology theories of symbolic interactionism (Becker 1963; Lemert 1967). Criminology has also been an aggregator of methodologies from varied academic disciplines, bringing quantitative and qualitative analytics from other fields to study the subject matter of crime and justice.

In its orthodox form, criminology, occupies the contradictory position of claiming to be an *independent* intellectual framework for inquiry into matters of crime and justice, while simultaneously being part of what Gramsci (1971) saw as the 'extended state'. The latter comprises key elements of civil society, including intellectuals, which play important roles in establishing and reproducing hegemonic concepts of appropriate social order favoured by the political state. As part of the extended state, orthodox criminology is more than a hybrid area of *academic* inquiry. It also serves the interests of the political state. The designation of behaviours, as legal or illegal and, among illegal activities, those deemed minor and major infractions by the criminal justice system, is shaped by political power. A basic proposition within critical criminology is that, in hierarchical societies, the dominant classes play a central role in determining what will and will not be criminalised and that these classes will rarely define the harms they commit as crimes (Chambliss and Seidman 1971; Platt 1974; Quinney 1974; Michalowski 1985). By focusing primarily on those acts criminalised by the state, orthodox criminology serves to reproduce existing distributions of power and wealth by validating hegemonic definitions of crime and social threat that give little attention to crimes by the powerful. For example, less than 10% of the content of major journals in the field address corporate or political crimes, with the remaining 90% devoted to aspects of routine street crimes against persons, property or public order, particular drug offenses (Michalowski 2013).

Critical criminologists challenge this orthodoxy by arguing for an approach that focuses on the *problem of crime* in its entirety. The problem of crime encompasses the ways in which law and justice systems do, and do not, address human behaviours and organisational arrangements that are *injurious to the well-being of humans*, *other living beings*, and the *biosphere*. Critical criminology holds that the field's subject matter must be expanded, to include analyses of *legal* social harms, if we are to understand and address the failure of legal systems to address many of the most serious threats to both human and planetary well-being (Hillyard et al. 2004; Presser 2013).

The first step away from orthodox criminology came in 1939 when Edwin Sutherland, in his presidential address to the American Sociological Association, argued that criminologists should add regulatory and civil violations of the 'white-collar' kind to their subject matter (Sutherland 1940, 1945). His subsequent book *White Collar Crime* (Sutherland 1949) pushed criminological boundaries further by suggesting that the level of *social injury* caused by businesses, rather than its legal status, should determine whether a topic was relevant for criminology. Most significantly, *corporations* should be the focus of corporate crime studies rather than individual wrongdoers (Kramer 1984).

By highlighting the wide disparity between punishments meted out for corporate and white-collar crime and those for street crimes, Sutherland's analyses opened the door to studying how social class and political power shape the probability of which acts and which individuals are criminalised. In doing so, he pointed towards a criminology focused, as much on the role of structural arrangements in generating social injury as, on individual miscreants.

CRIMINOLOGY AND CORPORATE ACTORS

The study of corporations by criminologists eventually led to the emergence of the concept of *state-corporate* crime. The integrated model of state-corporate crime is based on the proposition that, in market societies, many corporate crimes and social harms are either instigated by or made possible by political states. Conversely, most state crimes involve some degree of reliance on corporate capacity to provide the material, labour or knowledge needed to achieve state goals. While the typical distinction between state crimes and corporate crimes can be heuristically useful, it risks overlooking the fact that political actions always have economic consequences and involve economic interests, and that economic actions always have political consequences and engage political interests (Michalowski 2009). The concept of state-corporate crime sought to erase the line often drawn between economics and politics in social science analyses (see Chapter 3).

Kramer and Michalowski (1990, 3) initially defined state-corporate as 'illegal or socially injurious actions that occur when one or more institutions of political governance pursue a goal in direct cooperation with one or more institutions of economic production and distribution'. This emphasis on 'direct cooperation', however, was better suited to analyses of specific instances of state-corporate engagement, such as the production of nuclear weapons (Kauzlarich and Kramer 1998) or military drones (Kramer and Smith 2013), than on harms arising from broader structural arrangements through which the intersecting pursuits of business and government organisation generate ongoing environments for the production of social harm. In response, Aulette and Michalowski (1993, 175) redefined state-corporate crimes as

> illegal or socially injurious actions that result from a mutually reinforcing interaction between (1) policies and/or practices in pursuit of the goals of one or more institutions of political governance and (2) policies and/or practices in pursuit of the goals of one or more institutions of economic production and/or distribution.

Applying this definition to the deadly 1991 fire at the Imperial chicken processing plant in Hamlet, North Carolina, Aulette and Michalowski (1993) further argue for a distinction between *state-initiated* and *state-facilitated* forms of state-corporate crime. This distinction is based on whether the initial goals leading to eventual harms originated within institutions of government, and then relied on corporate assistance to achieve their aims, as in the case of the *Challenger* space shuttle explosion (Kramer 1992), or whether the initial impetus resided within some corporate goal that was advanced by government acts of commission or omission, such as the case of North Carolina creating a 'business-friendly' climate amid profoundly lax enforcement of the safety regulations that could have prevented the fire.

The integrated model of state-corporate crime directs attention to specific catalysts for action (motivations, opportunity and controls) as they operate at three levels of analyses (the societal, the organisational and the interactional). Table 6.1 offers one example of the particular social forces at play in the two case studies of state-corporate crime (the Imperial chicken plant fire and the space shuttle *Challenger* explosion). The *specific* social dynamics, belonging in the cells shown in Table 6.1, would vary depending on the harm being analysed, and the social, economic and political contexts within which it took place. What the model offers is a taxonomic framework within which analysts of the relationship between corporations and GHG can begin to identify the forces generative of any particular health outcome.

Table 6.1. An integrated theoretical model of state–corporate crime

	Catalysts for action		
Levels of analysis	*Motivation*	*Opportunity*	*Control*
Societal	Culture of competition Economic pressures Organisational goals Performance emphasis	Availability of legal means Obstacles and constraints Blocked goals/strain Availability of illegal means Access to resources	International reaction Political pressure Legal sanctions Media scrutiny Public opinion Social movements
Organisational	Corporate culture Operative goals Subunit goals Managerial pressures	Instrumental rationality Internal constraints Defective SOPs Creation of illegal means Task segregations Role specialisation Communications technology Normalisation of deviance	Culture of compliance Cultures of resistance Codes of conduct Reward structure Safety/quality control Transparency
Interactional	Socialisation Social meaning Individual goals Competitive individualism Material success emphasised	Definitions of situations Perceived of means availability Attractiveness of illegal means	Personal morality Neutralisation Diffuse responsibility Obedience to authority Remote consequences Groupthink

Source: Kramer, Ronald C. and Raymond Michalowski. 2006. 'The Original Formulation'. In *State-Corporate Crime: Wrongdoing at the Intersection of Business and Government*, edited by Raymond Michalowski and Ronald C. Kramer. New Brunswick, NJ: Rutgers University Press, p. 25.

STATE-CORPORATE CRIME AND GLOBAL HEALTH

The subject matter of state-corporate crime inquiry would appear to differ significantly from traditional public health research in two ways. First, public health (as distinct from clinical) research focuses on *the public*, that is health determinants and outcomes that have the potential to impact whole populations, from local communities to the entirety of the human species. By contrast, state-corporate crime analyses, as discussed later, address harms that affect more limited numbers of victims.

Second, while public health is typically defined as the protection and promotion of population health (Beaglehole and Bonita 1997), diseases have historically received far more attention than injuries despite the latter causing 5.8 million deaths annually. Because injuries and deaths from violent causes *appear* to be neither contagious nor amenable to the kinds of larger-scale interventions typical of public health projects, they play a lesser role in public health research. For instance, in 2013 only 1 of the top 13 public health issues listed by the US Centers for Disease Control – the global problem of violence against children – involves injury (listed as number 13). Even then, the reason given for this concern is not the violence and subsequent injuries per se, but that children who experience violence in homes 'are at greater risk HIV, chronic diseases, crime and drug abuse, as well as serious mental health problems' (CDC 2013). Similarly, in 2015 the only health threat involving injury listed by the US Association of Public Health Officials as a key issue was traffic mishaps (Esworthy 2015).

In contrast, state-corporate analyses typically focus on injuries and violence. These studies can be divided into two broad groups – those that examine *acute events* (e.g. factory fire) and those concerned with *destructive conditions* (e.g. ongoing toxic releases). The surface appearance of these acute events and destructive conditions can make them seem as if they are relatively self-contained occurrences. However, one of the core findings of state-corporate crime studies is that these singularly appearing events most often result from *systemic patterns and practices* that increase the likelihood of continued occurrence of substantively similar events (Kramer and Michalowski 2012; Stretesky, Long and Lynch 2014; Bradshaw 2015). Herein lies the key similarity between public health research and state-corporate crime studies, *to wit*, the identification and disruption of systemic forces responsible for *ongoing* risks of actions and outcomes that compromise human and planetary well-being.

State-corporate crime studies of violent *events* examine discrete occurrences that take place within a relatively brief timeframe and whose consequences are (usually) limited to immediate victims. Examples are the *Challenger* explosion (Kramer 1992), Imperial chicken plant fire (Aulette and Michalowski 1993), crash of *ValuJet* Flight 592 (Matthews and Kauzlarich 2000) and release of toxic gases from the Union Carbide plant in Bhopal, India (Walters 2009).

Destructive conditions differ from violent events, in that the harm-generating actions are often ongoing, rather than singular catastrophic moments. The resulting consequences radiate outwards, from the core actors and actions, to affect a socially and geographically wider range of people and other life forms. Destructive conditions can be further subdivided into *relatively bounded* and *relatively unbounded* conditions. Relatively bounded conditions, studied as state-corporate crimes, often involve environmental events that cause significant harm but whose reach can be approximately identified and whose consequences can be approximately ameliorated or compensated. Classic cases of relatively bounded state-corporate crimes include the *Exxon-Valdez* oil spill (Cruciotti and Matthews 2006) and the *DeepWater Horizons* blowout and subsequent pollution of the Gulf Coast of Louisiana and Mississippi (Bradshaw 2012). In cases such as these, a specific event initiated a chain of consequences that harm humans, animals and sea life well beyond both the time and place of the original cause. Even though it is possible to map the temporal and geographical scope of these events, they are only *relatively* bounded because they may also have more subtle, far-reaching effects that will manifest only years or decades later. For instance, it will be many decades before we can fully calculate the environmental and human toll of the despoliation of the shore and offshore waters of the Gulf of Mexico by the *DeepWater Horizons* blowout (Plaisance and McGill 2014; Mole 2015).

Studies of acute events and relatively bounded destructive conditions, as state-corporate crimes, differ from routine criminology studies because, as noted earlier, they focus on organisations rather than individuals. Nevertheless, these inquiries still fit within a general investigative framework that begins with asking 'who did what to whom, and when did they do it', even if the 'who' may be an aggregate of organisational actors. By contrast, the analysis of relatively *unbounded* destructive conditions moves beyond examining organisations, whose specific actions cause harm, by interrogating how these organisations are embedded in social *systems* that magnify, and sometimes even require that they engage in, actions that will result in harm. It is here that we find particularly useful concepts for understanding and analysing the context within which global health threats emerge.

EXAMPLES OF STATE-CORPORATE CRIMES IN THE GLOBAL HEALTH ARENA

During the 20-year Vietnam War (1955–1974), there was a popular anti-war poster drawn as if by a young child with a box of crayons. It pictured a flower and the words, 'War is not healthy for children and other living things.' In their immediacy, given their wide-ranging harms with undeniable public health consequences, wars are an excellent example of unbounded destructive conditions. As Epstein (1997) observes, 'While it is axiomatic that war involves killing . . . war also leaves wounds, infections, and suffering lingering for years, poisoning relationships, psyches, soils, forests, and underground water systems.' Moreover, state-corporate organisations that supply the machinery of war are embedded in social systems that bind them politically and economically to these harms (Levy and Siedel 2007).

Another example is the far-reaching harms to global health from climate change. The strong consensus among independent scientists is that our carbon-dependent world economy is creating systemic changes that will have devastating impacts, not only on climate but also on long-term human and planetary well-being and even survival (Klein 2014; Kolbert 2014). Importantly, climate change is not the natural or inevitable consequence of market forces, as neoliberal economists claim (Friedman 2002; Hayak 2011). It is the result of political and economic *choices*, made at the intersection of the corporate pursuit of profit and state policies and practices developed to facilitate that pursuit (Livingston 2011; Robinson 2014; Kotz 2015; Reich 2015). In many parts of the world, the twin effects of war and climate change are coming together. Desertification is already causing public health crises of starvation, disease, death and war. Meanwhile, wealthier and as yet less-affected countries have begun militarising their borders against refugees fleeing the 'catastrophic convergence' of overstressed economies, climate change and militarism. If continued, it is a strategy that will ensure that the poorest nations and populations will bear a disproportionate burden of the health harms generated, what Parenti (2011) terms the *politics of the armed lifeboat*.

What do large-scale processes like armed violence or climate change have to do with the application of a state-corporate crime model to the study of global health? Put simply, harms such as war, exploitation, inequality and climate change are grounded in the decisions and actions undertaken within economic (i.e. corporate) organisations and political (i.e. government) systems to facilitate their growth and protect their interests. Similarly, the production and hyper-marketing of health-harming products (e.g. tobacco, high fat, high sugar) and the continued corporate efforts to weaken the ability of governments to effectively control the pollution of air, soil and water are *routine and legal activities* whose consequences for human and planetary health are at least, if not more, devastating for human health than contagious disease.

CONCLUSION

If we are to understand the gravest threats to global health, we must undertake careful and systematic analyses not just of the patterns and consequences of disease and injury but of how corporate and political interests intersect in ways that promote unbounded destructive conditions and thwart efforts to curtail them. For every epidemic, there are profits to be made and political advantages to be gained or lost. For every increase in inequality, with all of its harmful human health consequences, there are corporations and governmental officials who benefit. For every regulation of harmful products or practices that is defeated, there are those who win either financially or politically by that defeat. Bringing the state-corporate nexus into research on GHG can provide the critical context and background needed to fully understand what is happening on the ground in many situations where human and planetary well-being are threatened.

FURTHER READING

Kassirer, Jerome. 2005. *On the Take: How Medicine's Complicity with Big Business Can Endanger Your Health*. New York: Oxford University Press.

Klein, Naomi. 2016. 'Let Them Drown: The Violence of Othering in a Warming World'. *London Review of Books* 38(11): 11–14.

Laslett, Kristian. 2015. *State Crime at the Margin of Empire: Rio Tinto, the War on Bougainville and Resistance to Mining*. London: Pluto Press.

REFERENCES

Aulette, Judy R. and Raymond Michalowski. 1993. 'Fire in Hamlet: A Case Study of State-Corporate Crime'. In *Political Crime in Contemporary America: A Critical Approach*, edited by Kenneth D. Tunnell, 170–206. London: Garland Publishing Incorporated.

Bandura, Albert and Richard H. Walters. 1963. *Social Learning and Personality Development*. New York: Holt Rinehart and Winston.

Beaglehole Robert and Ruth Bonita. 1997. *Public Health at the Crossroads, Achievements and Prospects*. Cambridge, UK: Cambridge University Press.

Becker, Howard. 1963. *Outsiders: Studies in the Sociology of Deviance*. Glencoe, IL: The Free Press.

Bradshaw, Elizabeth. 2012. 'Deepwater, Deep Ties, Deep Trouble: A State-Corporate Environmental Crime Analysis of the 2010 Gulf of Mexico Oil Spill'. PhD Thesis, Western Michigan University.

Bradshaw, Elizabeth. 2015. 'Blacking Out the Gulf: State-Corporate Environmental Crime and the Response to the 2010 BP Oil Spill'. In *The Routledge International Handbook of the Crimes of the Powerful*, edited by Gregg Barak, 363–72. New York: Routledge.

CDC (Centres for Disease Control). 2013. 'CDC Looks Ahead: 13 Public Health Issues in 2013'. Accessed September 19, 2016. http://blogs.cdc.gov/cdcworksforyou24-7/2013/01/cdc-looks-ahead-13-public-health-issues-in-2013/.

Chambliss, William and Robert Seidman. 1971. *Law, Order, and Power*. Reading, MA: Addison-Wesley.

Cruciotti, Tricia and Rick Matthews. 2006. 'The *Exxon-Valdez* Oil Spill'. In *State Corporate Crime: Wrongdoing at the Intersection of Business and Politics*, edited by Raymond J. Michalowski and Ronald C. Kramer, 116–33. New Brunswick, NJ: Rutgers University Press.

Epstein, Paul. 1997. 'War and Public Health'. *Journal of the American Medical Association* 277(18): 1479–80.

Esworthy, Jane. 2015. 'Public Health Issues to Watch in 2015'. *State Public Health*, 3 March. http://www.astho.org/StatePublicHealth/Public-Health-Issues-to-Watch-in-2015/3-3-15/.

Frankel, Glenn. 1996. 'U.S. Aided Cigarette Firms in Conquests across Asia'. *Washington Post*, 17 November. Accessed September 19, 2016. http://www.washingtonpost.com/wp-srv/national/longterm/tobacco/stories/asia.htm.

Friedman, Milton. 2002. *Capitalism and Freedom*. Chicago, IL: University of Chicago Press.

Gramsci, Antonio. 1971. *Selections from the Prison Notebooks*. Edited and translated by Quintin Hoare and Geoffrey Nowell Smith. New York: International Publishers.

Hayak, Fredrick. 2011. *The Constitution of Liberty*. Chicago, IL: University of Chicago Press.

Hillyard, Paddy, Christina Pantazis, Dave Gordon, Steve Tombs and Daniel Dorling. 2004. *Beyond Criminology: Taking Harm Seriously*. London: Pluto Press.

Kauzlarich, David and Ronald C. Kramer. 1998. *Crimes of the American Nuclear State: At Home and Abroad*. Boston, MA: Northeastern University Press.

Klein, Naomi. 2014. *This Changes Everything: Capitalism vs. the Climate*. New York: Simon & Schuster.

Kolbert, Elizabeth. 2014. *The Sixth Extinction: An Unnatural History*. New York: Henry Holt.

Kotz, David. 2015. *The Rise and Fall of NeoLiberal Capitalism*. Cambridge, MA: Harvard University Press.

Kramer, Ronald C. 1984. 'Corporate Criminality: The Development of an Idea'. In *Corporations as Criminals*, edited by Ellen Hochstedler, 13–33. Beverly Hills, CA: Sage Publications.

Kramer, Ronald C. 1992. 'The Space Shuttle Challenger Explosion'. In *White Collar Crime Reconsidered*, edited by Kip Schlegel and David Weisburd, 214–34. Boston, MA: Northeastern University Press.

Kramer, Ronald C. and Raymond Michalowski. 1990. 'Toward an Integrated Theory of State-Corporate Crime'. Presented at the American Society of Criminology, Baltimore, Maryland.

Kramer, Ronald C. and Raymond Michalowski. 2012. 'Is Global Warming a State-Corporate Crime?' In *Climate Change from a Criminological Perspective*, edited by Rob White, 71–88. New York: Springer.

Kramer, Ronald C. and Amanda Marie Smith. 2013. 'Death Flies Down: The Bombing of Civilians and the Paradox of International Law'. In *Towards a Victimology of State Crime*, edited by Dawn L. Rothe and David Kauzlarich, 110–30. New York: Routledge.

Lemert, Edwin. 1967. *Human Deviance, Social Problems, and Social Control.* Englewood Cliffs, NJ: Prentice Hall.
Levy, Barry S. and Victor W. Siedel. 2007. *War and Public Health,* 2nd edition. New York: Oxford University Press.
Livingston, James. 2011. *Against Thrift.* New York: Basic Books.
Matthews, Rick and David Kauzlarich, David. 2000. 'The Crash of Valujet Flight 592: A Case of Study in State-Corporate Crime'. *Sociological Focus* 3(3): 281–98.
Michalowski, Raymond. 1985. *Order, Law and Crime: An Introduction to Criminology.* New York: Random House.
Michalowski, Raymond. 2009. 'Power, Crime and Criminology in the New Imperial Age'. *Crime, Law and Social Change* 51(3): 303–25.
Michalowski, Raymond. 2013. 'What Is Crime? Why Is Criminology?' Presidential Panel Address, American Society of Criminology Annual Meeting, Atlanta, GA. https://asc41.com/Annual_Meeting/2013/Presidential%20Papers/Michalowski,%20Raymond.pdf.
Michalowski, Raymond and Ronald C. Kramer. 2006. *State-Corporate Crime: Wrongdoing at the Intersection of Business and Politics.* New Brunswick, NJ: Rutgers University Press.
Mole, Beth. 2015. 'Five Years on, Deepwater Horizon Oil Spill's Impact Lingers'. *Science News,* 3 April. https://www.sciencenews.org/article/five-years-deepwater-horizon-oil-spills-impact-lingers.
Parenti, Christian. 2011. *Tropic of Chaos: Climate Change and the New Geography of Violence.* New York: Nation Books.
Plaisance, Stacey and Kevin McGill. 2014. 'Nearly Four Years after the BP Oil Spill, Long-Term Health Impacts Remain Unclear'. *Huffington Post,* 11 April.
Platt, Tony. 1974. 'Prospects for a Radical Criminology in the United States'. *Crime and Social Justice* 1 (Spring–Summer): 2–10.
Presser, Lois. 2013. *Why We Harm.* New Brunswick, NJ: Rutgers University Press.
Quinney, Richard. 1974. *Critique of Legal Order: Crime Control in Capitalist Society.* Boston, MA: Little, Brown and Company.
Reich, Robert. 2015. *Saving Capitalism: For the Many, Not the Few.* New York: Knopf.
Robinson, William. 2014. *Global Capitalism and the Crisis of Humanity.* New York: Cambridge University Press.
Stretesky, Paul, Michael Long and Michael Lynch. 2014. *The Treadmill of Crime: Political Economy and Green Criminology.* New York: Routledge.
Sutherland, Edwin. 1939. *Criminology.* Philadelphia, PA: J.B. Lippincott.
Sutherland, Edwin. 1940. 'White-Collar Criminality'. *American Sociological Review* 5(1): 1–12.
Sutherland, Edwin. 1945. 'Is "White Collar Crime" Crime?' *American Sociological Review* 10(2): 132–39.
Sutherland, Edwin. 1949. *White Collar Crime.* New York: Dryden Press.
Walters, Reece. 2009. 'Bhopal, Corporate Crime and Harms of the Powerful.' *Global Social Policy* 9(3): 324–7.
Zimring, Franklin and Gordon Hawkins. 1973. *Deterrence: The Legal Threat in Crime Control.* Chicago, IL: University of Chicago Press.

Chapter 7

Anthropology

Richard G. Parker and Nora J. Kenworthy

Anthropology is the study of humans, examining both the origins and the structures, forms and practices of contemporary cultures. The discipline is traditionally divided into four substantive areas – sociocultural anthropology, linguistic anthropology, physical or biological anthropology and archaeology – which are further broken down into an extensive range of subfields such as political and medical anthropology. This chapter focuses on sociocultural anthropology as most relevant to the study of corporations and their impacts on global health governance (GHG). Sociocultural anthropology focuses on the practices, social relations, meanings and institutions that shape the world, and the ways people live within particular social and political contexts. By examining these worlds in detail, and over extended periods of time, anthropologists seek to understand how cultural meanings, ideas and practices, forms of social organisation and hierarchies and tensions and conflicts within societies impact people's lives.

Anthropologists generally agree that scholars must look beyond individual practices to focus on shared meanings, patterns of behaviour and collective practices that reveal insights about a society. As Geertz (1973) noted, culture cannot exist solely within the mind of an individual, but is intersubjective, 'constructed' through the interactions and communicative exchanges between individuals. Whereas earlier work in anthropology focused on small-scale, non-Western societies, by the mid-twentieth century, anthropologists extended efforts to study more complex social groups and to depart from conceptions of culture as static, bounded and uniformly distributed within groups. In the late twentieth century, postmodernist and poststructuralist perspectives underscored the hierarchical ways in which anthropology itself constructed knowledge and texts, prompting calls for more polyvocal accounts offering multiple views from researchers, informants and even onlookers.

This chapter focuses on the contributions of anthropologists to scholarship on corporations and GHG. This is achieved through a review of the literature on anthropology and global health, and on corporations. Theoretical and methodological progress in anthropology lays the crucial groundwork for innovative and expanding research on global health, global institutions and elites in the private and public spheres. Chapter 12 provides an overview of ethnography as the primary method used in anthropological research.

ANTHROPOLOGY AND GLOBAL HEALTH

Drawing on two important subfields – medical anthropology and the anthropology of development – research on global health has typically been grounded in critical social theories of globalisation, challenging the ways neoliberalism and neo-colonialism shape health and politics. This approach focuses on the role of power and inequalities in producing conditions of health across populations. Janes and Corbett (2009, 170) identify four major contributions that anthropological studies have made to global health research: (1) ethnographic studies of health inequities in diverse political and economic contexts; (2) analysis of the impact of the forms of science and technology that circulate globally on local worlds and experiences; (3) interrogation, analysis and critique of international health policies and programmes; and (4) analysis of the health consequences from the reconfiguration of the social relations of international health development.

Anthropology's extensive use of ethnographic research and methods (see Chapter 12) makes it especially well suited to highly detailed and nuanced descriptions of health inequalities in different social and cultural settings (Briggs and Mantini-Briggs 2003; Maternowska 2006; Biehl 2007). This work has been especially important because it captures the lived experience of human suffering. While much global health research provides important data on epidemiologic trends, or large-scale patterns of health behaviour, it does not offer insights into the subjective realities of the people that policies and programmes are intended to serve (Nguyen and Peschard 2003).

Anthropological studies also play a key role in documenting the negative local consequences of development policies, such as privatisation of health financing and services (Foley 2010) and the related effects of structural adjustment programmes (Pfeiffer and Chapman 2010). By focusing on detailed descriptions and analyses of the political economy within which health and illness are experienced, an ethnographic record of what Paul Farmer (2004) characterises as an anthropology of structural violence is produced. This research documents how historical and political forces driving social inequalities produce physical and mental harms.

Because this research is deeply grounded in local communities and their experiences, anthropology provides an important foundation and point of departure for 'studying up' from local domains to examine powerful actors and global phenomena (Nader 1972), investigating institutions and processes through which global health policies and programmes operate. A wave of research has emerged since the 2000s that gives critical attention to global health practices and institutions as objects of study in their own right. Described as critical studies of global health, or critical anthropologies of global health, this work uses ethnographic and related methods to examine the activities of intergovernmental organisations, civil society groups, aid agencies and other institutions engaged in shaping global health practices (Pfeiffer and Nichter 2008; Biehl and Petryna 2013). Drawing on anthropology's strong emphasis on reflexivity and social criticism, this research turns a critical lens to analysing the field of global health itself, examining the social, political and economic dimensions of what might be described as a global health 'industry', a system that itself produces and reproduces the very health inequalities it seeks to redress.

The production and experience of health inequalities is perhaps the most important work in the anthropology of global health; within this domain, research on the politics of global health, GHG and the diverse institutional settings within which GHG is produced, implemented and contested is crucial. This work has tended to question and critique systems of power and domination that are produced and reproduced by the institutional architecture, policy processes and programmatic assemblages that are often uncritically designated as GHG.

Anthropological studies examine the institutional arenas and policy debates that shape the field of global health, such as the response to HIV and AIDS (Parker 2000; Hardon 2005). They also explore mobilisations such as the global responses to non-communicable diseases (Livingston 2012; Sivaramakrishnan and Parker 2012) and the 2014 West African Ebola outbreak (Ebola Response Anthropology Platform 2015). Anthropological studies also critically examine what is novel about public–private partnerships, such as the Global Fund to Fight AIDS/HIV, Tuberculosis and Malaria, and other global health innovations (Kapilashrami and Hanefeld 2014).

Anthropological research on GHG is also innovative in moving beyond analyses of institutional architectures, to investigate the processes by which policy decisions are operationalised, such as the implementation of neoliberal reforms within local health systems (Janes 2004), and the local impact of scaling up anti-retroviral treatments (Kalofonos 2014; Kenworthy 2014). The growing role and influence of non-state actors such as non-governmental organisations, charitable foundations and corporations in GHG are also investigated (Adams, Novotny and Leslie 2008; Nichter 2008; Redfield 2013).

Increasing awareness of how weak health systems may threaten global health goals has supported the need for ethnographic studies that go beyond a focus on technological, vertical and biomedical solutions. Anthropology emphasises the complex political forces that affect health service delivery and the social relations that shape health systems (Storeng and Mishra 2014). Attention is given to the social production of global health science and knowledge production, which are considered key aspects of GHG but are largely overlooked by other disciplines. Anthropology has made especially important contributions to developing critical appraisals of what constitutes 'evidence' in global health and how such evidence is put to use (Erikson 2012). In examining the shift from 'international health' in the latter part of the twentieth century to what is reconceived as 'global health' since the beginning of the twenty-first century, anthropological analyses have highlighted a growing emphasis on what Adams, Craig and Samen (2016) describe as 'evidence-based metrics', the use of experimental research platforms such as randomised controlled trials and cost-effectiveness rubrics such as Disability-Adjusted Life Years to assess interventions and programmes. Such shifts are linked, in turn, to changes in administrative procedures and auditing practices, justifying patterns of funding, programme design and evaluation in ways that transform the science and practice of global health (Adams 2013).

This very emphasis on certain types of metrics also opens alternative forms of investigation. In a world increasingly dominated by quantitative evidence related to outcomes, qualitative anthropological research can strategically position what anthropologists traditionally define as 'local knowledge' (Geertz 2000) about why people do the things they do. This contributes crucial perspectives to GHG by giving policymakers and programme staff new insights into how global health interventions are interpreted and experienced at the local level by the people that they are intended to serve.

Finally, anthropological studies of global health science interrogate the ways in which 'biological sciences are mobilized and stabilized in global health endeavours' and how 'global biomedicine serves as a planetary sociotechnical system for calibrating interventions on bodies and populations' (Brotherton and Nguyen 2013, 287). They also examine how dominant intellectual paradigms, primarily developed in high-income countries, have begun to shift research collaborations. In her work on the science of HIV in the United States and in Uganda, for example, Crane (2013) uses ethnographic research to track how some low-income countries have moved from being excluded from medical advancements to becoming key locations for scientific research. This is creating a new global landscape of 'postcolonial science' that involves new forms of collaboration and contestation among researchers from high-income countries and low- and middle-income countries (LMICs) (Geissler and Molyneux 2011; Crane 2013).

ANTHROPOLOGY AND CORPORATIONS

While anthropological engagement with issues concerning GHG is diverse and robust, the corporate form has not always been recognised as a key topic for anthropology. While it is tempting to imagine that corporations exist above, or outside of, culture, corporations are indeed a key component of societies, shaping publics, discourses, values and meanings, in addition to policies and politics (Welker, Partridge and Hardin 2011). Anthropology offers key insights into how corporations function as institutions in broader social environments. In addition to influencing cultures among consumers, corporations work to develop 'symbolic building blocks . . . charged with cultural meaning', to cultivate 'corporate personas' (Bashkow 2014, 298). Anthropology's focus on shared meanings, social processes, hierarchies and practices also underscores why corporate appeals to personhood are so problematic. Corporations claim legal personhood (see Chapter 15) and insist that they are simply made up of individual employees and shareholders (Bashkow 2014, 304). By focusing on corporate social systems, discourses and legacies of harm to the public, anthropology reveals that corporations are far more than their constituent parts (Geertz 1973). Indeed, what is most notable about the corporation, in a globalised era, are the myriad social systems with which it is engaged: networks of shareholders, activist-critics and other corporations; auditing systems; supply chains; and multiple levels of government. It is within these dynamic social systems that corporate power is exercised, and anthropology is particularly nimble at revealing and documenting these forms of governance (Tsing 2004; Rajak 2011).

Though anthropology's engagement with the corporation has been limited to date, rich ethnographies of diverse corporations are not lacking. Anthropologists have studied industries such as mining in diverse sites around the world (Ferguson 1999; Kirsch 2007; Welker 2009). They have traced products and their meanings in an increasingly globalised world, examining how fair trade tea (Besky 2013) and flowers (Dolan 2007) gain additional value as ethical products, and how complex commodity chains deliver broccoli (Fischer and Benson 2006) or sugar (Mintz 1985) to our tables. Following Nader's (1972) invocation to 'study up', anthropology has sustained a rich engagement with companies like IBM (Cefkin 2009) and studied corporate influence over perceptions of cancer mortality (Jain 2011) and the administration of universities (Strathern 2000). Petryna (2009) finds that private medical research companies can exploit global inequities, searching out host countries with lower standards of ethical oversight for drug trials, a contemporary corollary of manufacturing industries' preferences for countries with lax labour laws.

Benson and Kirsch (2010, 459) make a strong argument for scholars to 'reorient the study of power in anthropology' to include corporations and, in particular, to analyse corporate discourses responding to accusations of harm. Many of these studies uncover the inner workings and public manoeuvres of what are called 'harm industries' (Benson and Kirsch) or 'killer commodities' (Singer and Baer 2009). Crucially, theories of structural violence (see earlier) have enabled anthropologists to link large-scale corporate processes (along with structural dynamics like neoliberalism, structural adjustment and privatisation) with bodily harms (e.g. see Holmes 2013). Benson and Kirsch (2010, 461–62) argue that harmful industries require special attention, not just because of the harms they produce but because corporate powers act as a 'mode of discipline and control that seeks to inoculate the body politic against critique and to promote satisfaction with consumer choice and flexible modes of accumulation'. Harm industries' disproportionate influence in policy making and governance, often motivated by their attempts to minimise regulation, is thus as important as more direct harms and externalities they cause.

Perhaps the most exciting work on corporations in anthropology focuses on industries as moral arbiters and institutions whose 'corporate social responsibility' (CSR) projects constitute new forms of governance. Dolan and Rajak (2011, 4) argue that 'ethics . . . have increasingly become the province of corporate capitalism, as the market supplants politico-judicial and religious domains as society's ethical arbiter'. Corporations' 'ethical turn' introduces alternate modes by which they influence public opinion, change consumption practices, avoid conflict and influence governance. Consumers may now actively purchase goods from brands whose CSR projects they perceive to be in line with their own values (Dolan 2007). Studies of CSR practices also underscore the importance of attention to corporate discourse and messaging, which powerfully influences consumer choices, and often changes the terms of the debate about corporate responsibility for harm (Benson and Kirsch 2010; Rajak 2011).

Many corporations now take on or supplant state functions, particularly where the capacity of LMICs to provide public services is limited. As Ferguson (2005) notes, corporations can mimic certain state functions, and even impose elaborate security apparatuses, while creating corporate enclaves removed from the state itself. Not all corporate efforts to seal off their activities from the purviews of governance, or the 'interference' of the public, necessarily succeed. Tsing's (2004) pioneering work on globalisation describes the productive 'frictions' of global connection that emerge among village residents, local environmental activists, transnational campaigners and extractive industries in Indonesian rainforests. Similarly, Welker (2009) describes the localised hierarchies exploited by a mining corporation in Indonesia while attempting to demonstrate more socially responsible practices. In this setting, activists and village elites play a crucial role in determining the success and salience of corporate efforts at CSR on the ground. Both studies underscore how communities impacted by corporations are not simply victims or recipients of corporate practices, but key interlocutors whose complex social worlds mediate corporate practices, discourses and impacts.

As anthropological research has tended to examine global health and the corporate world separately, it has given minimal attention to date to the role of corporations in GHG. Nevertheless, two lines of inquiry are especially fruitful. The first examines corporations as producers, whose practices can be studied by tracing the circulation, meaning and appropriation of the material goods they produce. Some of the most studied corporate products in this regard are pharmaceuticals (Petryna, Lakoff and Kleinman 2006). Studies of pharmaceutical use, resale and exchange in Chile (Han 2013) and India (Das and Das 2006) demonstrate that consumers are not just recipients of marketed goods but active participants in the construction of product meanings, corporate image and the problems products purport to solve. Second, research on the involvement of corporations in pharmaceutical governance, particularly relating to intellectual property, is crucial (see Petryna, Lakoff and Kleinman 2006). Anthropologists' efforts to document activist demands for access to medicines, particularly relating to anti-retroviral drugs, have been especially important (Biehl 2008; Upton 2014).

Two further works present interesting anthropological perspectives on corporations and GHG. Peter Benson's *Tobacco Capitalism* (2011) is a remarkable example of the dynamic and multi-level perspectives anthropology can offer. Although the ethnography is situated within the North Carolina tobacco farming industry, Benson's inquiry extends to the unhealthy working conditions migrant workers encounter on farms; the racial tensions embedded within tobacco farm histories; the economic hardships of farmers struggling to maintain livelihoods in the face of industrialisation and foreign production; and tobacco corporations' efforts to shape discourses about harm, heritage and blame. In doing so, Benson's ethnography reveals the multiple spheres of tension, meaning and health risks embedded within production chains. Similarly, in her study of Anglo American's CSR programmes, Dinah Rajak (2011) employs what might be termed a *multiscalar* ethnography, moving between corporate headquarters and glitzy global meetings, and the hostels where miners live and seek treatment for HIV in South Africa's mining areas. At the heart of the book is an insightful study of how corporate ethics are crafted and deployed, and how they impact GHG. As Rajak argues, CSR is effective not simply because it provides an ethical veneer to cover corporate harms but because ‘it provides [corporations] with a moral mechanism through which their authority is extended over the social order’ (Rajak 2011, 13).

CONCLUSION

Despite limited anthropological research to date on the impacts of corporations on global health, research on the separate topics of corporations and global health is central to some of the most robust, innovative and rapidly changing fields of inquiry within anthropology. Anthropology offers detail-rich perspectives, on such topics as how the poor experience disease or global health programmes, or how power hierarchies limit the voices of the marginalised, that are gaining growing attention (Pfeiffer and Nichter 2008; Ebola Response Anthropology Platform 2015). Anthropology offers a set of particularly unique perspectives on power, hierarchies, organisational structures, knowledge production, informal forms of governance and the viewpoints of marginalised people that promise to add much-needed intellectual depth and richness to scholarship on the impacts of corporations on GHG.

FURTHER READING

Benson, Peter and Stuart Kirsch. 2010. ‘Capitalism and the Politics of Resignation’. *Current Anthropology* 51(4): 459–86.

Biehl, João and Adriana Petryna, eds. 2013. *When People Come First: Critical Studies in Global Health*. Princeton, NJ: Princeton University Press.

Janes, Craig R. and Kitty K. Corbett. 2009. ‘Anthropology and Global Health’. *Annual Review of Anthropology* 38: 167–83.

REFERENCES

Adams, Vincanne. 2013. ‘Evidence-Based Global Public Health’. In *When People Come First*, edited by João Biehl and Adriana Petryna, 54–90. Princeton, NJ: Princeton University Press.

Adams, Vincanne, Sienna R. Craig and Arlene Samen. 2016. ‘Alternative Accounting in Maternal and Infant Global Health’. *Global Public Health* 11(3): 1–19.

Adams, Vincanne, Thomas E. Novotny and Hannah Leslie. 2008. ‘Global Health Diplomacy’. *Medical Anthropology* 27(4): 315–23.

Bashkow, Ira. 2014. ‘Afterword: What Kind of a Person Is the Corporation?’ *PoLAR: Political and Legal Anthropology Review* 37(2): 296–307.

Benson, Peter. 2011. *Tobacco Capitalism: Growers, Migrant Workers, and the Changing Face of a Global Industry*. Princeton, NJ: Princeton University Press.

Benson, Peter and Stuart Kirsch. 2010. 'Capitalism and the Politics of Resignation'. *Current Anthropology* 51(4): 459–86.

Besky, Sarah. 2013. *The Darjeeling Distinction: Labor and Justice on Fair-Trade Tea Plantations in India*. Los Angeles: University of California Press.

Biehl, João. 2007. *Will to Live: AIDS Therapies and the Politics of Survival*. Princeton, NJ: Princeton University Press.

Biehl, João. 2008. 'Drugs for All: The Future of Global AIDS Treatment'. *Medical Anthropology* 27(2): 99–105.

Biehl, João and Adriana Petryna, eds. 2013. *When People Come First: Critical Studies in Global Health*. Princeton, NJ: Princeton University Press.

Briggs, Charles L. and Clara Mantini-Briggs. 2003. *Stories in a Time of Cholera: The Transnational Circulation of Bacteria and Racial Stigmata in a Venezuelan Epidemic*. Los Angeles: University of California Press.

Brotherton, P. Sean and Vinh-Kim Nguyen. 2013. 'Revisiting Local Biology in the Era of Global Health'. *Medical Anthropology* 32(4): 287–90.

Cefkin, Melissa. 2009. *Ethnography and the Corporate Encounter: Reflections on Research in and of Corporations*. New York: Berghahn Books.

Crane, Johanna. 2013. *Scrambling for Africa: AIDS, Expertise, and the Rise of American Global Health Science*. Ithaca, NY: Cornell University Press.

Das, Veena and Ravendra K. Das. 2006. 'Urban Health and Pharmaceutical Consumption in Delhi, India'. *Journal of Biosocial Science* 38(1): 69–82.

Dolan, Catherine S. 2007. 'Market Affections: Moral Encounters with Kenyan Fairtrade Flowers'. *Ethnos* 72(2): 239–61.

Dolan, Catherine S. and Dinah Rajak. 2011. 'Introduction: Ethnographies of Corporate Ethicizing'. *Focaal: Journal of Global and Historical Anthropology* 60: 3–8.

Ebola Response Anthropology Platform. 2015. Accessed 25 September. http://www.ebola-anthropology.net/.

Erikson, Susan L. 2012. 'Global Health Business: The Production and Performativity of Statistics in Sierra Leone and Germany'. *Medical Anthropology* 31(4): 367–84.

Farmer, Paul. 2004. 'An Anthropology of Structural Violence'. *Current Anthropology* 45(3): 305–17.

Ferguson, James. 1999. *Expectations of Modernity: Myths and Meanings of Urban Life on the Zambian Copperbelt*. Los Angeles: University of California Press.

Ferguson, James. 2005. 'Seeing Like an Oil Company: Space, Security, and Global Capital in Neoliberal Africa'. *American Anthropologist* 107(3): 377–82.

Fischer, Edward F. and Peter Benson. 2006. *Broccoli and Desire: Global Connections and Maya Struggles in Postwar Guatemala*. Redwood City, CA: Stanford University Press.

Foley, Ellen E. 2010. *Your Pocket Is What Cures You: The Politics of Health in Senegal*. New Brunswick, NJ: Rutgers University Press.

Geertz, Clifford. 1973. *The Interpretation of Cultures: Selected Essays*. New York: Basic Books.

Geertz, Clifford. 2000. *Local Knowledge: Further Essays in Interpretive Anthropology*. New York: Basic Books.

Geissler, P. Wenzel and Catherine Molyneux, eds. 2011. *Evidence, Ethos and Experiment: The Anthropology and History of Medical Research in Africa*. New York: Berghahn Books.

Han, Clara. 2013. 'Labor Instability and Community Mental Health: The Work of Pharmaceuticals in Santiago, Chile'. In *When People Come First: Critical Studies in Global Health*, edited by João Biehl and Adriana Petryna, 276–301. Princeton, NJ: Princeton University Press.

Hardon, Anita. 2005. 'Confronting the HIV/AIDS Epidemic in Sub-Saharan Africa: Policy versus Practice'. *International Social Science Journal* 57(186): 601–8.

Holmes, Seth M. 2013. *Fresh Fruit, Broken Bodies: Migrant Farmworkers in the United States*. Los Angeles: University of California Press.

Jain, S. Lochlann. 2011. 'Survival Odds: Mortality in Corporate Time'. *Current Anthropology* 52(S3): S45–55.

Janes, Craig R. 2004. 'Going Global in Century XXI: Medical Anthropology and the New Primary Health Care'. *Human Organisation* 63(4): 457–71.

Janes, Craig R. and Kitty K. Corbett. 2009. 'Anthropology and Global Health'. *Annual Review of Anthropology* 38: 167–83.

Kalofonos, Ippolytos. 2014. '"All They Do Is Pray": Community Labour and the Narrowing of "Care" during Mozambique's HIV Scale-Up'. *Global Public Health* 9(1–2): 7–24.

Kapilashrami, Anuj and Johanna Hanefeld. 2014. 'Meaningful Change or More of the Same?: The Global Fund's New Funding Model and the Politics of HIV Scale-Up'. *Global Public Health* 9(1–2): 160–75.

Kenworthy, Nora J. 2014. 'Participation, Decentralisation and Déjà Vu: Remaking Democracy in Response to AIDS?'. *Global Public Health* 9(1–2): 25–42.

Kirsch, Stuart. 2007. 'Indigenous Movements and the Risks of Counter-Globalisation: Tracking the Campaign against Papua New Guinea's Ok Tedi Mine'. *American Ethnologist* 34(2): 303–21.

Livingston, Julie. 2012. *Improvising Medicine: An African Oncology Ward in an Emerging Cancer Epidemic*. Durham, NC: Duke University Press.

Maternowska, M. Catherine. 2006. *Reproducing Inequities: Poverty and the Politics of Population in Haiti*. New Brunswick, NJ: Rutgers University Press.

Mintz, Sidney W. 1985. *Sweetness and Power: The Place of Sugar in Modern History*. New York: Penguin.

Nader, Laura. 1972. 'Up the Anthropologist: Perspectives Gained from Studying Up'. In *Reinventing Anthropology*, edited by Dell Hymes, 284–311. New York: Pantheon Books.

Nguyen, Vinh-Kim and Karine Peschard. 2003. 'Anthropology, Inequality, and Disease: A Review'. *Annual Review of Anthropology* 32(1): 447–74.

Nichter, Mark. 2008. *Global Health: Why Cultural Perceptions, Social Representations, and Biopolitics Matter*. Tucson, AZ: University of Arizona Press.

Parker, Richard G. 2000. 'Administering the epidemic: HIV/AIDS policy, models of development, and international health.' In Global Health Policy, Local Realities:

The Fallacy of the Level Playing Field, edited by Lenore Manderson and Linda Whiteford. Boulder, CO: Lynne Rienner.

Petryna, Adriana. 2009. *When Experiments Travel: Clinical Trials and the Global Search for Human Subjects*. Princeton, NJ: Princeton University Press.

Petryna, Adriana, Lakoff, Andrew, and Kleinman, Arthur, eds. 2006. Global Pharmaceuticals: Ethics, Markets, Practices. Durham, North Carolina: Duke University Press.

Pfeiffer, James and Rachel Chapman. 2010. 'Anthropological Perspectives on Structural Adjustment and Public Health'. *Annual Review of Anthropology* 39(1):149–65.

Pfeiffer, James and Mark Nichter. 2008. 'What Can Critical Medical Anthropology Contribute to Global Health?' *Medical Anthropology Quarterly* 22(4): 410–15.

Rajak, Dinah. 2011. *In Good Company: An Anatomy of Corporate Social Responsibility*. Redwood City, CA: Stanford University Press.

Redfield, Peter. 2013. *Life in Crisis: The Ethical Journey of Doctors without Borders*. Los Angeles: University of California Press.

Singer, Merrill and Hans Baer. 2009. *Killer Commodities: Public Health and the Corporate Production of Harm*. Lanham, MD: AltaMira.

Sivaramakrishnan, Kavita and Richard Parker. 2012. 'The United Nations High Level Meeting on the Prevention and Control of Noncommunicable Diseases: A Missed Opportunity?' *American Journal of Public Health* 102(11): 2010–12.

Storeng, Katerini T. and Arima Mishra. 2014. 'Politics and Practices of Global Health: Critical Ethnographies of Health Systems'. *Global Public Health* 9(8): 858–64.

Strathern, Marilyn, ed. 2000. *Audit Cultures: Anthropological Studies in Accountability, Ethics and the Academy*. London: Routledge.

Tsing, Anna Lowenhaupt. 2004. *Friction: An Ethnography of Global Connection*. Princeton, NJ: Princeton University Press.

Upton, Mike. 2014. 'HIV/AIDS, "TRIPS Plus" and "Knowledge Ecology": Unpacking the Semantics of Transnational Intellectual Property "Harmonisation"'. *Anthropology Matters* 15(1): 115–40.

Welker, Marina. 2009. '"Corporate Security Begins in the Community": Mining, the Corporate Social Responsibility Industry, and Environmental Advocacy in Indonesia'. *Cultural Anthropology* 24(1): 142–79.

Welker, Marina, Damani J. Partridge and Rebecca Hardin. 2011. 'Corporate Lives: New Perspectives on the Social Life of the Corporate Form'. *Current Anthropology* 52(S3): S3–16.

Chapter 8

Public Health

Heather Wipfli and Alexandra Mack

In its landmark report *The Future of Public Health*, the US Institute of Medicine defined public health as the actions society takes collectively to assure the conditions for people to be healthy (IOM 1988). Similarly, the American Public Health Association stresses the role of public health in protecting the health of people and communities where they live, learn, work and play (American Public Health Association 2016). The three main functions of public health are assessment, including surveillance and monitoring of communities and populations at risk to identify health problems; policy development to solve identified local and national health problems; and assurance that all populations have access to appropriate and cost-effective care (Centers for Disease Control and Prevention 1994). In carrying out these functions, contemporary public health is a multidisciplinary field, incorporating the natural and social and behavioural sciences. Traditionally focused on epidemiology, the field has broadened to embrace biostatistics, economics, law, communications, public policy, anthropology and other disciplines (Table 8.1). The breadth of the field comes, in part, from the sweeping definition of health put forth in the preamble of the World Health Organization's (WHO) constitution, which reads: 'Health is a state of complete physical, mental, and social wellbeing and not merely the absence of disease or infirmity' (WHO 1948).

Over the past century, the focus of public health has evolved from predominantly large-scale hygiene and vaccine interventions focused on preventing infectious diseases towards behavioural change programmes often related to modern lifestyles (tobacco control, obesity prevention) (Koplan, Thacker and Lezin 1999). These shifts in public health programming reflect and respond to the epidemiological transition occurring worldwide from communicable, maternal, neonatal and nutritional causes of deaths to non-communicable diseases (i.e. cancer, diabetes, heart diseases and chronic respiratory diseases)

Table 8.1. Core approaches to public health research

Approach	*Definition*
Biostatistics	The collection, organisation, analysis and interpretation of numerical data as applied to the biological and health sciences (Pagano and Gauvreau 2000)
Epidemiology	The study of factors determining the distribution and determinants of disease frequency in human populations and the application of this study to prevent and control health problems (Aschengrau and Seage 2014)
Qualitative research	The collection and analysis of data using ethnography, observation, interviews, focus groups, document analysis, grounded theory and other methods in an attempt to gain an in-depth understanding of structures, orders and broad patterns found within specific populations (Ulin, Robinson and Tolley 2004)
Behavioural science	The study of psychological and social influences on health with the goal of designing, implementing and evaluating programmes that promote optimum health practices (Glanz, Rimer and Viswanath 2008)
Policy analysis	The synthesis of elements from disciplines including economics, politics and various sciences in order to create, critically assess, improve and communicate courses of action for policymakers (Dunn 2012)

Sources: Aschengrau, Ann and George R. Seage. 2014. *Essentials of Epidemiology in Public Health*, CSZA, 3rd edition. Burlington, MA: Jones & Bartlett Learning; Dunn, William N. 2012. *Public Policy Analysis: An Introduction*, 2nd edition. Englewood Cliffs, NJ: Routledge; Glanz, Karen, Barbara K. Rimer and K. Viswanath. 2008. *Health Behavior and Health Education: Theory, Research, and Practice*, 4th edition. San Francisco, CA: Jossey-Bass; Pagano, Marcello and Kimberlee Gauvreau. 2000. *Principles of Biostatistics*, 2nd edition. Pacific Grove, CA: Duxbury; Ulin, Pracilla R., Elizabeth T. Robinson and Elizabeth E. Tolley. 2004. *Qualitative Methods in Public Health: A Field Guide for Applied Research*. San Francisco, CA: Jossey-Bass.

and injuries (Mortality and Causes of Death Collaborators 2015). This shifting disease burden is driven by a number of factors, including greater life expectancy, ageing populations, rapid urbanisation and environmental degradation (Wagner and Brath 2012). The latter are associated with the expansion of Western corporations expanding beyond their traditional markets in Europe and North America to new, emerging markets in low and middle-income countries (LMICs). This has led, among other consequences, to increases in the consumption of alcohol and processed food, marketed by these companies as status symbols and aspirational symbols of desirable Western lifestyles. Regular surveillance and reports of causes of death and disease have allowed public health professionals to identify and re-prioritise the health issues most in need of attention and develop new ways of addressing these.

In an effort to address the evolving burden of disease, public health researchers have increasingly shifted away from targeting individual behaviours in favour of altering environments in which individuals live, work and make decisions. This 'social determinants of health' approach entails environmental assessments, which require consideration of a vast number of risk factors that are entwined with corporate behaviours, motivations and output (Marmot 2005). Risk factors vary widely by population and may include contaminants in the air and/or water from natural sources or nearby industrial operations; the availability and quality of regionally available fresh and processed foods and drinks; the condition and usability of nearby parks and open spaces; and access to local jobs, housing and health care services.

As social, political and economic globalisation increasingly link the determinants of health and health outcomes of individuals and communities worldwide, the field of public health has grown increasingly global. What was once termed *Tropical Medicine*, involving the delivery of clinical interventions in low-income countries, evolved into *International Health* programmes in the 1970s. These programmes expanded the range of research collaboration between public health professionals in high-income countries and those in LMICs, but largely remained tied to the unilateral transfer of international aid, technologies and interventions. Over the past decade, a growing number of International Health programmes (and even schools of public health) have been re-labelled 'Global Health' programmes. With this name change came recognition of the multi-directional nature of transnational collaborations in public health and the growing interdependence of health worldwide irrespective of traditional geographic, political and cultural barriers. In 2010, the deans of seven prestigious schools of public health wrote to the *Lancet*, arguing that global health and public health are indistinguishable, and that attempts to distinguish differences between them conflict with the key tenets of global health strategy (Fried et al. 2010). Public health schools, they argued, are the primary structure through which to educate global health leaders and prepare them to confront the global burden of disease, while medicine, law, international relations and other natural and social science programmes can strengthen the capacity of future global public health leaders. While there is no question that public health approaches provide fundamental building blocks in achieving global health, the disciplines and approaches contributing to this book exemplify the challenge public health programmes face when addressing current global health crises alone.

RESEARCH ON PUBLIC HEALTH AND CORPORATE ACTORS

The influence of corporations on public health has long been recognised. Initially, public health research related to corporate activity was largely driven by occupational health concerns. The poor conditions experienced by factory workers at the turn of the twentieth century, for example, led to surveillance and regulatory protections. Leaded petroleum (TEL) provides one example of early public health efforts to document large-scale negative health effects on employees and, eventually, the public. Despite the known neurologic and physiologic health risks of lead poisoning, General Motors, DuPont and Standard Oil manufactured and sold TEL (innocuously dubbed ethyl gasoline) in the early 1900s (Kitman 2000). In October 1924, five workers in an ethyl gas production facility died after experiencing symptoms that included visual and auditory hallucinations, delirium and disorientation. After the Chief Medical Examiner of New York found the cause of these deaths to be lead poisoning, a panel of experts recommended that workers use gloves and masks and take other precautions to protect themselves during TEL production (US Public Health Service 1926). Despite evidence of additional public health harm, industry obfuscation and lobbying postponed the banning of leaded gasoline in the United States for over half a century, and leaded gasoline is still sold in a handful of LMICs (Kitman 2000). Today, there are extensive national and international regulations and guidelines to assist corporations in improving employee health and safety, although the health of millions of workers globally remains at risk while at work. A number of recent crises involving harsh working conditions have been in the news, including suicides and explosions at iPhone manufacturing facilities in China and deadly fires in textile factories in Bangladesh (Harris 2013; Bilton 2014).

During the twentieth century, the advancement of epidemiology helped improve the understanding of the relationship between corporate activity and public health. The global tobacco pandemic represents one of the best-documented cases of public health harm resulting from corporate activity. Tobacco use is the leading cause of premature mortality worldwide and is projected to kill over one billion people in the twenty-first century (WHO 2013). Just five transnational tobacco companies, Philip Morris International, British American Tobacco, Imperial Tobacco Group, Japan Tobacco International and China National Tobacco Corporation (a state monopoly), control the world tobacco market (Eriksen et al. 2015). The vast wealth of the consolidated transnational tobacco companies dwarfs many low- and middle-income countries' economies (Eriksen et al. 2015). The tobacco industry has used numerous strategies to avoid regulation and expand its markets. The release of millions of internal industry documents in 1998, as a result of US litigation, provided a unique opportunity to research and better understand the industry's decades-long campaign to deceive the public and target vulnerable consumers. This research found the industry deliberately created doubt concerning the scientific evidence on the health consequences of active and passive smoking (Yach and Bialous 2001); intentionally undermined tobacco control strategies (Francey and Chapman 2000); marketed products with lower machine-measured yields of tar and nicotine with the implication of less risk than higher-yield products (Etter, Kozlowski and Perneger 2003); and targeted high-risk consumers, including children, adolescents, young adults and minorities (Moore, Williams and Qualls 1996).

In 2003, WHO member-states unanimously adopted the Framework Convention on Tobacco Control (FCTC) (WHO 2003a). The treaty includes restrictions on tobacco company activities and specifically calls on governments to protect their public health policies from industry influence. Despite the treaty, tobacco companies continue to challenge laws and trade agreements in order to block core tobacco control measures around the globe, including plain packaging laws, regulation of flavoured cigarettes, use of warning labels, elimination of point-of-sale product materials and taxation on tobacco (Sud, Brenner and Shaffer 2015). Adding to the complexity of the issue is the rapid development by tobacco companies and others of alternative nicotine delivery devices such as e-cigarettes, which carry health risks of their own and have the potential to reinforce smoking acceptability and undermine the efforts and progress of smoke-free policies (Grana, Benowitz and Glantz 2014). Moreover, the rapid investment of the tobacco industry in e-cigarette companies offers the tobacco industry a potential way of attempting to regain access to policy-making forums and decision makers in contravention of Article 5.3 of the FCTC which explicitly wards against industry influence over policy.

Other industries subjected to research related to the population impacts of their products include alcohol, food and non-alcoholic beverage corporations. In the case of food companies, all along the supply chain appear public health hazards for workers and consumers alike – chemicals and pesticides used in producing fresh and processed foods, pathogens and substandard food handling causing foodborne illnesses and deceptive sales and marketing practices targeting vulnerable populations (IOM 2015). The size of food corporations enables them to alter entire national economies by changing suppliers or by entering local food markets and exposing those communities to supply, demand and price instabilities (Hawkes and Ruel 2006). The food companies are directly implicated in the global epidemic of obesity. While once affecting mainly wealthy nations, the worldwide rate of obesity has nearly doubled since 1980, affecting all age groups, with increasing prevalence in countries at all prosperity levels (WHO 2012). Studies of food companies have consistently found that 'food and beverage marketing practices geared to children . . . contribute to an environment that puts their health at risk' (IOM 2006; Harris, Bargh and Brownell 2009; Kunkel, Castonguay and Filer 2015). In an environment of self-regulation, the food industry advertising and marketing practices have included television and radio ads, adver-gaming, toy manufacture, character licensing and creation, celebrity endorsement, product placement and sports sponsorships (Brownell and Horgen 2004). Reminiscent of past tobacco industry tactics to deceive the public, in 2014 Coca-Cola launched the Global Energy Balance Network, a non-profit organisation run by scientists funded by Coca-Cola. The Global Energy Balance Network consistently blamed the obesity epidemic on a lack of physical activity rather than caloric intake (O'Conner 2015). In 2015 the *New York Times* published an exposé on the organisation, resulting in its dismantling and the retirement of the executives responsible for the association (Taylor 2015).

A third area of public health research related to corporations pertains to pharmaceutical and medical device industries. While both are technically in the 'health care' sector, decisions related to which treatments to invest in, and who to make drugs available at what prices, have resulted in contestation with the public health community. Despite the public health benefits that their products could deliver, research on medical device and pharmaceutical corporate actors has indicated that patient access and experiences matter little and decisions related to investment and price are often regarded as purely market related. The industries' influence on policymakers is also evidenced by their ability to shape national and international policies and regulations of intellectual property protection in the interest of international trade as opposed to health (Sell 2003; Nestle 2007). The interaction of both industries directly within the health system is a key area of research as both influence purchasing decisions, price controls and reimbursements.

Another intersection between corporations and public health is the growing number of social enterprises (D.C. Central Kitchen, Toms), which use commercial strategies to encourage human and environmental well-being. Methods of doing business within traditional corporations are also evolving in regard to health. Influential global organisations such as the European Investment Bank have adopted tenets such as corporate responsibility governance as core business principles (EIB 2005). Transnational corporations (e.g. PepsiCo, Nestlé) are investing in outward-facing departments such as Sustainability and Corporate Social Responsibility and developing executive positions such as director of global health and chief scientific officer. A number of corporations are increasingly instituting wellness programmes to improve the health of their workforce. Such programmes include tobacco cessation, physical activity promotion, cancer screenings and other preventative services. The incentives for, and outcomes of, these programmes are currently the subject of extensive public health research efforts (Mattke et al. 2013). Many of the actions mentioned earlier are viewed with scepticism by some in the public health community and warrant close surveillance.

PUBLIC HEALTH APPROACHES TO STUDYING CORPORATIONS

A number of public health models have been used to investigate the activities and influence of corporate actors in global health. Three common public health models are described in this section. They provide frameworks for investigating the pathways by which corporations make decisions and the resulting consequences for downstream disease production.

Surveillance and monitoring systems

Public health surveillance is 'the continuous, systematic collection, analysis and interpretation of health-related data needed for the planning, implementation, and evaluation of public health practice' (WHO 2016) (Figure 8.1). Public health surveillance comes in many forms depending on the disease(s) involved and the conditions under which it is being done. Some methods include mandatory reporting of specific diseases; mortality tracking through death certificates; and tracking through national health insurance data, household surveys, cancer registries and field reports (Nsubuga et al. 2006). While the terms *surveillance* and *monitoring* are often used interchangeably, there are distinct differences between the two within public health. Both involve routine and ongoing collection of data, although surveillance is focused on the impact of disease, and monitoring evaluates public health interventions or action (WHO 2003b). The public health campaigns against lead poisoning,

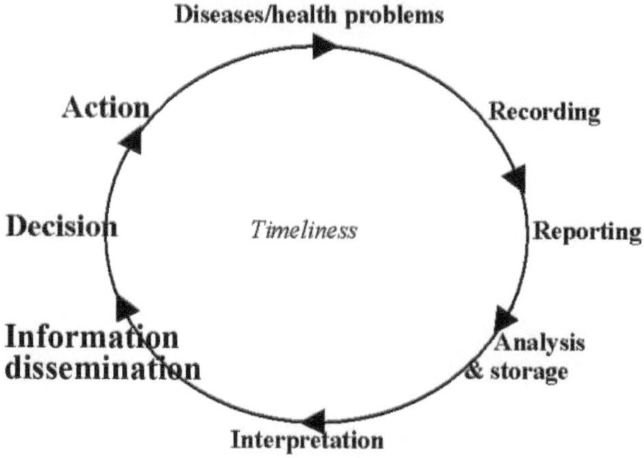

Figure 8.1. The public health surveillance loop

Source: Pacific Public Health Surveillance Network. 'Why Public Health Surveillance?' http://www.pphsn.net/Background/SurveillanceWheel.htm.

tobacco-related diseases and obesity owe an understanding of these products' direct and indirect impacts on global health. Because surveillance systems are better designed to measure diseases and clinical outcomes, they may not pick up the impact of corporate activity on health until it is too late to impose regulations on corporations to prevent negative health outcomes (Jahiel 2008). Robust surveillance and monitoring systems also involve costs that corporations may be resistant to cover and that researchers may be unable to fund independently.

Epidemiology (The Disease Triangle)

The Epidemiologic Triangle is a widely used agent-host-vector model originally applied to the study of infectious diseases (Figure 8.2). It can also be usefully applied to illustrate the role corporations play in the global spread of disease (Gordis 2014). The traditional understanding of the model was applied to infectious diseases such as malaria in which the agent was the malaria pathogen, the environment was the tropical conditions where the disease was endemic, the vector was the mosquito that spreads the disease and the host was the affected population. The model has more recently been extended to non-communicable diseases in which corporations are embedded in the triad as the vector, while drugs, tobacco and processed foods laden with salt and refined carbohydrates are the disease-causing agents; the environment is the broad social and policy context related to the marketing, availability and use of the products; and populations remain the host (Wipfli and Samet 2016). Conceptualising corporations in relation to the public health triangle allows for the identification of interventions targeting each element of the model as is done with other public health challenges.

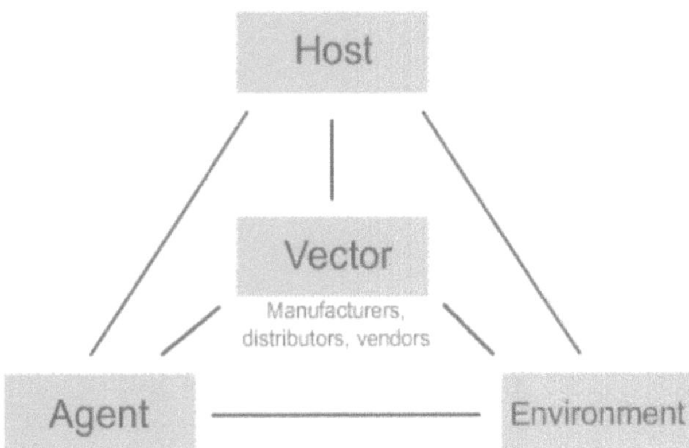

Figure 8.2. The agent-host-vector model of disease
Source: Gordis (2014).

Multi-levelled determinants

It has now become implicit within public health that a multi-levelled, life course perspective capturing determinants of health overlies the Epidemiologic Triangle's triad interaction (Figure 8.3). Returning to the examples of tobacco and processed foods, vulnerabilities to corporate output and practices exist all along the life course, from before birth to adolescence when the peer environment and social norms are critical to adopting health behaviours (Wipfli and Samet 2016). The long-term accumulation of negative health implications, beginning from prenatal exposures, has the potential to prevent longevity for individuals and deteriorate overall well-being. The nesting of a lifespan approach to health within complex understandings of covering political, economic and social contexts from global to the local requires nuanced considerations of reflect relational responses and mixed methodologies (Glass and McAtee 2005).

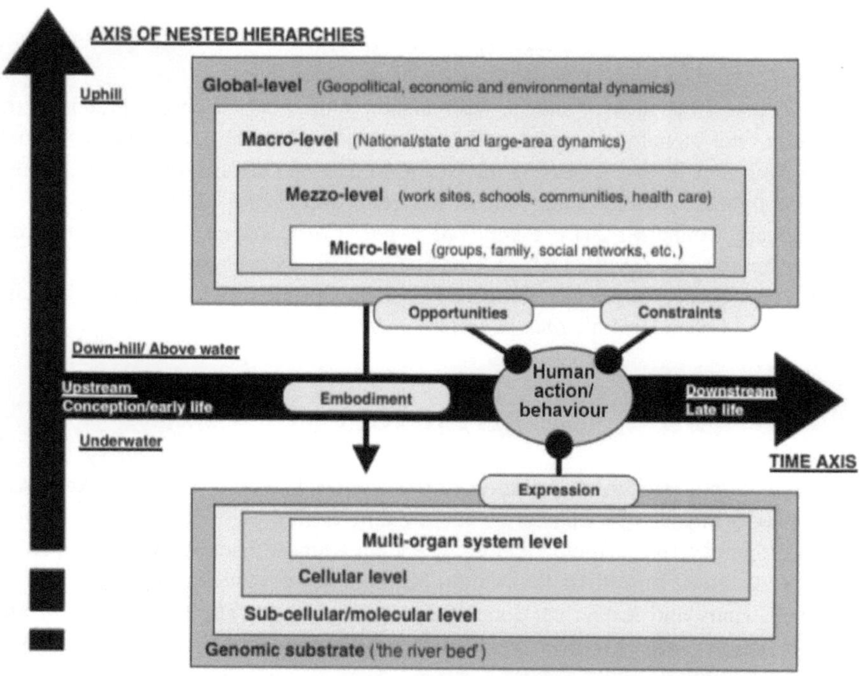

Figure 8.3. Model of multi-levelled determinants of health

Source: Glass and McAtee (2005).

CONCLUSION

The contributions of corporations to public health over the past 100 years have not been auspicious. Public health has long recognised the impact of corporate activity on community health and continues to struggle with how to manage the negative health externalities resulting from corporate activity. While public health approaches often focus on diseases and clinical outcomes, corporate activity is often set at very high levels of organisational behaviour, including shaping the economic and regulatory environment within which they operate. New measurement methods and transparency of corporate data are needed to better monitor the impact of corporations on health and to achieve positive outcomes for populations. In addition, in order to realise preventive benefits the public health community requires partnerships with workers from other disciplines to analyse complex determinants of disease as opposed to the diseases and clinical outcomes traditionally measured. With proper application, public health research and measurement methods can be used to improve corporate transparency, support global surveillance, promote public policy, plan and build healthy environments and robustly engage the community in order to encourage corporations to make choices consistent with public health.

FURTHER READING

Baum Frances, David M. Sanders, Matt Fisher, Julia Anaf, Nicholas Freudenberf, Sharon Friel, Ronald Labonté, Leslie London, Carlos Monteiro, Alex Scott-Samuel and Amit Sen. 2016. 'Assessing the Health Impact of Transnational Corporations: Its Importance and a Framework'. *Globalization and Health* 12: 27–33.

Freudenberg, Nicholas. 2014. *Lethal but Legal: Corporations, Consumption, and Protecting Public Health*. Oxford, UK: Oxford University Press.

Jahiel René. 2008. 'Corporation-Induced Diseases, Upstream Epidemiologic Surveillance, and Urban Health'. *Journal of Urban Health* 85(4): 517–31.

REFERENCES

American Public Health Association. 2016. 'What Is Public Health?' Accessed June 2016. https://www.apha.org/what-is-public-health.

Bilton, Richard. 2014. 'Apple "Failing to Protect Chinese Factory Workers"'. *BBC News*. Accessed June 2016. http://www.bbc.com/news/business-30532463.

Brownell, Kelly and Katherine Horgen. 2004. *Food Fight: The Inside Story of the Food Industry, America's Obesity Crisis, and What We Can Do about It*. Chicago, IL: Contemporary Books.

Centers for Disease Control and Prevention. 1994. 'The Public Health System and the 10 Essential Public Health Services'. Accessed June 2016. http://www.cdc.gov/nphpsp/essentialservices.html.

Eriksen, Michael, Judith Mackay, Neil Schluger, Farhad Islami Gomeshtapeh and Jeffrey Drope. 2015. *The Tobacco Atlas*, 5th edition. Atlanta, GA: The American Cancer Society.

Etter, Jean-François, Lynn T. Kozlowski and Thomas V. Perneger. 2003. 'What Smokers Believe about Light and Ultralight Cigarettes'. *Preventive Medicine* 36(1): 92–98.

European Investment Bank Group (EIB). 2005. *Statement on Corporate Social Responsibility*. Luxembourg: EIB Document Production Services.

Francey, Neil and Simon Chapman. 2000. '"Operation Berkshire": The International Tobacco Companies' Conspiracy'. *British Medical Journal* 321(7257): 371.

Fried, Linda, Margaret Bentley, Pierre Buekens, Donald S. Burke, Julio J. Frenck, Michael J. Klag and Harrison C. Spencer. 2010. 'Global Health Is Public Health'. *Lancet* 375(9714): 535–37.

Glass, Thomas A. and Matthew J. McAtee. 2005. 'Behavioral Science at the Crossroads in Public Health: Extending Horizons, Envisioning the Future'. *Social Science and Medicine* 62(7): 1650–71.

Gordis, Leon. 2014. *Epidemiology*, 5th edition. Philadelphia, PA: Elsevier.

Grana, Rachel, Neal Benowitz and Stanton A. Glantz. 2014. 'E-cigarettes: A Scientific Review'. *Circulation* 129(19): 1972–86.

Harris, Gardiner. 2013. 'Bangladeshi Factory Owners Charged in Fire That Killed 112'. *New York Times*. http://www.nytimes.com/2013/12/23/world/asia/bangladeshi-factory-owners-charged-in-fatal-fire.html?_r=0. Accessed September 19, 2016.

Harris, Jennifer, John Bargh and Kelly Brownell. 2009. 'Priming Effects of Television Food Advertising on Eating Behavior'. *Health Psychology* 28(4): 404–13.

Hawkes, Corinna and Marie Ruel. 2006.'Links between Agriculture and Health: An Intersectoral Opportunity to Improve the Health and Livelihoods of the Poor'. *Bulletin of the World Health Organization* 84 (12): 984–90.

Institute of Medicine (IOM). 1988. *The Future of Public Health*. Washington, DC: The National Academies Press.

Institute of Medicine (IOM). 2006. *Food Marketing to Children and Youth: Threat or Opportunity?* Washington, DC: The National Academies Press.

Institute of Medicine (IOM). 2015. *A Framework for Assessing Effects of the Food System*. Washington, DC: The National Academies Press.

Jahiel René. 2008. 'Corporation-Induced Diseases, Upstream Epidemiologic Surveillance, and Urban Health'. *Journal of Urban Health* 85(4): 517–31.

Kitman, Jamie Lincoln. 2000. 'The Secret History of Lead'. *The Nation*, 20 March. https://www.thenation.com/article/secret-history-lead/.

Koplan, Jeffrey P., Stephen Thacker and Nicole A. Lezin. 1999. 'Epidemiology in the 21st Century: Calculation, Communication, and Intervention'. *American Journal of Public Health* 89(8): 1153–55.

Kunkel, Dale, Jessica Castonguay and Christine Filer. 2015. 'Evaluating Industry Self-Regulation of Food Marketing to Children'. *American Journal of Preventive Medicine* 49(2): 181–87.

Marmot, Michael. 2005. 'Social Determinants of Health Inequalities'. *Lancet* 365(9464): 1099–104.

Mattke, Soeren, Hangsheng Liu, John P. Caloyeras, Christina Y. Huang, Kristin R. Van Busum, Dmitry Khodyakov and Victoria Shier. 2013. *Workplace Wellness Programs Study, Final Report*. US Department of Labor and the US Department of Health and Human Services. Arlington, VA, and Santa Monica, CA: RAND Corporation.

Moore, David, Jerome Williams and William Qualls. 1996. 'Target Marketing of Tobacco- and Alcohol-Related Products to Ethnic Minority Groups in the United States'. *Ethnicity and Disease* 6(1–2): 83–98.

Mortality and Causes of Death Collaborators. 2015. 'Global, Regional, and National Age–Sex Specific All-Cause and Cause-Specific Mortality for 240 Causes of Death, 1990–2013: A Systematic Analysis for the Global Burden of Disease Study'. *Lancet* 385(9963): 117–71.

Nestle, Marion. 2007. *Food Politics: How the Food Industry Influences Nutrition and Health*. Berkeley, CA: University of California Press.

Nsubuga, Peter, Mark E. White, Stephen B. Thacker, Mark A. Anderson, Stephen B. Blount, Claire V. Broome, Tom M. Chiller, Victoria Espitia, Rubina Imtiaz, Dan Sosin, Donna F. Stroup, Robert V. Tauxe, Maya Vijayaraghavan and Murray Trostle. 2006. 'Public Health Surveillance: A Tool for Targeting and Monitoring Interventions'. In *Public Health Surveillance in Disease Control Priorities in Developing Countries*, 2nd edition, edited by Dean T. Jamison, Joel G. Breman, Anthony R. Measham, George Alleyne, Mariam Claeson, David B. Evans, Praghat Jha, Anne Mills and Philip Musgrove. Washington, DC: World Bank and Oxford University Press.

O'Conner, Anahad. 2015. 'Coca-Cola Funds Scientists Who Shift Blame for Obesity Away from Bad Diets'. *New York Times*, 9 August. http://well.blogs.nytimes.com/2015/08/09/coca-cola-funds-scientists-who-shift-blame-for-obesity-away-from-bad-diets/. Accessed September 19, 2016

Sell, Susan. 2003. *Private Power, Public Law: The Globalization of Intellectual Property Rights*. Cambridge, UK: Cambridge University Press.

Sud, Sohil, Joseph Brenner and Ellen Shaffer. 2015. 'Trading Away Health: The Influence of Trade Policy on Youth Tobacco Control'. *Journal of Pediatrics* 166(5): 1303–7.

Taylor, Kate. 2015. 'The $1.5 million Health Research Group Coca-Cola Helped Fund – and Influence — Disbands after the Soda Giant Cuts Ties'. *Business Insider*, 1 December. http://www.businessinsider.com/coke-funded-research-group-disbands-2015-12. Accessed September 19, 2016.

US Public Health Service. 1926. *The Use of Tetraethyl Lead Gasoline in Its Relation to Public Health*. Public Health Bulletin No. 163. Washington, DC: Government Printing Office.

Wagner, Karl-Heinz and Helmut Brath. 2012. 'A Global View on the Development of Noncommunicable Diseases'. *Preventive Medicine* 54(Supplement 1): S38–41.

WHO. 1948. *Constitution of the World Health Organization*. Geneva: WHO.

WHO. 2003a. *Framework Convention on Tobacco Control*. Geneva: WHO Document Production Services.

WHO. 2003b. *STEPS: A Framework for Surveillance*. Geneva: WHO Document Production Services.

WHO. 2012. *Population-Based Approaches to Childhood Obesity Prevention*. Geneva: WHO Document Production Services.

WHO. 2013. *WHO Report on the Global Tobacco Epidemic, 2013: Enforcing Bans on Tobacco Advertising, Promotion and Sponsorship*. Geneva: Tobacco Free Initiative.

WHO. 2016. 'Public Health Surveillance'. Accessed September 19, 2016. http://www.who.int/topics/public_health_surveillance/en/.

Wipfli, Heather and Jonathan Samet. 2015. 'Framing Progress in Global Tobacco Control to Inform Action on Noncommunicable Diseases'. *Health Affairs* 34(9): 1480–508.

Yach, Derek and Stella Aguinaga Bialous. 2001. 'Junking Science to Promote Tobacco'. *American Journal of Public Health* 91(11): 1745–48.

Chapter 9

Development Studies

Michelle Carnegie

Development studies is a multi-disciplinary field that draws on the insights of several social science disciplines, including human geography, sociology, anthropology, political science and economics. One central concern of development studies is to understand patterns of uneven development under conditions of ongoing change (McMichael 2008). Analyses may cover demographic, political, socioeconomic and environmental change, and how this shapes economies and societies at local, national, regional and global levels. Development studies research often aims explicitly to inform development policy and practice.

Developing countries are defined, in the mainstream development literature, as having high absolute poverty rates and low incomes per capita (Sumner and Tribe 2008, 17). The term assumes temporal differences in the trajectory of economic development on a global scale, positioning 'developing' countries as less advanced and sophisticated compared with 'developed' countries. This conceptualisation stems from modernisation theory, which posits that developing countries and regions need to make the transition, from traditional to modern societies, through technological and industrial change (Peet and Hartwick 2009). Modernisation theory underpinned the post–Second World War development project, of high-income donor (or 'First World') countries and multilateral agencies, intervening in what was known as the 'Third World' or 'Global South' (McMichael 2008). The underlying assumptions of modernisation theory, however, are now critiqued as highly problematic by scholars for perpetuating a Western-centric development model that undermines local visions and aspirations, and degrades physical environments (see Escobar 1995; Baker 2006).

Amid these shifting paradigms, conceptualisations of poverty changed, from a narrow focus on patterns of income and consumption to encompass multidimensional, non-economic aspects, such as physical and mental health and well-being, social relations, empowerment and political freedoms (Hulme and McKay 2005).

Another key area of contemporary development studies focuses on the influence of different policy regimes on poverty reduction. Since the 1990s, developing countries around the world – following the lead of the Group of Seven countries and multilateral financial institutions such as the World Bank and International Monetary Fund (IMF) – have adopted neoliberal policies which prioritise market-led development. According to this approach, developing countries are called upon to open their economies and liberalise their trade relations. While mainstream development agencies have promoted export-led growth to address poverty (Veltmeyer 2009), substantial debate has arisen over evidence that poverty reduction benefits have been realised in only a limited number of countries that have integrated into the world economy. Trade and export-led development has not alleviated poverty in sub-Saharan Africa, for example, where the number of extremely poor living on less than US$1 per day rose by 60 million over the 1998–2007 period to 350 million people (Dicken 2011, 483).

This chapter locates research on corporations and global health governance (GHG) within these debates in development studies. It begins by reviewing the development studies literature on global health.

DEVELOPMENT STUDIES AND GLOBAL HEALTH

From a development studies perspective, 'global health' pertains to health needs in the developing world and, in particular, inequalities within developing countries, or between the developing and developed worlds. Moreover, studies conceptualise health as 'both the cause and the consequence of development' (Gaimard 2014). The ability of disease-affected working-age people to contribute to gross domestic product (GDP) is significantly reduced (for HIV/AIDS, see Cahu and Fall 2011; for malaria, see Gallup and Sachs 2000). Health is also a consequence of development. If development is narrowly defined as economic growth, the assumption is that higher levels of growth lead to higher household incomes, which in turn facilitates improvements in living conditions and many of the environmental and structural determinants of health. Potentially this includes improvements in diet and nutrition, although increased wealth may also be accompanied by transitions to unhealthy consumption patterns, including processed food, sugar-sweetened beverages and alcohol. This reciprocal link between health and development is examined in the WHO Commission on Macroeconomics and Health (1999, 10), which states:

> Until recently, economic growth was seen as a precondition for real improvements in health. But the Commission turned this notion around and provided evidence that improvements in health are important for economic growth. It confirmed that in countries where people have poor health and the level of education is low it is more difficult to achieve sustainable economic growth.

Importantly, there is evidence that people living in poverty in developing countries are more vulnerable, not just to communicable diseases (e.g. malaria and tuberculosis) but also to non-communicable diseases (e.g. heart disease, cancer and hypotension). The latter diseases are linked to lifestyle factors arising from industrialised food production and the globalised marketing of tobacco and alcohol products. This double disease burden is also reflected in the coincidence of undernutrition among the poor and substantial increase in 'overnutrition' (i.e. overweight and obesity) among more affluent population segments within the same geographies (Amuna and Zotor 2008).

Finally, development studies research has analysed how greater affluence may translate into greater ability to access health care services in developing countries. Over time, economic growth can increase the resources available for health care provision, and can be translated into more investment in health systems, with subsequent population-level health improvements. Achieving this in a way that benefits all members of society, however, presents many political and institutional challenges (Szreter 1997; Obeng-Odoom 2012). The literature on health and development covers topic areas that analyse these challenges in developing countries, for example, how health system strengthening can increase service delivery that meets the needs of poor and vulnerable populations (Bloom and Wolcott 2013), and that increases their access to health services (Peters et al. 2008); and how health sector reforms and trends in health expenditure impact poverty, equity and health (Simms et al. 2005).

DEVELOPMENT STUDIES AND CORPORATE ACTORS

Development studies seek to answer questions about how key actors, such as intergovernmental organisations, aid agencies, non-governmental organisations (NGOs) and private sector actors, including corporations, contribute to or hinder development goals. They are also concerned with assessing whether corporations 'can make a contribution, and on *which* and *whose* terms' (Newell 2008, 1070, emphasis in original). With the deregulation of markets, and a more limited role for the state, under the neoliberal development agenda, powerful multilateral financial institutions such as the World Bank and IMF, together with bilateral aid agencies such as the UK Department for International Development, have allowed, and perhaps even expected, corporations and other private sector actors to play a more prominent role in development (Newell and Frynas 2007, 672). At the same time, corporations have been criticised for harmful global environmental and labour practices and a lack of operational transparency (Jenkins 2005, 527). Corporations have responded by espousing and widely publicising Corporate Social Responsibility (CSR) programmes. Jenkins (2005, footnote 1, 525) defines CSR as 'voluntary corporate initiatives aimed at improving the social and environmental impacts of a company's business activities, but excludes philanthropy which arises after profits are made'. Study of the role of corporations in development is therefore embedded in debates about the role of the state and the market. Since the 1990s, during which market-led development approaches have been dominant, development studies research has also been exploring the impacts of inadequately regulated corporations on poor and marginalised populations who are not able to compete fairly in labour or commodity markets.

Wach and Thorpe (2015) identify three approaches that reflect different perspectives on the potential for corporations to contribute to development outcomes and the different roles of states and markets within each approach (see also Humphrey et al. 2014). The first perspective views corporations as part of the solution to poverty through their ability to boost economic growth under conditions of minimal interference from the state. The second perspective argues that profit-seeking corporations are part of the problem because they are exploitative and must be regulated by the state in ways that mitigate their potential harms. The third perspective accepts that corporations can be part of a solution if novel ways are found of including them in collaborative efforts, with states and other development actors (Humphrey et al. 2014, 13).

The first approach is focused on economic growth alone as the pathway to development. Corporations are seen as alleviating poverty because their core business activities as investors, employers and tax payers contribute to the growth of national economies (Newell and Frynas 2007, 671; Wach and Thorpe 2015, 1). According to this view, governments' primary role in an economy is to ensure favourable conditions for private sector investment, including foreign direct investment, and to correct 'market failures' that undermine efficiency. The emphasis is on facilitating business activity and creating growth with the underlying assumption that increased business activity will have a multiplier effect, producing benefits that 'trickle down' to everyone in society, including the poor.

The second approach sees economic growth as insufficient on its own to achieve development. Corporations are viewed as problematic development actors because their end goals are to maximise profits and accumulate wealth through processes that are at odds with the greater public good goals of sustainability and equity. Corporations are understood to be 'rapacious and exploitative, with business activities imposing social costs that are not reflected in the costs facing the business itself' (Wach and Thorpe 2015, 2). Here the emphasis shifts, from a narrow focus on creating economic growth through increased business activity, which does not necessarily lead to better development outcomes or an equitable distribution of economic gains throughout society, to an increased focus on the 'quality' of development. This includes the distributional affects of business activity and the potential negative externalities of economic growth such as environmental degradation and the associated health impacts. From this perspective, corporations need to be held in check by the state and other development actors, such as NGOs, which seek to highlight the negative side effects of the private sector activity and hold corporations and politicians to account for their effects on health and society.

The third approach occupies the middle ground between these opposing views, recognising the potential for corporations to bring about positive development outcomes if their activities are supported and leveraged in more inclusive ways by state and civil society actors. Some examples of inclusive collaborations include public–private partnerships; large businesses developing business models (known as 'base of the pyramid') that are profitable and give more access to goods and services for poor consumers; and value chain development and market system initiatives that involve corporations modifying their business operations to benefit poor producers or entrepreneurs in commodity and supply chains (Wach and Thorpe 2015, 2). It is this latter approach that offers, perhaps, the most promising avenue of research on corporations and GHG.

AGRIBUSINESS, CSR AND RURAL PRODUCERS IN DEVELOPING COUNTRIES

Much of the CSR-related research in development studies has focused on the struggles for environmental protection, livelihoods and human rights of the poor related to the activity of global mining companies (see e.g. Gardner 2012; Imbun, Duarte and Smith 2015). This section focuses on the activities of transnational tobacco companies (TTCs) and supermarket retailers involved in agribusiness and, in particular, their impact on rural development. The discussion highlights the empirical findings of two key articles which explore corporate actors' claims to improve poor rural producer livelihoods, particularly in relation to food security, in Malawi and Nicaragua. The discussion draws on Wach and Thorpe's approaches to understanding the role and influence of corporations in development described earlier. Many developing countries have largely agrarian economies, with a sizeable proportion of their GDP derived from agriculture, with large numbers of smallholder farmers engaged in agricultural production. A central policy instrument of national governments (in their attempts to achieve economic growth) is to emphasise export-oriented intensification of agriculture via cash crops. This can elevate corporations to a powerful position in agricultural supply chains where they can dominate certain commodities and supply chains.

Otañez and Graen (2014) critique the export-led growth approach to development in Malawi whereby the government allows the tobacco industry to operate with few regulations in exchange for foreign earnings they generate. The tobacco industry includes leaf merchants Limbe Leaf and Alliance One (subsidiaries of US-based leaf buyers) and global cigarette manufacturers, including Philip Morris International and British American Tobacco (BAT). The Malawian economy is heavily dependent on tobacco as a cash crop, accounting for 52% of export earnings in 2010. Malawi has a majority rural agrarian population, mostly smallholders with family farms of whom '48 percent own less than 0.5 hectares of land' (Otañez and Graen 2014, 68). Approximately 60% of tobacco exports are grown by smallholder farmers (Otañez and Graen 2014, 67). The industry argues that smallholders have no economically sustainable or alternative cash crops, and tobacco is thus of national significance. The industry cites loss of jobs, revenues and livelihoods if it were to cease its operations in Malawi (Otañez and Graen 2014, 61).

Despite decades of growing and exporting tobacco in Malawi, and being the recipients of CSR programmes, Otañez and Graen (2014) argue that most smallholder households still experience high rates of poverty, chronic food insecurity and child undernutrition. Wiggen, Henley and Keats (2015) found that introducing industrial crops alone, to low-income farmers with limited access to land, labour and capital, will not reduce poverty and food insecurity. They point out that farmers also need to obtain a fair return through crop prices and effective supply chains (Wiggen, Henley and Keats 2015, 4). However, Otañez and Graen (2014) document how TTCs control prices in the supply and sale of tobacco leaf in Malawi, through contract farming, to the detriment of smallholders. They argue that measures to improve the livelihoods of poor farmers must include fairer pricing, diversifying food crops and non-agricultural livelihood pursuits and valuing subsistence production (Otañez and Graen 2014, 68).

TTCs have attempted to respond to concerns about child labour, which is widely used in tobacco farming in Malawi, resulting, among other things, in high rates of stunting (Otañez and Graen 2014, 68). During the early 2000s, several TTCs partnered with international unions and national governments to establish the Eliminating Child Labour in Tobacco Growing Foundation (ECLT). In Malawi, BAT built schools and planted trees through the ECLT fund. However, Otañez et al. (2006) found this served to distract attention from the problem of children's low wages and unpaid work. Other ECLT partners have funded community-based initiatives since the mid-2000s. For example, Alliance One funded an orphanage for vulnerable children (Otañez and Graen 2014, 87). Otañez and Graen (2014, 87) argue that TTCs have done nothing meaningful to improve the livelihoods of poor tobacco farmers. They remain critical of CSR initiatives and caution the acceptance of industry claims at face value. CSR activities are designed to enhance corporate reputation while the business model based on profiting from unfair leaf prices continues. More development studies research, which independently assesses the impacts of the ECLT on livelihoods, health and well-being of local populations and indeed CSR claims by the tobacco industry in developing countries overall, is needed.

Similarly, Elder and Dauvergne (2015) examine the outcomes of an 'inclusive collaboration' between the Nicaraguan government, NGOs and Walmart as the world's largest retailer. According to the World Bank (2016), Nicaragua is 'one of Latin America's least developed countries, where access to basic services is still a daily challenge. Poverty, although declining steadily in recent years, remains high'. Walmart's Direct Farm programme aims to source fruit and vegetables from small- and medium-sized farmers, and provide training in sustainable agricultural practices to improve productivity, market access, incomes and food security. From a business perspective, this CSR initiative is seen as a win–win. Walmart ultimately seeks to enter markets in the developing world, as well as gain control over supply chains. To achieve this, Walmart has offered contracts to farmers 'stipulating product volumes and price, quality standards, and frequency of delivery' (Elder and Dauvergne 2015, 1038).

In studying the effectiveness of the Direct Farm programme, however, Elder and Dauvergne (2015) found that many farmers, once selling to Walmart, no longer were, and had gone back to selling in local markets. Over a six- to seven-year period, in a sample of 70 farmers, the number of farmers supplying Walmart declined by more than two-thirds (Elder and Dauvergne 2015, 1036). The reasons included higher prices in local markets, lack of capital to grow vegetables, cooperatives that stopped working and farmers who simply no longer wanted to sell to Walmart because of company practices. The study showed, for example, that 20% of farmers had stopped selling to Walmart because the company purchased only produce that meets its standards, with farmers bearing the loss of the rejected produce. The farmers regarded this as unfair, and feelings of distrust towards Walmart were generated. In general, many farmers perceived Walmart to be more concerned with increasing sales and profits, through savings and efficiencies, than genuinely entering into agreements of mutual benefit.

Furthermore, the authors found no evidence that Walmart's Direct Farm programme in Nicaragua had an 'effect on wealth, food security, or agricultural sustainability' (Elder and Dauvergne 2015, 1039). Most families surveyed were already food secure, and this did not change whether or not they entered into agreements with Walmart. Overall, the study found that the CSR initiative was not achieving the company's objectives of controlling supply chains or fulfilling its promises to farmers. This raised questions about Walmart's motives. Rather than Walmart fundamentally changing its practices to meet its stated aim of improving farmer livelihoods, Elder and Dauvergne (2015, 1030) argue that their real aim was to secure 'high-quality and inexpensive food from dependable sources'. In this sense, the study is an example of how development studies research can provide closer interrogation of the claims of corporate actors in the developing world, in terms of how they conduct their businesses and their actual impacts on economic development of local people and communities.

CONCLUSION

There is an emerging body of development studies research that explores the relationship between development and health, mostly undertaken by political scientists and development economists. There is a similarly small, but growing, body of development studies research on development and corporate actors. This chapter sets out two examples of research that investigate the impact of corporate activity on smallholder farmers or 'poor producers' in developing countries. The studies provide empirical evidence and important insights on how corporations that wish to appear to be contributing to development instead exploit and impact negatively on the livelihoods and food security of smallholder farmers in developing countries. The critique offered by the authors of both key articles aligns with Wach and Thorpe's second approach to understanding corporations in development. Corporations that claim to be advancing the interests of smallholder farmers need to be held accountable, not only to ensure they 'do no harm' but also to ascertain whether through CSR they actually 'do more good' (Sayer 2005). Elder and Dauvergne (2015, 1042) go further, arguing that 'instead of relying on CSR, the global community should be looking at much stronger state and international regulation of multinational corporations to protect the independence and values of smallholder farmers. CSR governance is not a solution for the needs of agrarian societies in the global South'.

It is likely that many corporations will position themselves in future as development actors which contribute to poverty reduction. Development studies scholars are well placed to contribute research which interrogates such claims, drawing on evidence of the impacts of market-led development.

To fully understand CSR initiatives, surveys and interviews with all development stakeholders are essential, including the intended beneficiaries. A livelihoods focus and placed-based approach can help illuminate what happens at the household level when corporations attempt to mediate (or deny) poor rural producers' access to market opportunities and resources. In addition, analyses of changes to people's income or wealth in the form of assets, food security and related aspects of health and well-being are important to consider.

FURTHER READING

Elder, Sara and Peter Dauvergne. 2015. 'Farming for Walmart: The Politics of Corporate Control and Responsibility in the Global South'. *The Journal of Peasant Studies* 42(5): 1029–46.

Otañez, Marty and Laura Graen. 2014. '"Gentlemen, Why Not Suppress the Prices?": Global Leaf Demand and Rural Livelihoods in Malawi'. In *Tobacco Control and Tobacco Farming: Separating Myth from Reality*, edited by Wardie Leppan, Natacha Lecours and Daniel Buckles, 61–95. London: Anthem Press and International Development Research Centre, Ottawa.

Wach, Elise and Jodie Thorpe. 2015. 'Introduction: Changing Perspectives in Business and Development'. *IDS Bulletin* 46(3): 1–6.

REFERENCES

Amuna, Paul and Francis B. Zotor. 2008. 'Epidemiological and Nutrition Transition in Developing Countries: Impact on Human Health and Development'. *Proceedings of the Nutrition Society* 67(1): 82–90.

Baker, Susan. 2006. *Sustainable Development*. London: Routledge.

Bloom, Gerald and Sara Wolcott. 2013. 'Building Institutions for Health and Health Systems in Contexts of Rapid Change'. *Social Science and Medicine* 96: 216–22.

Cahu, Paul and Falilou Fall. 2011. 'Accounting for the Effects of AIDS on Growth in Sub-Saharan Africa'. CES Working Papers, Centre d'Economie de la Sorbonne, Université Paris, Paris, France.

Dicken, Peter. 2011. *Global Shift: Mapping the Changing Contours of the World Economy*, 6th edition. London: Sage.

Elder, Sara D. and Peter Dauvergne. 2015. 'Farming for Walmart: The Politics of Corporate Control and Responsibility in the Global South'. *The Journal of Peasant Studies* 42(5): 1029–46.

Escobar, Arturo. 1995. *Encountering Development: The Making and Unmaking of the Third World*. Princeton, NJ: Princeton University Press.

Gaimard, Mary. 2014. *Population and Health in Developing Countries*. Dordrecht: Springer.

Gallup, John Luke and Sachs, Jeffrey D. 2000. 'The Economic Burden of Malaria'. Working Paper No. 52, Centre for International Development, Harvard University, Cambridge.

Gardner, Katy. 2012. *Discordant Development: Global Capitalism and the Struggle for Connection in Bangladesh*. London: Pluto Press.

Hulme, David and Andrew McKay. 2005. 'Identifying and Measuring Chronic Poverty: Beyond Monetary Measures'. Working Paper 30, Chronic Poverty Research Centre and Indian Institute of Public Administration.

Humphrey, John, Stephen Spratt, Jodie Thorpe and Spencer Henson. 2014. 'Understanding and Enhancing the Role of Business in International Development: A Conceptual Framework and Agenda for Research'. IDS Working Paper 440, Business and Development Centre, Institute of Development Studies, Sussex, UK.

Imbun, Benedict Y., Fernanda Duarte and Paul Smith. 2015. ' "You Are Not Our Only Child": Neoliberalism, Food Security Issues and CSR Discourse in the Kutubu Oilfields of Papua New Guinea'. *Resources Policy* 43: 40–49.

Jenkins, Rhys. 2005. 'Globalization, Corporate Social Responsibility and Poverty'. *International Affairs* 81(3): 525–40.

McMichael, Philip. 2008. *Development and Social Change: A Global Perspective*, 4th edition. Thousand Oaks, California: Pine Forge Press.

Newell, Peter. 2008. 'CSR and the Limits of Capital'. *Development and Change* 39(6): 1063–78.

Newell, Peter and Jedrzej George Frynas. 2007. 'Beyond CSR? Business, Poverty and Social Justice: An Introduction'. *Third World Quarterly* 28(4): 669–81.

Obeng-Odoom, Franklin. 2012. 'Health, Wealth and Poverty in Developing Countries: Beyond the State, Market, and Civil Society'. *Health Sociology Review* 21(2): 156–64.

Otañez, Marty and Laura Graen. 2014. ' "Gentlemen, Why Not Suppress the Prices?": Global Leaf Demand and Rural Livelihoods in Malawi'. In *Tobacco Control and Tobacco Farming: Separating Myth from Reality*, edited by Wardie Leppan, Natacha Lecours and Daniel Buckles, 61–95. London: Anthem Press and International Development Research Centre, Ottawa.

Otañez, Marty G., Stanton A. Glantz, Monique E. Muggli and Richard D. Hurt. 2006. 'Eliminating Child Labour in Malawi: A British American Tobacco Corporate Responsibility Project to Sidestep Tobacco Labour Exploitation'. *Tobacco Control* 15(3): 224–30.

Peet, Richard and Elaine Hartwick. 2009. *Theories of Development. Contentions, Arguments, Alternatives*. New York: Guilford Press.

Peters, David, Anu Garg, Gerry Bloom, Damian G. Walker, William R. Brieger and Hafizur M. Rahman. 2008. 'Poverty and Access to Health Care in Developing Countries'. *Annals of the New York Academy of Sciences* 1136: 161–71.

Sayer, John. 2005. 'Guest Editor's Introduction: Do More Good, Do Less Harm: Development and the Private Sector'. *Development in Practice* 15(3/4): 251–68.

Simms, Christine, Michael Rowson, Rachel Marcus and Anthony Costello. 2005. *Do No Harm: The Human Impact of Economic and Health Policy Reforms*. London: Zed Books.

Sumner, Andy and Michael Tribe. 2008. *International Development Studies: Theories and Methods in Research and Practice*. London: Sage.

Szreter, Simon. 1997. 'Economic Growth, Disruption, Deprivation, Disease and Death: On the Importance of Public Health for Development'. *Population Development Review* 23(4): 693–728.

Veltmeyer, Henry. 2009. 'The World Bank on "Agriculture for Development": A Failure of Imagination or the Failure of Ideology?' *The Journal of Peasant Studies* 36(2): 393–410.

Wach, Elise and Jodie Thorpe. 2015. 'Introduction: Changing Perspectives in Business and Development'. *IDS Bulletin* 46(3): 1–6.

WHO Commission on Macroeconomics and Health. 1999. *Investing in Health: A Summary of the Findings of the Commission on Macroeconomics and Health*. Geneva: World Health Organisation. Accessed 21 June 2016. http://www.who.int/macrohealth/infocentre/advocacy/en/investinginhealth02052003.pdf.

Wiggen, Steve, Giles Henley and Sharada Keats. 2015. 'Competitive or Complementary? Industrial Crops and Food Security in Sub-Saharan Africa', *ODI Report*, Overseas Development Institute, London. Accessed 2 March 2016. http://www.odi.org/sites/odi.org.uk/files/odi-assets/publications-opinion-files/9633.pdf.

World Bank. 2016. 'Nicaragua. Overview'. Accessed 21 June 2016. http://www.worldbank.org/en/country/nicaragua/overview.

Chapter 10

Media Analysis and Corporate Communication

Stephen Kline

This chapter focuses on the role that media analysis can play in helping health researchers understand the ideational power of corporations, particularly their use of marketing and public relations (PR) strategies, as a tool for influencing global health governance (GHG). The chapter begins by outlining the historical development of commercial speech. It then highlights the growing sophistication of corporate communication strategies which target public opinion and policy making. The final section outlines key ways that health researchers can use media analysis approaches to understand the growing impact of corporate communications on risk perception, consumer behaviour, public opinion and health policy making. The analysis that follows focuses principally on the development of commercial speech in the United States because it is the domain in which the communications industry first emerged and is most developed. However, these same techniques and practices are increasingly being deployed by corporations operating worldwide in an increasingly globalised marketplace. The intent of this chapter is not only to argue that health researchers must take account of the complex panoply of corporate communication strategies employed today but also to acknowledge their impact on GHG (Coates and Fein 2015).

MEDIA HISTORY AND CORPORATE ACTORS: THE EXPANSION OF COMMERCIAL SPEECH

Media historians such as Marshall McLuhan (1951), Roland Marchand (1998) and Stuart Ewen (1996) have contributed significantly to our understanding of the communication dynamics underpinning the emerging global economy, by drawing attention to the historical development of advertising and PR as two key aspects of corporate ideational power. *Ideational power* refers to the ability of powerful actors, including corporations, to shape the views, opinions and ideas and values of citizens and consumers. These innovations in marketing and PR were initially motivated by the desire to 'educate' the potential consumer about the relative benefits and uses of new products that were increasingly competing for buyers. Communication history has highlighted how, as national markets emerged in the eighteenth century in Britain, France and the United States, print posters, newspapers and magazines became increasingly important tools for selling. Industrialisation further galvanised mass advertising as an evolving but legitimate form of commercial speech practised by merchants attempting to sell their expanding range of mass-produced wares.

Lears (1994) highlighted the role played by American purveyors, of 'health tonics' (e.g. Coca-Cola) and food products (e.g. Uneeda biscuits), as among the first to use media marketing to motivate purchases through brand recognition. By the late nineteenth century, however, display advertising in newspapers and illustrated magazines was subsidising the expansion of mass journalism and entertainment media, reinforcing the idea of 'free speech' as the pillar of modern democracies. The expansion of corporate ideational power, in turn, coincided with this expansion of commercial media and their mass audiences. Media historians have also documented the growth in advertising spending in the twentieth century, from US$700 million annually before the First World War to about US$3 billion by the Great Depression when advertising investment peaked at about 3% of US gross domestic product.

With the rapid expansion of commercial media, full-service advertising agencies emerged as the creative middle men, responsible for the negotiations between producers and consumers, on the one hand, and media and audiences, on the other (Leiss et al. 2005). Three innovations in communication practices fostered expansion of advertising agencies. The first was the 'marketing concept': the firm belief that corporate speech must be based on a precise understanding of what the consumer wants and thinks. The second was the evolution of visualised design and storytelling about branded products and their users as a commercial genre. Based on his analysis of 25,000 magazine ads in the 1920s and 1930s, Marchand (1986) portrayed corporate advertisers, not just as the purveyors of goods but as the 'apostles' of the modern way of life. The third was the formalisation of audience evaluation methods based on circulation metrics, copy testing and opinion change measurement techniques into a science of marketing.

FROM BRANDED MARKETING TO CORPORATE COMMUNICATION

Abraham Lincoln had a prescient understanding of the changing role of public opinion in American politics, recognising that 'he who moulds public sentiment, goes deeper than he who enacts statutes or pronounces decisions. He makes statutes and decisions possible or impossible to be executed' (Zarefsky 1994). However, it took marketing communication professionals like Sigmund Freud's nephew, Edward Bernays, to forge this insight into a generalised corporate strategy for public opinion management (Ewen 1996). Since stories in the press or popular magazines could damage a business's reputation, Bernays argued that the vigilant corporate citizen must not only track public opinion but also respond directly to it. The PR professional, he insisted, 'interprets the client to the public which he is enabled to do in part because he interprets the public to the client'. Bernays (2004) called the emerging practice of public opinion management the 'engineering of consent', which, he argued, must exploit all media possibilities to win acceptance of the corporation and its products.

The increasing influence of corporate America did not go unnoticed by policymakers in these expansionary years for the PR industry. The need for the advertising and PR industries to establish their right to market products on behalf of their corporate clients and to avoid regulatory limits being placed on this became clearly apparent to the industry. Their strategy was twofold. First, pre-empting calls for legislated limits to commercial speech, advertising agencies formed an industry association in 1926. They began lobbying legislators that corporations, selling legal products, had the right to communicate with consumers as long as their claims were not misleading or false. They also mobilised PR efforts in an attempt to forestall limits to commercial speech rights. Second, the industry association called for self-regulation among its membership 'to promote public confidence in advertising and advertised goods'. This approach to heading off regulation, through the promotion of industry codes of practice and voluntary standards, is now a well-established practice across controversial industries.

CORPORATE COMMUNICATION, PUBLIC POLICY AND HEALTH

The history of tobacco illustrates how brand marketing and PR, fostered by full-service advertising agencies, directly impacted public health. Until the 1920s, smoking or chewing tobacco was largely a male prerogative, with only rare and brave women willing to try what was marketed as a masculine habit. Realising such social mores excluded 50% of their potential market, the Lord & Thomas Advertising Agency advised the American Tobacco Company (ATC) to redress this gender-based taboo with a campaign that potentially could double their market.

ATC achieved this by investing heavily in advertising in female magazines. Bernays strategically directed the marketing campaign, reframing a woman's decision to smoke as alluring and glamorous. For example, the campaign featured attractive young, female smokers, often in bathing suits, accompanied by the slogan 'Reach for a Lucky instead of a sweet'. Smoking was depicted as sophisticated and modern. Wealthy celebrities endorsed *Luckies*' smoothness, while film stars puffed on cigarettes in front of admiring males. To further win the 'consent' of female consumers, tobacco marketing used medical spokespersons to overcome any public concerns about smoking as a social irritant or smelly habit. These campaigns also sponsored radio programmes and helped to make the 'soap opera' a key vehicle for selling on the back of entertainment. Marketers even branded programmes with the names of their products, with shows featuring ubiquitous advertisements. For example, on *The Lucky Strike Radio Show*, female listeners heard the sponsor's jingles ('So round, so firm, so fully packed, so free and easy on the draw') repeated after every second song.

Bernays famously broadened this female-focused strategy further by associating smoking, and *Lucky Strike* in particular, with the suffragette movement. Bernays encouraged ATC to pay young debutantes to smoke their 'torches of freedom' in New York's Easter Day Parade in 1929. He also used celebrity endorsement by giving female film stars free cigarettes, in the hope that they would smoke them on camera or when photographed. By 1929, the *Lucky Strike* campaign contributed 25% of Lord & Thomas' US$40 million annual billings, pushing the advertising agency into the higher echelons of the industry. Million more American women also became regular smokers.

Tobacco was not the only product sector to demonstrate the power of strategic corporate communication. In the late 1920s, corporations like General Motors (GM), which were increasingly concerned about brand loyalty and winning national market share, refocused their marketing efforts on company reputation to win customer loyalty. To guide the brand strategy, GM extensively used consumer surveys, media monitoring and public opinion polling to identify the key characteristics of its customer base. It then designed products which could be marketed in ways that appeal to customer desires and preferences. In this way, products, advertising and PR were brought into alignment to target particular consumers within a unified corporate marketing strategy. As Marchand (1998) shows, in his meticulous historical analysis, a 'unified imagery of corporations at the service of the nation' underwrote

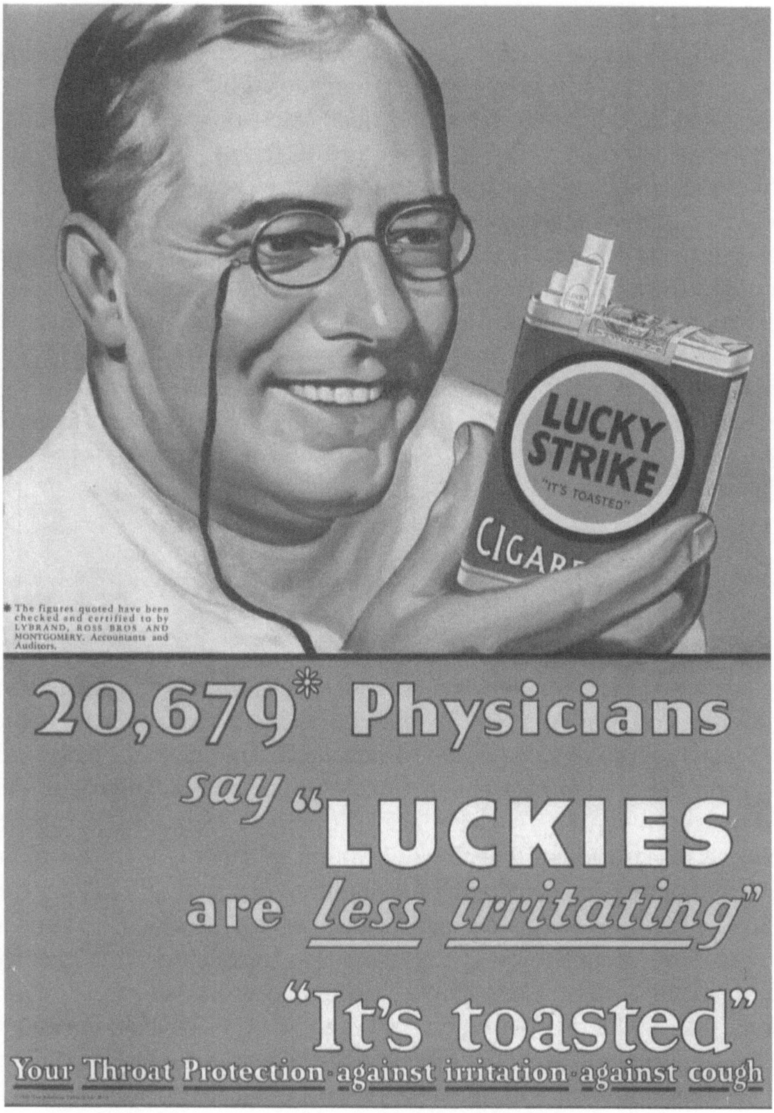

LUCKY STRIKE
"IT'S TOASTED"
CIGAR
* The figures quoted have been checked and certified to by LYBRAND, ROSS BROS AND MONTGOMERY, Accountants and Auditors.
20,679* Physicians
say "LUCKIES
are less irritating"
"It's toasted"
Your Throat Protection against irritation against cough

Figure 10.1. *Lucky Strikes* advertisement from the 1930s
Source: Stanford Research into the Impact of Tobacco Advertising.

modern corporate advocacy. Branding thus became a means of both selling goods and defending the corporate world's right to do so.

This success in influencing consumer behaviour focused public apprehension on the growing role that corporate interest groups, and their PR consultants, were playing in debates about health policy (Nelson 2015). Calls for legislated limits to corporate speech gained momentum, especially in relationship to drugs, foods and alcohol, which together accounted for almost 25% of total US advertising spends annually. Following the 1933 repeal of prohibition, the newly created Federal Alcohol Control Administration proposed a 'fair trade code' that governed false and misleading advertising, unfair trade practices and prices that were 'oppressively high or destructively low'. Given the known risks associated with the marketing of foods and drugs, the Roosevelt administration also signed the Food, Drug, and Cosmetic Act in 1938, which prohibited false therapeutic claims for drugs. The Federal Trade Commission (FTC) was then granted jurisdiction over the assessment of drug advertising's claims. In the same year, the FTC enacted legislation that proscribed 'unfair and deceptive' advertising practices generally to all products. However, by legitimising the principle of commercial free speech, these restrictions did little to diminish the enthusiasm of corporations for advertising and PR.

CORPORATE COMMUNICATION IN THE AGE OF TELEVISION

The advent of television brought a radical transformation in social communication in post-war America. By the mid-1950s, American mass audiences were watching up to three hours of news and entertainment daily, making television the pre-eminent channel of public communication with citizen-consumers. Given the avid embrace of this new medium, US advertising spending rose steadily from US$5.7 billion in 1950 to US$280 billion in 2007, with television accounting for one-third of total corporate investment in 'above-the-line' (targeting mass consumer audience) public persuasion. As with radio, the diffusion of television also led to innovation in corporate communication approaches. Orchestrated under the banner of marketing science and media relations, advances in the field of psychology and methods of audience research, consumer focus groups, systematic copy testing and scientific opinion polling, corporate communication was progressively forged into a more effective instrument for promoting corporate interests (Schroder et al. 2003). McLuhan's (1951) *Mechanical Bride* renewed attention to the part played by corporate communication (what he called 'commercial education') within the post-war expansion of the consumer economy. His critical analysis of advertisements, news stories and corporate proclamations, drawn from popular culture during the post-war years, led him to declare that 'ours is the first age in which many thousands of the best-trained individual minds have made it a full-time business to get inside the collective public mind. To get inside in order to manipulate, exploit, control is the object now'.

These marketing and communication strategies also transformed political communication after the war. Under the tutelage of the advertising agency Batten, Barton, Durstine & Osborn, Dwight Eisenhower's 1952 US presidential campaign decided to experiment in political marketing on television. The agency employed a series of short political announcements, purchasing spots in prime time during the final weeks of the campaign, to focus on personae rather than policy. For instance, it highlighted Eisenhower's humble roots and wartime accomplishments. The campaign's success made television advertising specialists as essential as press agents to political strategists. Investment in political advertising rose dramatically, in turn, making politicians more financially dependent on interest groups, like the National Rifle Association, and their supporters, to help fund campaigns.

The adjustment to television occurred, not only in Washington, DC, and on New York's Madison Avenue (where the headquarters of major US advertising firms are located) but throughout the news and entertainment industries. During the Cold War years, television supplanted newspapers as the main source of news. By the 1960s, television was not only the most widely consumed medium but also the most trusted source of information with a demonstrable impact on public opinion. In this context, PR professionals recognised the increasing need to influence television news coverage. Ross (1959) notes, for example, how Whitaker and Baxter, a California-based team of PR specialists, who cut their teeth writing speeches and favourable editorials for pharmaceutical companies, applied PR principles in an effort to shape health policy debates on behalf of the American Medical Association (AMA). Combining press releases with an advertising campaign, they successfully reframed US president Harry Truman's health policy reforms as 'socialised' medicine (Ross 1959). The AMA's campaign was critical in preventing the introduction of universal health insurance in America.

Another example, of the importance of television, is how the tobacco industry countered health research which linked smoking with lung cancer. Amid renewed calls for bans on television advertising of unhealthy products, PR firm Hill and Knowlton used media relations tactics to reposition the tobacco industry as responsible and public-minded. Faced with growing evidence of the health risks of tobacco use, science advocacy became an important extension of the tobacco industry's marketing and PR efforts. To enhance lobbying efforts, the industry funded the Tobacco Industry Research Committee, an ostensibly autonomous research group dedicated to communicating tobacco and health science in the media. To ensure positive coverage of their products and scientific debates, many companies threatened to withdraw advertising from magazines and papers that gave too much editorial space to risks of smoking.

What ensued was a 50-year-long policy debate, between Big Tobacco and the medical establishment, over the public health impacts of smoking. Many see the discursive politics of tobacco as a victory for public health or, at least, a turning point in public health policy because it alerted the medical world to the need to confront the ideational power of corporations (Glantz and Balbach 2000). Slowly the advertisements disappeared from television screens. As governments spent heavily on health promotion campaigns, to deter smoking and encourage quitting, smoking became inextricably linked with ill health in the public mind. Yet the principles regulating commercial speech, and the right to market a legal product, established by the tobacco companies in the 1930s, remained intact. Cigarette marketing shifted to science advocacy, sponsorship and, more recently, the Internet (Smith 2012) to maintain sales. In the United States, the mandate of commercial communication was extended to other health-harming and controversial industries, enabling, for example, alcohol producers to advertise in mainstream media and prescription drug advertisers to sell their products directly to consumers on television as long as contraindications are included (Mintzes 2009).

USING MEDIA ANALYSIS TO STUDY CORPORATE IDEATIONAL POWER

By the 1990s, the contribution of marketing and corporate communications professionals had left its mark in the commercial media. Not only were politicians being sold like branded goods, but elections were being won or lost by advertising spending. Media analysts have detailed the panoply of techniques that marketing and PR professionals employ to influence public opinion and policy making through their corporate communications strategies. Moreover, the case of tobacco had taught health researchers about not only the implications of corporate marketing and PR for health policy but also the importance of social marketing and health advocacy in the media (Wallack et al. 1993). Public health initiatives now employ similar strategies, and the research techniques and metrics that corporations used to monitor and evaluate the effectiveness of their investment in marketing and PR (Schroder et al. 2003). These insights of communication researchers have provided health researchers with a range of analytical tools for understanding the exercise of corporate ideational power.

Dubbed the 'new tobacco', the obesity epidemic revealed how important research into mediated corporate communication has become for GHG. Using a content analysis of news coverage of the obesity epidemic in the quality media in the United States, Canada and the United Kingdom, to track the discursive politics of this epidemic between 1997 and 2007, Kline (2011) notes how World Health Organization (WHO) studies documenting population weight gain initially received little public attention. However, as this analysis shows, growing documentation of Big Food's escalating marketing of 'junk food', especially on children's television, helped to focus researchers' attention on the rising incidence of child obesity. Prompted by the intensified public attention to 'globesity', and faced with calls for a 'ban on food advertising to kids', public health agencies commissioned research into the content of food marketing (Hastings et al. 2003); the nutritional limits of the television diet (Linn 2004); and children's exposure to food advertising and its impact on children's weight gain (FTC 2006).

Big Food responded to this threat to its marketing with both advertising and PR efforts (Lewin, Lindstorm and Nestle 2006). As soft drinks were implicated in the WHO's report (WHO/FAO 2003), Coca-Cola funded obesity researchers, who emphasised inactivity rather than diet as the leading cause of obesity and helped publicise this research. As content analysis of food advertising reveals, health claims were then added and active lifestyles were emphasised as a way of mitigating child obesity (Kline 2009). In addition, Big Food publicly contested the threatened ban on television marketing in the press by claiming, first, that there is no evidence that exposure to food advertising is associated with weight gain; second, that socially responsible food advertising is important in promoting healthy lifestyles; and third, that children's television would be underfunded under a ban (Kline 2009). However, resisting an advertising ban was only part of Big Food's PR strategy. Tracing McDonald's changing PR strategies in the news, Botterill and Kline (2007) show how the obesity panic helped reframe the company's PR strategies towards responsible marketing.

The ways that media monitoring and content analysis can help reveal the impact of corporate communication within public policy debates are demonstrated by the opposition to US president Barack Obama's health insurance initiative (dubbed ObamaCare). The media became saturated with corporate advocacy around the bill. In 2014, over 1.3 million health insurance and political ads that referenced health care issues aired across the United States, largely divided between those aimed at getting people to sign up and those using advertising as a political tool to influence voters against the Affordable Care Act (ACA). Researchers at the Kaiser Foundation (2014) analysed the communications developed by a US$465 billion campaign, funded by the health insurance industry, to defeat ObamaCare. Between 2010 and 2014, an estimated US$418 million was spent on 880,000 negative television spots opposing the law, compared to US$27 million on 58,000 positive spots. A majority of these advertisement spots promoted insurance products or encouraged people to enrol in coverage (56%), including 28% that specifically mention the ACA. The other 44% were political advertisements that mention health care issues, including 24% that specifically mention the ACA. Nearly all of the spending was on local television stations, so it could both undermine public support and target party candidates in races ranging from governor to Congress.

CONCLUSION

Corporate actors have forged product advertising, social marketing and corporate responsibility campaigning into a powerful approach for corporate advocacy, which needs to be acknowledged in the context of GHG. Building on the cultural-historical analysis of commercial speech in the United States, this chapter has outlined the ways that corporate actors exert influence in market democracies, both through branded advertising and corporate advocacy campaigns and through PR and media relations. Public health researchers have increasingly realised the need to understand, and document, how these practices impact global health policy. To do so, health communication researchers can draw on the key approaches of media researchers, which focus on corporate actors' investment in, and content of, mediated communication, as well as its impact on public opinion. To the degree that media institutions legitimise corporate rights of commercial and political speech, GHG has few means available for restraining, or holding corporations to account, for health risks intensified by corporate communication. Nor can GHG limit the indirect influences that corporations have on health. This is particularly true in national settings, such as the United States, where there is a robustly defended constitutional right to free speech. Ironically, advertising research, branding techniques and media relations strategies employed by corporate communicators have now become important tools for health promotion advocates seeking to mitigate the health impacts of corporations. Research can provide better understanding and support the deployment of such methods as public information messaging and social marketing (e.g. anti-smoking, don't drink and drive campaign) in the public interest.

FURTHER READING

Ewen, Stuart. 1996. *PR: A Social History of Spin*. New York: Basic Books.

Marchand, Roland. 1986. *Advertising the American Dream: Making Way for Modernity, 1920–1940*. Berkeley: University of California Press.

Schroder, Kim, Kirsten Drotner, Stephen Kline and Catherine Murray. 2003. *Researching Audiences*. London: Arnold.

REFERENCES

Bernays, Edward. 2004. *Crystallizing Public Opinion*. New York: Kessinger.
Botterill, Jacqueline and Stephen Kline. 2007. 'From McLibel to McLettuce: Childhood, Spin and Re-branding'. *Society and Business Review* 2(1): 74–97.
Coates, John and Ron Fein. 2015. 'Corporations Are Perverting the Notion of Free Speech'. *Newsweek*, 4 August. Accessed September 19, 2016. http://www.newsweek.com/corporations-are-perverting-notion-free-speech-359785.
Ewen, Stuart. 1996. *PR: A Social History of Spin*. New York: Basic Books.
FTC. 2012. *A Review of Food Marketing to Children and Adolescents: Follow-Up Report*. Washington, DC: US Federal Trade Commission.
Glantz, Stan and Edith D. Balbach. 2000. *Tobacco War. Inside the California Battles*, Berkeley: University of California Press.
Hastings, Gerard, Martine Stead, Laura McDermott, Alasdair Forsyth, Anne Marie MacKintosh, Mike Rayner, Christine Godfrey, Martin Caraher and Kathryn Angus. 2003. *Review of Research on the Effects of Food Promotion to Children*. Glasgow, UK: Centre for Social Marketing, University of Strathclyde.
Kaiser Foundation. 2014. 'ACA Advertising in 2014 – Insurance and Political Ads'. Accessed September 19, 2016. http://kff.org/health-reform/report/aca-advertising-in-2014-insurance-and-political-ads/.
Kline, Stephen. 2009. 'Ronald's New Dance: A Case Study of Corporate Rebranding in the Age of Integrated Communication'. In *The Advertising Handbook*, edited by Helen Powell, 24–33. London: Routledge.
Kline, Stephen. 2011. *Globesity, Food Marketing, and Family Lifestyles*. Basingstoke, UK: Palgrave Macmillan.
Lears, Jackson. 1994. *Fables of Abundance: A Cultural History of Advertising in America*. New York: Basic Books.
Leiss, William, Stephen Kline, Sut Jhally and Jacqueline Botterill. 2005. *Social Communication in Advertising*. New York: Routledge.
Lewin, Alexandra, Lauren Lindstrom and Marion Nestle. 2006. 'Food Industry Promises to Address Childhood Obesity: A Preliminary Evaluation'. *Journal of Public Health Policy* 27(4): 327–48.
Linn, Susan. 2004. 'Food Marketing to Children in the Context of a Marketing Maelstrom'. *Journal of Public Health Policy* 25(3/4): 367–78.
Marchand, Roland. 1986. *Advertising the American Dream: Making Way for Modernity 1920–1940*. Berkeley: University of California Press.
Marchand, Roland. 1998. *Creating the Corporate Soul, The Rise of Public Relations and Corporate Imagery in American Big Business*. Berkeley: University of California Press.
McLuhan, Marshall. 1951. *Mechanical Bride: The Folklore of Industrial Man*. Berkeley, CA: Ginko Press.
Mintzes, Barbara. 2009. '"Ask Your Doctor": Women and Direct-to-Consumer Advertising'. In *The Push to Prescribe: Women and Canadian Drug Policy*, edited by Anne Rochon Ford and Diane Saibil, 17–46. Toronto: Women's Press.
Nelson, J. May 20, 2004. 'Advertising Bans in the United States'. Economic History Association. Accessed September 19, 2016. https://eh.net/encyclopedia/nelson-adbans.

Ross, Irwin. 1959. *The Image Merchants: The Fabulous World of American Public Relations*. New York: Doubleday.
Schroder, Kim, Kirsten Drotner, Stephen Kline and Catherine Murray. 2003. *Researching Audiences*. London: Arnold.
Smith, Elizabeth. 2012. 'Corporate Image and Public Health: An Analysis of the Philip Morris, Kraft, and Nestlé Websites'. *Journal of Health Communication* 17(5): 582–600.
Wallack, Lawrence, Lori Dorfman, David Jernigan and Makani Themba-Nixon. 1993. *Media Advocacy and Public Health*. Newbury Park, CA: Sage.
WHO/FAO 2003. *Diet, Nutrition and the Prevention of Chronic Diseases: Risks, Promoting Healthy Life*. Technical Report Series 916, Geneva: WHO.
Zarefsky, David. 1994. '"Public Sentiment Is Everything": Lincoln's View of Political Persuasion'. *Journal of Abraham Lincoln Association* 15(2): 23–40.

Part II

METHODS AND DATA SOURCES FOR ANALYSING CORPORATIONS

Chapter 11

Interviewing Key Informants from the Corporate Sector

Benjamin Hawkins and Rebecca Cassidy

Interviewing key informants is a well-established research method used to document, and understand, the motivations, goals and activities of organisations. There are three main types of research interview – structured, unstructured and semi-structured (see Brinkman 2013). In structured interviews, the interview is closely controlled by the interviewer and content is strictly limited to pre-designed questionnaire in order to facilitate comparison between respondents. To control for bias questions may be read verbatim by the interviewer from a script. In unstructured interviews, general themes are identified by the interviewer, but the specific content and direction of the interview is allowed to flow organically. Open questions are used to prompt respondents to share their account and generate narratives. Unstructured interviews often take the form of life stories or personal accounts of events and experience and are thus widely used in the field of oral history (see Chapter 13). Semi-structured interviews combine elements of both: using interview guides to shape the content and flow of the interview but allowing flexibility to pursue new issues and lines of questioning which may arise in the interview itself.

In this chapter, we focus on semi-structured interviews, which have been widely deployed in the field of policy analysis to understand the process of policy change and the role of key actors in bringing about this change. Interviews provide new, sometimes unique, primary data sources derived from key actors such as policymakers, or those otherwise engaged in the policy process, including civil society representatives and corporate actors. Semi-structured interviews also allow researchers to examine issues in depth, to seek clarification and additional details and to probe issues with respondents to develop more nuanced understandings of complex processes. The process of conducting interviews may also reveal additional lines of inquiry, areas of interest and research questions which augment or deepen understandings of an organisation.

There is now a sizeable literature on elite interviewing, which guides the process of arranging, conducting and analysing interviews (see e.g. Rubin and Rubin 2012; Brinkman 2013; Bryman 2015). However, interviewing has arguably been underutilised to date in researching corporations and global health governance. This chapter sets out the specific issues which arise when doing interviews with corporations, and the types of research questions to be answered through them. This is achieved by discussing how semi-structured interviews have been used to study the alcohol and gambling industries, and then how they might be applied to corporate actors in other contexts.

USING INTERVIEWS TO STUDY CORPORATIONS

Interviews with key informants about corporations present challenges associated with elite interviewing more generally (Mikecz 2012). Identifying key informants with the ability, and willingness, to speak candidly and knowledgably about a corporation can be the first challenge. Potential key informants can be identified through an initial stakeholder mapping exercise, which identifies key actors involved in a policy debate, along with their perceived interests and attitudes (Brugha and Varvasovszky 2000; Varvasovszky and Brugha 2000). Typical stakeholders include civil servants, politicians and policymakers, public interest groups and private sector actors such as lobbyists and industry associations.

Given the nature of some business activities, and the perception that public health researchers may be antithetical to their interests, business representatives may be reluctant to participate. Individuals may be inhibited to speak about existing or former employers, or be subject to confidentiality agreements. Where an interview is granted, the researcher may be directed to an individual not well placed to answer research questions or lacking relevant experience or insights. Researchers may also not be able to control and manage the dynamics of the interview to ensure key issues are covered and useful data is generated.

The identity of the key informant interviewed will determine the type of data generated and the nature of the claims that can be made. It may be possible to secure an interview with the head of government affairs in a particular corporation, for example, who orchestrates the company's lobbying strategy. Alternatively, you may find yourself face to face with a public relations (PR) spokesperson whose role it is to deflect attention away from issues deemed sensitive to corporate interests. A meeting with researchers might even be approached as an opportunity to promote the company's corporate messaging. Rather than unearthing information about corporate political strategy, researchers may risk becoming an unwitting conduit for publicising this strategy.

Apart from current employees of corporations, there are other key informants who can be considered as, or provide useful insights on, corporate actors. These include industry association representatives, business analysts and scholars, private consultants, lobbyists and former and retired employees. The advantage of speaking to trade associations is that representatives may be easier to gain access to and may wish to help you understand the overall activities and perspectives of a specific industry, as well as specific position on a given issue. If the trade association's membership covers corporations with different interests, it might be a useful source to understand potential tensions or competing goals within an industry.

As in all social science research, it is vital to combine industry interviews with other data sources (e.g. policy documents and industry publications) in a process known as 'triangulation' (Skeggs 1997) in order to gain a full and accurate account of corporate behaviour. Finally, since interview-based research involves human subjects, it is vital to adhere to recognised research ethics standards of practice. How data is recorded, stored and analysed poses important ethical and legal issues concerning confidentiality and anonymity (see Chapter 22).

USING INTERVIEWS TO STUDY THE GLOBAL ALCOHOL INDUSTRY

A study of how alcohol industry actors attempted to influence policy debates on pricing policy in the United Kingdom demonstrates the wide range of insights to be generated with semi-structured interviews and the issues researchers need to be aware of at different stages of the research process (McCambridge, Hawkins and Holden 2014). The aim of the research is to identify the positions adopted by alcohol industry actors on pricing, explore their rationale for these positions and investigate the ways in which they sought to articulate their preferences to government and influence the policy process. Thirty-five qualitative interviews were conducted with representatives of transnational alcohol companies (TACs), trade associations, public health advocates, civil society organisations and policymakers, including civil servants and parliamentarians identified from responses to the Scottish government's 2008 alcohol policy consultation. Key informants were identified through purposive sampling (i.e. seeking interviewees with specific expertise on the issue at hand), and those initially contacted were then asked to suggest further respondents (i.e. snowball sampling). While around half the industry actors approached declined to participate in the study, interviews were eventually conducted with all key stakeholder groups, and with representatives of all sectors of the alcohol industry.

Interviewees were recruited by email and telephone, and through the researchers' attendance at events (e.g. seminars and policy forums) in which industry and other policy actors were present. Face-to-face contact proved the most effective way of gaining access to industry respondents, although effort was often needed to follow up initial contacts to secure an interview. The response of industry actors to interview requests varied. Almost all trade association representatives agreed to participate in the study, while only half of those corporations provided respondents.

Each interview was roughly one hour and mainly took place in the offices of the organisations in question. Complete anonymity was offered to respondents, who could select how the data they provided could be used and attributed to them, as set out in a consent form. Offering anonymity in this way can be vital to recruiting respondents and assuring candid responses. The interview drew on stakeholder mapping and document analysis to set out the main research questions, and potential follow-up questions and probes to delve deeper into issues which emerge during the course of the interview (Rubin and Rubin 2012). This allowed actors' positions to be explored further in a way which is impossible with document analysis. Having a semi-structure to the interview, while allowing space to explore unexpected angles and responses, is a key strength of this approach to data gathering.

The researchers found that many respondents were highly skilled at dealing with the questions asked. They appeared to have predetermined answers to certain types of questions, or potential criticisms of their businesses, which often closely mirrored positions stated in company publications and other documents. They sometimes repeated these carefully crafted phrasings when pushed on a subject. At times, inconsistencies in the arguments presented, or between the interview transcript and the published position of the companies, emerged. In several cases, respondents sought to control the dynamic of the interview, even steering conversation to favoured topics. It is thus important for the researcher to prepare ahead of time different ways of addressing key themes and issues at different points during the interview.

For this study, the key informants ranged from a chief executive to government affairs actors at the heart of the organisation's political strategy to PR officers who had limited insights into the company's policy engagement. As described earlier, the data generated from interviews with PR spokespersons (and those with government and public health actors) had a different status, and offered insights into different areas of interest, to actors more directly involved in corporate-government affairs. While PR officers told us little about policy-influencing strategies, they were vital in understanding attempts by industry actors to 'frame' the debate on alcohol-related harm or to shape perceptions of their organisations as part of the solution to these problems. Framing refers to the way in which policy problems and their solutions are presented by policy actors. Attempts to frame policy debates – to shape the terms in which they are couched and which aspects of the issue are given most attention – are key components of corporate political strategy (Hawkins and Holden 2013). Different types of interviews will be useful for answering different types of research questions, and the researcher needs to reflexively engage with the status of the data generated and the insights they offer.

To facilitate the analysis, all interviews were recorded (none of the participants declined this request) and then transcribed by an external transcription agency. Transcripts were then coded thematically using Nvivo coding software. The interview transcripts were initially read by the researcher who conducted the interviews, and recordings were listened to by a second researcher to identify the key themes which emerged. From this, the researchers identified and agreed on the key themes that emerged from the interviews, and these served as the basis for the codes used for systematic analysis of the transcripts. For example, it was a common element of industry responses to try to play down the extent of alcohol-related harm, so 'Claims about Alcohol Harms' was used as a code and all examples of this were recorded. During the analysis phase, additional codes and patterns between codes emerged.

The analysis of responses by key stakeholders to the Scottish consultation, on the proposed introduction of minimum unit pricing, facilitated triangulation between interviews and other data sources (Holden, Hawkins and McCambridge 2012). By triangulating industry interview responses, against those from respondents in other sectors and documentary sources, the study was able to build a picture of the points of access available to industry actors in the policy process and the methods they use to influence policy (Holden and Hawkins 2013; Hawkins and Holden 2014), as well as the internal dynamics of the alcohol industry as they sought a co-ordinated response to the pricing issue (Holden, Hawkins and McCambridge 2012).

USING INTERVIEWS TO STUDY THE GAMBLING INDUSTRY

The size of the global market for regulated gambling has more than doubled during the past 13 years, from just over US$200 billion in 2001 to US$450 billion in 2014 (GBGC 2015). In the United States, this expansion can be traced to the 1970s and the growth of casinos (Schüll 2012). The gambling market in Europe is more diverse, and the industry has expanded primarily through sports betting and online gambling, both of which are illegal in the majority of US states. Industry growth in Asia has been driven by tourists from China, where gambling is illegal, visiting casinos in Macau and Singapore. Regulated gambling has taken diverse forms across these regions, but in all cases, expansion has been accompanied by efforts from corporate actors to redefine gambling as a leisure activity rather than an illicit or immoral activity (Cassidy 2016).

Policymakers and gambling scholars argue that we lack high-quality evidence about gambling behaviour on which to base policy. A recent project (Cassidy, Loussouarn and Pisac 2014) set out to ask academics, policymakers and gambling treatment providers why they thought this was the case, and how they produced and made use of particular kinds of evidence. The project focused principally on the United Kingdom, the most diverse regulated gambling market in the world, but included interviews with participants in important emerging markets in Europe, Hong Kong and Macau.

Multiple methods, including interviews, participant observation at industry conferences and work shadowing, were used in an iterative process, with each of these methods serving a particular purpose within the overall research design. The value of interviewing, in this case, was that it enabled researchers to get beyond public representations of gambling to more nuanced and complex positions. Most important, interviewees were provided with anonymity, which allowed them to share information that would not otherwise have entered the public domain.

First, a focus group of potential respondents was convened, to develop and refine a specific set of interview questions. Once the core questions were agreed, the project team conducted semi-structured interviews with 109 active participants in gambling research, including users (policymakers, treatment providers, regulators), producers (in academia, the gambling industry and research institutes) and members of the gambling industries, both traditional (including sports betting and casinos) and new forms of gambling (including online and mobile gambling). An initial group of participants was selected based on their senior positions in the gambling industry and/or gambling research community. This included actors sitting on commercial, regulatory and public health boards; those contributing authoritative pieces of research in the field; and those supported by prestigious funding bodies, including national research councils.

Subsequent interviewees were identified using the snowball sampling method (also known as 'chain' or 'chain referral' sampling) whereby each participant was invited to recommend others he or she felt might make a valuable contribution to the study (Atkinson and Flint 2004). This was complemented by a randomly selected group of additional respondents from within the field, included to ensure that we consulted as widely as possible with members of different networks and at different stages of their careers. This allowed us to gather what might be called 'outlier' experiences. A random number generator was used to select potential respondents from, for example, a list of participants at a gambling conference, who were then approached to participate in the study.

Negotiating access to corporate actors working in gambling is extremely difficult and often unsuccessful. Many gambling operators simply do not respond to requests for access. Even where access is granted, this may be a long, time-consuming process. Approximately six months were spent negotiating, unsuccessfully, for access to one corporation, for example. However, this is not always the case; an offhand remark to a bookmaker during a boisterous industry event, for instance, yielded unconditional and instant access to workers in a chain of shops.

Interviews took place in a variety of settings, including the respondents' workplaces, coffee shops and pubs. Each took around one hour to complete. Some participants chose to meet on multiple occasions, and one respondent generated more than six hours of data. Interviews were sound recorded and transcribed and entered into qualitative data analysis software for thematic coding. The project focused on sensitive information that could affect career progression, reputation and commercial practices, meaning that the researchers' responsibilities to participants were extensive. In accordance with the Association of Social Anthropologists of the UK and Commonwealth guidelines (ASA 2014), consent was conceived of as an ongoing process. This included guarantees that their participation, or the content of their interview, would not be discussed with other members of the target group and that they would not be identifiable in the report.

Participants were briefed about the purpose of the study and how their data would be used prior to the interview. Throughout the process, participants were assured that they were free to withdraw from the study at any point. We asked permission to categorise them by gender, role, location and years of experience. They were also given the option not to be quoted, to speak entirely off the record and to stop the recording at any time. All data was managed and stored according to UK rules on data protection.

All data produced through interviews is dialogic, a product of the relationship between the interviewer and his or her subject. Trust and even rapport takes a great deal of time to build up and can be easily lost. As with TACs, all participants in the gambling study had a position that they wished to present. It was up to the researcher to ask questions that were sufficiently stimulating or unexpected to avoid receiving routine, premeditated or superficial answers. Findings were triangulated with other data sources, including research outputs; industry documents and publications; communications from research centres, research councils, regulators, government departments and funding bodies; and participant observation at conferences and meetings.

Similar to the alcohol study discussed earlier, it was evident, on triangulating our interviews, that attempts had been made by some informants – both senior researchers and members of the industry – to shape and guide the interviews towards certain topics and away from others. There was also evidence of collusion between interviewees in their responses, which was uncovered by careful comparison of the interview transcripts. This was again important data. Participants were asked about it and produced a justification which focused on reputation management.

The interviews produced unprecedented insights into the operations of the gambling industry and its attitudes towards research and regulation. The data suggested an alternative explanation for the dearth of high-quality evidence in the gambling field – the result of structural issues (including the funding of research by industry and its control over access to data) rather than due to the difficulty of studying gamblers as a hard-to-reach group. This conclusion was supported by the number and range of informants interviewed, and their insider status.

CRITICAL REFLECTIONS ON USING INTERVIEWS TO STUDY CORPORATIONS AND HEALTH

These case studies demonstrate how confidential, anonymised interviews can reveal crucial information about corporations' activities. They can provide insights into businesses' 'real' agenda, which may differ from the official accounts found on company websites or in publications. Interviews can also reveal inconsistencies within companies' publicly stated positions, which are, in themselves, interesting findings that may suggest areas for further investigation. At all times, however, it was vital to be aware that the responses may be designed to promote a particular image of the company or further a specific agenda. Responses of this kind may tell us little about the actual approach taken by corporations, but they are potentially helpful in understanding the way corporations attempt to frame policy debates and perceptions of their businesses and products.

The motivation for companies to participate in these particular studies is unclear, but in both studies, it was possible to gain access to industry respondents. The relative novelty of the research agenda on alcohol and gambling, and the limited public health research in these areas at the time, may partly explain the willingness of industry actors to engage in the studies documented earlier. It is uncertain, however, whether publication of these studies will affect future access to corporate actors in these and other fields. Our experiences suggest that interview-based studies may be most successful in subject areas that are currently under-researched. Given these obstacles, it is vital to use each interview opportunity to its fullest potential, by asking as wide a range of questions and establishing as extensive a data set as possible.

Interviews can produce unprecedented data about the alcohol and gambling industries. However, there are certain barriers which may limit the effectiveness of this approach when applied to the field of tobacco. The Framework Convention on Tobacco Control explicitly wards against the undue influence of the industry in the formulation of government policy in Article 5.3, and many academic institutions have policies of non-engagement with the tobacco industry. Some health journals refuse to publish tobacco industry–funded research. As a result of this, meeting with the tobacco industry, even for the purpose of conducting research interviews, is potentially politically problematic in a way which it may not yet be for researchers to meet with and engage with actors from other industries such as alcohol and gambling. Undertaking interviews with industry actors always has the potential of undermining the credibility of the researcher and the research in the eyes of the wider scholarly community. In the field of tobacco, this danger is especially pronounced.

CONCLUSION

This chapter demonstrates both the potential insights to be gained from and the challenges involved in conducting interview-based studies on corporations and global health. To date, interviews have been underutilised by researchers interested in corporations and global health. This chapter is intended to facilitate the use of interview-based studies to research other health-harming industries and different national contexts to which they have not to date been applied. Comparative analysis across both sectors and countries may also be undertaken using this methodology. The case studies presented here focus at the national level; interviews can be used to study corporate political influence at the regional or global levels, for example at the WHO. Working above the national level poses additional challenges as there may be language barriers and different cultural norms to negotiate, but in the context of globalisation, it is necessary to use the full range of methodologies at our disposal at all levels of governance in order to fully understand the political strategies, and impact on health, of transnational corporations.

NOTE

1. This chapter is based partly on fieldwork on gambling conducted by Rebecca Cassidy as part of a project funded by the European Research Council under the European Union's Seventh Framework Programme (FP/2007–2013)/ERC Grant Agreement no. 263443.

FURTHER READING

Irvine, Annie, Paul Drew and Roy Sainsbury. 2012. '"Am I Not Answering Your Questions Properly?" Clarification, Adequacy and Responsiveness in Semi-Structured Telephone and Face-to-Face Interviews'. *Qualitative Research* 13(1): 87–106.

King, Nigel and Christina Horrocks. 2010. *Interviews in Qualitative Research*. London: Sage.

Rubin, Herbert J. and Irene S. Rubin. 2012. *Qualitative Interviewing: The Art of Hearing Data*. London: Sage.

REFERENCES

ASA. 2014. 'Ethical Guidelines for Good Research Practice'. Accessed September 19, 2016. http://www.theasa.org/ethics/guidelines.shtml.

Atkinson, Rowland and John Flint. 2004. 'Snowball Sampling'. In *Encyclopedia of Social Science Research Methods*, edited by Michael S. Lewis-Beck, Alan Bryman and Tim Futing Liao, 1044–45. London: Sage. doi:http://dx.doi.org/10.4135/9781412950589.n931.

Brinkman, Svend. 2013. *Qualitative Interviewing: Understanding Qualitative Research*. Oxford, UK: Oxford University Press.

Brugha, Ruari and Zsuzsa Varvasovszky. 2000. 'Stakeholder Analysis: A Review'. *Health Policy and Planning* 15(3): 239–46.

Bryman, Alan. 2015. *Social Research Methods*, 5th edition. Oxford, UK: Oxford University Press.

Cassidy, Rebecca, Claire Loussouarn and Andrea Pisac. 2014. *Fair Game: Producing Gambling Research*. London: Goldsmiths College, University of London.

Cassidy, Rebecca. 'How Corporations Shape our Understanding of Problems with Gambling and their Solutions'. 2016. In Case Studies on Corporations and Global Health Governance Impacts, Influence and Accountability, edited by Nora Kenworthy, Ross MacKenzie and Kelley Lee. London: Rowman and Littlefield International.

GBGC. 2015. *Global Gambling Revenues Pass $450 billion in 2014*. 30 April. Accessed 29 June 2015. http://www.gbgc.com/global-gambling-revenues-pass-us-450-billion-in-2014/.

Hawkins, Benjamin and Christopher Holden. 2013. 'Framing the Alcohol Policy Debate: Industry Actors and the Regulation of the UK Beverage Alcohol Market'. *Critical Policy Studies* 7(1): 53–71.

Hawkins, Benjamin and Christopher Holden. 2014. '"Water Dripping on Stone?": Industry Lobbying and UK Alcohol Policy'. *Policy and Politics* 42(1): 55–70.

Holden, Christopher and Benjamin Hawkins. 2013. '"Whisky Gloss": The Alcohol Industry, Devolution and Policy Communities in Scotland'. *Public Policy and Administration* 28(3): 253–73.

Holden, Christopher, Benjamin Hawkins and Jim McCambridge. 2012. 'Cleavages and Co-Operation in the UK Alcohol Industry: A Qualitative Study'. *BMC Public Health* 12: 483.

McCambridge, Jim, Benjamin Hawkins and Christopher Holden. 2014. 'The Challenge Corporate Lobbying Poses to Reducing Society's Alcohol Problems: Insights from U.K. Evidence on Minimum Unit Pricing'. *Addiction* 109(2): 199–205.

Mikecz, Robert. 2012. 'Interviewing Elites Addressing Methodological Issues'. *Qualitative Inquiry* 18(6): 482–93.

Rubin, Herbert J. and Irene S. Rubin. 2012. *Qualitative Interviewing: The Art of Hearing Data*, 3rd edition. London: Sage.

Schüll, Natasha Dow. 2012. *Addiction by Design: Machine Gambling in Las Vegas*. Princeton, NJ: Princeton University Press.

Skeggs, Beverly. 1997. *Formations of Class and Gender: Becoming Respectable*. London: Sage.

Varvasovszky, Zsuzsa and Ruari Brugha. 2000. 'How to Do (or Not to Do). . .a Stakeholder Analysis'. *Health Policy and Planning* 15(3): 338–45.

Chapter 12

The Role of Ethnography in Analysing Corporations

Natalia Carrillo Botero

Ethnography, the primary methodology of anthropology, is defined as the scientific study of the customs of individuals and groups of people. While contemporary use of ethnography is not exclusive to anthropology, its origins and development as a scientific method are deeply embedded with the discipline from its development from the late nineteenth century. This chapter provides an overview of what ethnography is, its primary methods and the main forms of data it generates – namely ethnographic text or ethnographic accounts. The chapter then discusses how ethnographic research can be used to expand understanding of the role of corporations in global health governance.

CONDUCTING ETHNOGRAPHIC RESEARCH

Ethnography is a 'research process in which the anthropologist closely observes, records, and engages in the daily life of another culture – an experience labelled as the fieldwork method – and then writes accounts of this culture, emphasizing descriptive detail' (Marcus and Fisher 1999, 18). Fieldwork, for this type of research, requires being physically present in the research environment, sharing the day-to-day life of people.

Ethnographic fieldwork uses various methods of data collection, with the most essential being participant observation. As DeWalt and DeWalt (2011, 1) describe, participant observation 'is a method in which a researcher takes part in the daily activities, rituals, interactions, and events of a group of people as one of the means of learning the explicit and tacit aspects of their life routines and their cultures'. Through *immersion* in their cultural environment, the researcher aims to *build rapport* with the subjects and to *experience* their lives first-hand (Bernard 2011). Traditionally, ethnography requires this immersion to be longer term and focused in a geographical location. Ethnographers thus could typically spend several years living within the same community. The contemporary use of participant observation, however, has adapted to the different settings and is now often of shorter duration and undertaken across multiple contexts. Nevertheless, time in the field remains an essential factor for building rapport with subjects and to observe any changes in cultural practices over time. This is, therefore, a key consideration when considering whether to use participant observation as a research method.

The core data produced through participant observation is the researcher's recorded observations and perceptions. The writing of detailed fieldwork notes (or fieldwork diary) is critical. The challenge for the ethnographic researcher lies in the transformation of observations into field notes and field notes that are usable data. The more complete, detailed and accurate the notes, the easier it is for the researcher to subsequently catalogue, code and use them (Schensul, Schensul and LeCompte 1999).

Other data collection methods used in ethnography include interviews, surveys, questionnaires, archival research, focus groups and, in some cases, quantitative methods like census and demographic data. The appropriate method(s) used depends on the research question posed and the nature of the field site under study. In all cases, when these methods are used within the framework of ethnographic research, they serve to complement the key method of participant observation as the primary source of data. Together, these methods allow ethnographers to produce an interpretative, first-hand account of the subject consisting of both a description and interpretation (by the researcher) of the cultural practices under study. Ethnographic accounts privilege the point of view of the subject, presenting an 'insider's point of view'.

The final product of the research process, the ethnographic account, can take many forms, from an extended written text to a video or other media. The scope and nature of ethnographic outputs have been at the centre of debates in anthropology since the mid-twentieth century. Concerns that the production of such accounts, in itself, reflects embedded power relationships which can 'invent', rather than objectively 'describe', culture opened the way to experimental forms of writing such as 'dialogic anthropology' and 'narrative ethnography' (Marcus and Fisher 1999).

Ethnography can be used to answer a broad range of research questions focused on the meaning and significance of culture (Geertz 1973). What meaning do subjects assign to their behaviour and beliefs? Ethnographers want not only to know *what* people do but also to interpret *why* they engage in such behaviours.

The concept of culture in anthropology (from which the term *ethnography* takes its meaning) has evolved alongside the theoretical and methodological features of the discipline. Beyond any specific definition of culture, the assumption in ethnography is that culture exists everywhere: within all institutional structures, commercial transactions, governance systems and other social arenas. As described by Rosaldo (1989, 26), 'Culture encompasses the everyday and the esoteric, the mundane and the elevated, the ridiculous and the sublime. Neither high or low culture is all-pervasive.'

Consequently, the subject matter of ethnography has broadened beyond classical ethnography's almost exclusive focus on isolated and so-called exotic cultures, as perceived by North American and European researchers. The twentieth century brought important methodological changes that extended ethnography's focus to include studies of Western societies, transnational or global cultural forms and diverse cultural phenomena. Ethnographers began to study other forms of culture such as those of commerce, institutions, material goods and transnational networks. In addition, important questions have been raised about how 'the other' is conceptualised and represented, with increased critical reflection on the Western perspective. An overview of these disciplinary and methodological changes is explored.

CLASSICAL AND NEW ETHNOGRAPHIES: REPRESENTATION OF THE OTHER

Ethnography emerged during the nineteenth century as a research methodology when scholars in the West became increasingly interested in cultural contact with non-Western cultures. Thus, classical ethnography has been used to answer questions regarding cultural practices, behaviours and beliefs of 'other' (non-Western) cultures. In the context of colonisation, classic ethnography sought to answer questions around the cultural differences between European/North American and 'exotic' non-Western societies. Understanding systems of kinship and marriage, or beliefs of witchcraft and magic, for example, were subjects that classic ethnography sought to pursue. The aim was a holistic knowledge of culture, comprising a detailed understanding of the practices, norms and values within a group unfamiliar to Western societies. Classical ethnography, in essence, represented a Westernised account of the other and generated understandings of non-Western peoples and groups from this perspective (Said 1978).

The first half of the twentieth century brought changes to anthropology, as a discipline, and ethnography as a method evolved, from an exclusive focus on non-Western cultures to a methodology for studying any society, including that of the researchers themselves. In the United States, ethnographic fieldwork was developed by the Sociology Department of the University of Chicago in the 1930s to study the city of Chicago. Urban studies focused on marginalised groups, arguably still conceptualised as 'others', such as the homeless, gangs, delinquents, sex workers, homosexuals, drug addicts, ethnic minorities or immigrants (Deegan 2001). The focus changed, from explaining unfamiliar cultural practices of non-Western societies to answering questions about subgroups or subcultures within Western cultural settings.

The global political economic shifts from the 1960s, particularly processes of decolonisation, development, human rights movement and the emerging processes of economic globalisation, called into further question the ethnographer's authority to speak for others (Rosaldo 1989). Critics began to recognise that ethnographic accounts and histories are invariably constructed from the point of view of the researchers, oftentimes from societal elites, and from a Eurocentric bias. The new project of ethnography became the creation of a space for historically subordinated perspectives (and subjects) previously excluded from or marginalised within the dominant, mainstream discourse (Rosaldo 1989). The 'subaltern' perspective (view from below) became a central ethnographic concept, giving a voice to those marginalised in terms of race, class, caste, gender, language and culture (Spivak 1994; Mignolo 2000).

The emergence of post-colonial and feminist studies brought important methodological changes to ethnography. As Clifford (1986, 10) writes, 'Anthropology no longer speaks with automatic authority for others defined as unable to speak for themselves ("primitive", "pre-literate", "without history").' Such reflections on ethnographic authority led to the 'postmodern turn' in anthropology and the emergence of the 'new' ethnography (Geertz 1973; Clifford and Marcus 1986; Marcus and Fisher 1999). Questions concerning how ethnographic writing constructed or perpetuated myths about the non-Western other brought important methodological changes to the construction of the ethnographic account. Reflections on the ethnographer, as an individual with his or her own subjectivities, raised new questions: 'Who speaks? Who writes? When and where? With or to whom? Under what institutional and historical constraints?' (Clifford and Marcus 1986, 13). These critical reflections meant the voice of the ethnographer was no longer privileged in the construction of the narrative. Instead, new ethnography emphasises the cooperative and collaborative nature of the ethnographic situation between researcher and subject (Tyler 1986).

In the 1980s questions began to be raised by ethnographers about institutions, organisations and corporations (Marcus 1998). Anthropology traditionally favoured the study of the vulnerable, the subjugated, what anthropologist Laura Nader calls a preference for 'studying down' (Nader 1972). The need to study individuals or groups in positions of power generated methodological discussions about 'studying up'. As Nader (1972, 289) writes, 'What if, in reinventing anthropology, the anthropologist were to study the colonizers rather than the colonized, the culture of power rather than the culture of the powerless, the culture of affluence rather than the culture of poverty?' Drawing analytical attention to these additional social groups, and their influence on everyday life, opened ethnography to the study of new relationships of power. This trend has included the study of corporations, and the political and economic elite, within them, what Shore (2002, 4) calls 'those who occupy the most influential positions or roles in the important spheres of social life'.

Finally, the level of analysis of ethnography also correspondingly shifted, from a highly localised intellectual gaze to include social groups and cultural practices at the global and transnational levels. This includes the study of global flows of ideas, values, beliefs and other cultural artefacts amid an increasingly porous world (Appadurai 1990, 1996; Tsing 2004). This further expansion and development of ethnography went beyond what was traditionally considered as 'culture', even extending beyond the human, to recognising how humans are connected with a broader world of life, an 'anthropology beyond the human' (Kohn 2013, 7).

USING ETHNOGRAPHY IN THE STUDY OF CORPORATIONS AND GLOBAL HEALTH

Ethnography has been widely applied in the study of global health, frequently within the subfields of medical anthropology and anthropology of development. In Chapter 7, Parker and Kenworthy review the contributions of anthropological studies to global health governance in which ethnography is the primary methodological approach. Further examples are Nancy Scheper-Huges's ethnographic work on child mortality in northeastern Brazil (1992) and Biehl and Petryna's edited volume *When People Come First* (2013). Scheper-Huges uses ethnographic methods to reveal political conditions that contribute to high child mortality and how mothers respond to such conditions in their relationship with their children. Biehl and Petryna present an ethnographic critique of medical, social, political and economic dimensions of the global health enterprise, and offer reflections on ethnography as a crucial methodological tool for achieving a critical global health perspective.

A key intersection between corporations and global health governance is the study of pharmaceuticals. Petryna, Lakoff and Kleinman (2006) use ethnography to explore pharmaceutical governance – trade and marketing practices, patent protection distribution channels and regulation in different countries – as well as discuss the ethics of international human testing and human subjects research. Similarly, João Biehl's *Will to Live* (2007) uses ethnography to analyse Brazilian AIDS policy through the stories and lives of patients. Demonstrating ethnography's applicability to crossborder populations and practices, Seth Holmes's *Fresh Fruit, Broken Bodies* (2013) follows Mexican fruit workers as they migrate into the United States, conducting ethnographic research on the migration process, the hierarchical social dynamics on farms and the embodied health impacts (both physical and emotional) of migration and working conditions. A relevant work on transnational corporations and governance is Dinah Rajak's *In Good Company* (2011), an ethnographic study of corporate social responsibility (CSR) by the mining company Anglo American. Rajak's fieldwork was conducted with miners in South Africa, senior executives and senior personnel in charge of CSR in the company.

Ethnography has been used to study corporations from other perspectives, not all related to their health impacts (Benson and Kirsch 2010; see Chapter 7, Parker and Kenworthy, for discussion of *harm industries*). Welker, Partridge and Hardin's (2011) introduction to a special supplement of *Current Anthropology* provides a comprehensive overview of ethnographic research on corporate forms. Michael Burawoy's (1979) studies of industrial workplaces in the 1970s use ethnography to understand conditions of industrial production in South Africa, Zimbabwe and Zambia and machine shops in Hungary and the United States.

Social scientists have used ethnography to study business, governmental and non-governmental organisations since the 1930s, known as applied anthropology (e.g. business anthropology, organisational anthropology). In the 1970s, a new form of contemporary ethnography emerged, *within* and *for* corporations, highlighted by the hiring of in-house anthropologists by Xerox PARC (Fisher 2009). This type of ethnography focused on two main areas: workplace studies and consumer studies (Cefkin 2009). Ann Jordan's *Business Anthropology* (2003) provides a good overview of how ethnographic methods have been used in areas such as product design, consumer behaviour and organisational change, and gives practical examples of ethnographic fieldwork in a business setting. While the focus of corporate ethnography is not concerned with health harms, this work offers opportunities to extend understanding of corporate forms and practices (Welker, Partridge and Hardin 2011). Melissa Cefkin's edited volume *Ethnography and the Corporate Encounter* (2009) provides similar insights into the challenges of doing ethnography in corporate settings. It is important to note ethical concerns regarding corporate ethnography, particularly the use of anthropological expertise to increase corporate profits or generate proprietary knowledge (Welker, Partridge and Hardin 2011), or 'risks of co-optation, because the tendency of ethnographers to empathize and identify with their subjects may limit their findings or critical stand' (Benson and Kirsch 2010, 464).

CRITICAL REFLECTIONS

Ethnographers listen to people in order to understand why they do things and observe behaviour to interpret its meaning. This approach can be very useful when studying corporations and global health governance. Corporate actors, organisations and institutions attempt to create public personas and to shape perceptions of their identity and impact on society, and participant observation can provide valuable insights into corporate life beyond this official discourse.

The nature of multi-sited ethnography is another strength when applied to these disciplines. Various examples mentioned in the previous section use multi-site ethnography; anthropologist George Marcus (1998) called this 'following the thing' (e.g. HIV medication or CSR programmes) or 'following the people' (workers of fruit farms) across geographies and contexts. This approach emerged from recognition amid globalisation that cultures are not isolated entities, but interconnected and changing, as they move across the globe. In some cases, ethnography may not move around literally but may be embedded in a multi-sited context. It is the case of Scheper-Huges's study in Brazil: she follows the mothers into the various scenarios where they move between private and public life (home, work, the municipality, the child care centre), to be able to define their role as woman. The applicability of this approach to research on transnational corporations whose activities may be multifaceted and are spread across geographical locations is obvious.

Ethnography privileges subjective viewpoints, whereas most other fields, including the natural sciences and much research in the field of public health, strive for objectivity. In the latter approach, the researcher attempts to shield the research process from his or her personal beliefs and ideas. He or she attempts to create methodologies which minimise sources of subjectivity and bias from influence research outcomes. Ethnographers, by contrast, explicitly embrace the subjective and interpretative nature of their research process. They reject the possibility of truly 'value-neutral', objective social science. According to Rosaldo (1989, xvii), 'The observer's point of view always influences the observations she makes . . . this perspective emphasizes human diversity, historical change, and political struggle.' By acknowledging and revealing one's beliefs and background, they argue, the ethnographer can convey to the public an interpretative account of the research object which aims to render it meaningful and comprehensible to the reader. A key concept for ethnographers working within this tradition is reflexivity. The reflexive practitioner makes explicit his or her own standpoint, views, beliefs and positions within the interpretative process, setting these out for the reader to acknowledge when considering the accounts he or she produces of his or her research objects. Margery Wolf's *A Thrice-Told Tale* (1992) illustrates the positioning and subjectivities of the ethnographer can significantly change the final outcome of a research process. The author makes three different accounts of the same fieldwork on a Taiwanese village 30 years ago, all from different points of view conditioned by individual and professional circumstances as well as different writing styles. Yet the key concepts and the norms of this type of research and the notion of reflexivity will be equally important when researching corporations and global health.

LIMITATIONS TO USING ETHNOGRAPHY TO STUDY CORPORATIONS AND GLOBAL HEALTH

There are potential limitations to the use of ethnography in the study of corporations and global health governance. On studying elites, Shore (2002, 10) points out that participant observation poses a challenge of access: 'One cannot simply pitch one's tent in the board room of the World Bank or the Pentagon, or unobtrusively observe the bargains being struck at the European Council Ministers' meeting.' Most elites are unlikely to grant open and uncensored access. Even if an individual agrees, observing the day-to-day life of a corporation can be restricted by concerns of privacy, privilege and confidentiality regarding business activities. Even corporate ethnographers, working in and for corporations, have highlighted the difficulties of conducting 'proper' participant observation on these arenas. Jordan and Lambert (2009) describe the problems of dealing with company secrets (industrial secrets), limited access to industrial production sites, complex and bureaucratic procedures for access to documents, restrictions to take images or video record and the fact the company needs to protect itself from unauthorised disclosure of how its operates. All ethnographic work has its restrictions of access/what can be observed, but in the case of corporations, these may be driven by concerns unfamiliar to the researcher, such as intellectual property, privacy and image, as well as health and safety standards. How can the researcher be a 'participant observer' when studying such subjects?

Anthropologists have sought to address the limitations of participant observation, when studying corporations, institutions and organisations since the 1970s. Nader (1972) argues that access to the powerful in the corporate world can be an issue, but it is certainly not an insurmountable obstacle. Any research site can present some form of access problem. While studying up may pose challenges to conventional participant observation, there are other forms of 'being there' that can replace limited access. As virtual ethnography has demonstrated, being there does not necessarily require physical presence (Boellstorff 2010). There are also alternative data sources for 'studying up' that do not involve placement within a corporation, such as ethnographic analysis of public relations campaigns, corporate interactions with external actors such as workers and labour unions and documentation of discrepancies between official policy statements and actual practices' (Benson and Kirsch 2012, 464). Textual analysis or critical readings of advertisement and marketing campaigns are also alternative tools. Anthropologist Peter Benson's work, on the impact of the transnational tobacco industry on the traditional tobacco-growing region of North Carolina in the United States, is based on ethnographic work on tobacco farms as workplaces, households, migrant labour camps and former tobacco-growing communities (Benson 2012). In addition to direct observation on farms, he conducted extensive archival research, interviews with farmers, farm employees, warehouse managers, labour organisers and public health advocates (Benson 2008). His work shows it is possible to conduct an ethnography of corporations using diverse data sources, without the researcher sitting in the boardroom or conducting observation inside company offices. Because the corporation is not an isolated actor, studying its networks and relationships with society more broadly can provide relevant insights into corporate cultural practices and behaviour. There are then different levels of engagement that should be considered when using ethnography to study corporations and global health governance. Finding different ways of 'being there', combined with the use of other techniques and methods to complement participant observation (interviews, personal documents, memoires, focus groups, etc.), can help the researcher overcome any access problems encountered on the site.

FURTHER READING

DeWalt, Kathleen and Billie E. DeWalt. 2010. *Participant Observation: A Guide for Fieldworkers*. Lanham, Maryland: Altamira Press.

LeCompte, M.D. and Jean J. Schensul. 1999. *Designing and Conducting Ethnographic Research. The Ethnographer's Toolkit*, Vol. 1. New York: Altamira Press.

Rajak, Dinah. 2011. *In Good Company: An Anatomy of Corporate Social Responsibility*. Stanford, CA: Stanford University Press.

REFERENCES

Appadurai, Arjun. 1990. 'Disjuncture and Difference in the Global Cultural Economy'. *Theory, Culture and Society* 7: 295–310. Accessed 3 February 2016. doi:10.1177/026327690007002017.

Appadurai, Arjun. 1996. *Modernity at Large: Cultural Dimensions of Globalization*. Minneapolis: University of Minnesota Press.

Benson, Peter. 2008. 'Good Clean Tobacco: Philip Morris, Biocapitalism, and the Social Course of Stigma in North Carolina'. *American Ethnologist* 35(3): 357–79.

Benson, Peter & Stuart Kirsch. 2010. 'Capitalism and the Politics of Resignation.' *Current Anthropology* 51(4): 459–86.

Benson, Peter. 2012. *Tobacco Capitalism: Growers, Migrant Workers, and the Changing Face of a Global Industry*. Princeton, NJ: Princeton University Press.

Benson, Peter and Stuart Kirsch. 2010. 'Capitalism and the Politics of Resignation'. *Current Anthropology* 51(4): 459–86.

Bernard, H. Russell. 2011. *Research Methods in Anthropology. Qualitative and Quantitative Approaches*, 5th edition. Lanham, Maryland: Altamira Press.

Biehl, João. 2007. *Will to Live: AIDS Therapies and the Politics of Survival*. Princeton, NJ: Princeton University Press.

Biehl, João and Adriana Petryna, eds. 2013. *When People Come First: Critical Studies in Global Health*. Princeton, NJ: Princeton University Press.

Boellstorff, Tom. 2010. *Coming of Age in Second Life*. Princeton, NJ: Princeton University Press.

Burawoy, Michael. 1979. *Manufacturing Consent. Changes in the Labour Process under Monopoly Capitalism*. Chicago, IL: University of Chicago Press.

Cefkin, Melissa. 2009. 'Introduction'. In *Ethnography and the Corporate Encounter: Reflections in and of Corporations*, edited by Melissa Cefkin, 1–37. New York: Berghahn Books.

Clifford, James. 1986. 'Introduction: Partial Truths'. In Writing Culture: The Poeteics and Politics of Ethnography, edited by James Clifford and George E. Marcus. Berkeley and Los Angeles, California: University of California Press.

Clifford, James and George Marcus, eds. 1986. *Writing Culture: The Poetics and Politics of Ethnography*. Berkeley: University of California Press.

Deegan, Mary Jo. 2001. 'The Chicago School of Ethnography'. In *Handbook of Ethnography*, edited by Paul Atkinson, Amanda Coffey, Sara Delamont, John Lofland and Lyn Lofland, 11–26. London: Sage. Accessed 5 August 2015. doi:http://dx.doi.org/10.4135/9781848608337.n1.

DeWalt, Kathleen and Billie E. DeWalt. 2011. *Participant Observation: A Guide for Fieldworkers*. Lanham, Maryland: Altamira Press.

Fisher, Michael M.J. 2009. 'Emergent Forms of Life in Corporate Arenas'. In *Ethnography and the Corporate Encounter: Reflections in and of Corporations*, edited by Melissa Cefkin, 227–38. New York: Berghahn Books.

Geertz, Clifford. 1973. *The Interpretation of Cultures: Selected Essays*. New York: Basic Books.

Holmes, Seth M. 2013. *Fresh Fruit, Broken Bodies: Migrant Farmworkers in the United States*. Berkeley: University of California Press.

Jordan, Ann T. 2003. *Business Anthropology*. Long Grove, IL: Waveland Press Inc.

Jordan, Brigitte and Monique Lambert. 2009. 'Working in Corporate Jungles: Reflections on Ethnographic Praxis in Industry'. In *Ethnography and the Corporate Encounter: Reflections in and of Corporations*, edited by Melissa Cefkin, 95–133. New York: Berghahn Books.

Kohn, Eduardo. 2013. *How Forests Think. Towards and Anthropology beyond the Human*. Berkeley: University of California Press.

Marcus, George E. 1998. 'Ethnography in/of the World System: The Emergence of Multi-Sited Ethnography'. In *Ethnography through Thick and Thin*, edited by George E. Marcus, 79–104. Princeton, NJ: Princeton University Press.

Marcus, George E. and Michael M.J. Fisher. 1999. *Anthropology as Cultural Critique: An Experimental Moment in the Human Sciences*, 2nd edition. Chicago, IL: University of Chicago Press.

Mignolo, Walter. 2000. *Local Histories/Global Designs: Coloniality, Subaltern Knowledges, and Border Thinking*. Princeton, NJ: Princeton University Press.

Nader, Laura. 1972. 'Up the Anthropologist. Perspectives Gained from Studying Up'. In *Reinventing Anthropology*, edited by Dell Hymes, 285–311. New York: Pantheon Books.

Petryna, Adriana, Andrew Lakoff and Arthur Kleinman, eds. 2006. *Global Pharmaceuticals: Ethics, Markets, Practices*. Durham, NC: Duke University Press.

Rajak, Dinah. 2011. *In Good Company: An Anatomy of Corporate Social Responsibility*. Stanford, CA: Stanford University Press.

Rosaldo, Renato. 1989. *Culture and Truth: The Remaking of Social Analysis*, 1993 edition. Boston, MA: Beacon Press.

Said, Edward. 1978. *Orientalism*. New York: Vintage Books.

Schensul, S.L., J.J. Schensul and M.D. LeCompte. 1999. *Essential Ethnographic Methods: Observations, Interviews, and Questionnaires*, Vol. 2. The Ethnographer's Toolkit, Book 2. New York: Altamira Press.

Scheper-Huges, Nancy. 1992. *Death without Weeping: The Violence of Everyday Life in Brazil*. Berkeley: University of California Press.

Shore, Chris. 2002. 'Introduction'. In *Elite Cultures: Anthropological Perspectives*, edited by Chris Shore and Stephen Nugent, 1–21. London: Routledge.

Spivak Chakravorty, Gayatri. 1994. 'Can the Subaltern Speak?' In *Colonial Discourse and Post-Colonial Theory: A Reader*, edited by Patrick Williams and Laura Chrisman, 66–111. New York, Columbia University Press.

Tsing, Anna. L. 2004. *Friction: An Ethnography of Global Connection*. Princeton, NJ: Princeton University Press.

Tyler, Stephen A. 1986. 'Post-Modern Ethnography: From Document of the Occult to Occult Document'. In *Writing Culture: The Poetics and Politics of Ethnography*, edited by James Clifford and George E. Marcus, 122–40. Berkeley: University of California Press.

Welker, Marina, Damani J. Partridge and Rebecca Hardin. 2011. 'Corporate Lives: New Perspectives on the Social life of the Corporate Form'. *Current Anthropology* 52(S3): S3–16.

Wolf, Margery. 1992. *A Thrice-Told Tale: Feminism, Postmodernism, and Ethnographic Responsibility*. Stanford, CA: Stanford University Press.

Chapter 13

Oral History

Michael Stevenson

Oral history is a qualitative research methodology that involves the recording, transcribing, analysing and archiving of face-to-face interviews. It is used to draw out memories of the lived experiences of interviewees (hereafter 'narrators') who have an expressed intention to preserve their understanding of the past for future interested parties (Oral History Association 2009, 1). As an analytical method, to build an account of past events, oral history requires a critical appraisal of this dialogue. Oral history begins with the assumption that an objective account of history is not attainable (Yow 1997). Instead, scholars must interpret multiple, subjective accounts, each from the perspective of the narrator in question. A narrator's experiences of a given issue may thus be limited in time and exposure to an issue. In addition, the sentiments of researchers and narrators, related to a given topic and to each other, function as filters, which inevitably shape both the questions asked and answers given (Grele 1998).

Oral history is inherently critical in its roots and orientation. It developed out of the modernist movement of the early twentieth century, which rejected traditional approaches to understanding the natural and social worlds, and the cultural history movement, which sought to incorporate anthropological methods oriented towards chronicling cultural practices and interpretations of past events into historical analysis (Evans 1956; Thomson 2007; Abrams 2010). Thus, oral history infers that traditional academic accounts of 'what happened', informed by the analysis of written documents (i.e. 'mainstream' history), are limited by their failure to explicitly acknowledge how their authors' biases have shaped the research and writing process (Crane 1996).

There are clear similarities between oral history and ethnographic approaches (Chapter 12), both of which share a common endeavour in personally recording the stories of society's 'voiceless' and making their documentation publicly available. However, Di Leondardo (1987) writes that the former differs in important ways. Oral historians focus solely on narrative, while ethnographers place equal value on observed behaviours. Moreover, while ethnographies typically include descriptions of, and narratives from, individuals whose identities are shielded through the use of pseudonyms, oral history tends to use individual narratives of named subjects to inform studies of groups or organisations. A further difference is that ethnography methodologically underpins anthropology. Mainstream historians, however, place greater value on written than oral evidence. This reticence stems from lingering questions about the validity of oral testimony – whether individual narrators are representative of social groups that researchers are seeking to understand – and thus a perceived lack of methodological rigour (Grele 1998; Errante 2000). Oral historians have responded to such criticisms by arguing that statistically representative samples and standardised questionnaires become irrelevant when one is looking at key decision makers (Errante 2000). To improve perceptions of rigour, the Oral History Association has since 1968 published a collection of principles and best practices. These cover key issues such as process, consent, copyright, misrepresentation, narrator anonymity and quality assurance related to the recording and archiving of oral documents (Oral History Association 2009).

This chapter sets out the use of oral history as a possible methodology for supporting research on corporations and global health governance (GHG). After reviewing how oral history has been applied, to date, to study corporations, the chapter considers how the methodology can be extended to GHG. This includes a discussion of the strengths and weaknesses of the approach.

ORAL HISTORY AND RESEARCH ON CORPORATIONS

The oral history method was embraced during the 1960s by socialist and feminist scholars seeking to document and validate the experiences of groups such as the working classes and women, traditionally excluded from mainstream historical texts, which prioritised the lives and institutions of elites (Thompson 2000; Perks 2010a). In the United Kingdom, where the majority of oral history research has been publicly funded, limited attention has been paid by oral historians to the private sector and corporate world. However, there are exceptions. Oral history documents relating to England's declining coal mining, textiles and auto manufacturing sectors and public bodies such as the National Health Service and Royal Mail are housed in the British Library (Perks 2010a).

The situation is very different in the United States, where the practice of commissioned, privately funded oral histories is well established (Gluck

1977; Perks 2010b). Documenting the voices of elites, including corporate decision makers, is deeply rooted in American history. Examples include initiatives to document the activities of the Carnegie, Rockefeller, Ford and Alfred Sloan Foundations, contracted to Columbia University's Oral History Research Office founded in 1948, the oldest university-based oral history research centre in the United States (Gardner 1992; Perks 2010a). Thus, while oral history has proven effective for revealing the overlooked experiences of the working poor and politically disenfranchised, it has also been used to present the stories of powerful actors at the opposite end of the socio-economic spectrum.

USING ORAL HISTORY TO STUDY CORPORATIONS AND GHG

Oral history documents events that shaped the life courses of narrators and how the narrators view themselves as affected by historical events. For researchers seeking to better understand the role of corporations in contemporary societies, including their impacts on global health, this might begin by documenting the experiences of marginalised groups adversely affected by corporate practices. For example, oral history could be applied to document the lived experiences of community residents subject to the illegal dumping of toxic waste (Margai and Fatoumata 2011), or contracted labourers working for transnational corporations required to work under hazardous conditions (Brown 2002). These applications would be consistent with how oral history has been traditionally employed in research.

In addition, there is potential for using oral history as a means of gaining greater understanding of the inner workings of corporations. The method could be used to illuminate the circumstances by which a senior executive, for instance, came to work at a particular company; his or her contribution to ideas informing company policies or strategies; how and why these changed over time; and what, from his or her perspective, the implications of these policies were for the company and wider world. For critical analyses of corporations, oral history's greatest utility may be to help showcase the individual logic guiding organisational decision making, or reactions to policies under which narrators worked during their tenure as corporate employees. Individuals holding senior roles within a corporation, or who have invested considerable time and energy into particular initiatives of interest, constitute particularly important sources of information on macro-level corporate policies and strategies. Oral history can also be used to capture understanding of the motivation and ideas of a corporation's leadership as well as the opportunity to gain anecdotal details useful for linking people or groups together.

Oral history also offers a means for gaining insights into emotional and cognitive dissonance held by those working in health-harming industries. This might mean, for example, probing whether people who work for tobacco companies experience moral conflicts or dilemmas. Researchers may seek out how middle-level managers, who have carried out policies that they did not agree with, understand the reasoning for doing so. The aim of oral history applied to corporations is thus to gain personal perspectives, which are different from the official positions of a firm and for which publicly available documents do not exist.

An interesting and significant variation of the oral history method, which is specifically tailored to bring new understanding to long-contested topics, was developed by Cold War scholars James Blight and Janet Lang. Termed *Critical Oral History*, individual decision makers during events of interest, including but not limited to the Cuban Missile Crisis and the Vietnam War, were brought together with academic experts to participate in structured meetings. Pertinent declassified documents were also made available for consultation (Blight and Lang 2005, 6; Blight 2010). While these events brought to light new factual revelations, the purpose of bringing together multiple sources of information in one place goes beyond attaining certainty about what transpired. Rather, the research sought to assemble and contrast as many relevant credible versions of the same event as possible. Coming from the decision makers themselves, this creates, in the words of Blight and Lang (2005, 9), 'a thickening of the texture of the historical narrative concerning how decisions were actually made'.

Critical oral history accounts are particularly insightful for understanding politically sensitive topics, which are often shrouded in secrecy and lack in formal records. It has been noted that this group variant of the oral history method decreases the likelihood of narrators becoming defensive, when questioned on polarising subjects (Blight and Lang 2005). This can be attributed to their responding equally to their engaged peers, as to the interviewers. Most important, it provides researcher(s) with the ability to hear the personal accounts of multiple narrators in the same sitting, while offering all participants the opportunity to seek clarification and/or revisit responses in the light of new information. This could not occur in traditional one-on-one interviews (Postel 2002).

Given the logical and financial requisites associated with staging a critical oral history event, in the style of Blight and Lang (2005), the approach is unlikely to be feasible for many researchers. Nevertheless, as a methodological approach, it has great potential utility for those seeking to bring new understandings to controversial events, including those involving corporate actors.

THE STUDY OF CORPORATIONS AND GHG USING ORAL HISTORY

Oral history has been employed to study GHG, but only to a limited extent, in conjunction with the role of corporations. The World Health Organization (WHO) Global Health Histories initiative, launched in 2004 to heighten awareness of the history of international health collaboration, is perhaps the best example (WHO 2004). The WHO Oral History Project was initiated in 2005, as part of this wider initiative, to record the perspectives of former WHO staff. The interviewers were themselves former WHO employees who operated under British Library Sound Archive guidelines. The project was intended to be a catalyst for individuals to write their own memoirs and a supplement to official WHO records regarding important health events. This was to be achieved by gathering the perspectives of retired staff, preserving their voices, personalities and varied perspectives unlikely to be sufficiently captured by written records. All of these oral documents have been subsequently housed in the WHO archive and are publicly available (WHO 2007). Another example of oral history in GHG research is *The Global Health Chronicles*, a digital repository conceived in 2005 by individuals involved in the smallpox eradication campaign. The repository contains interviews with key (predominantly American) figures involved in the global campaign to control and eventually eradicate the disease. The initiative is jointly run by Emory University and the US Centers for Disease Control and Prevention David J. Sencer Museum. The contents are accessible using a searchable database (see http://www.globalhealthchronicles.org).

The application of oral history, specifically to understanding the role of corporations in GHG, has so far been limited. The use of in-depth interviews by Muraskin (1995, 1998, 2005), in his insightful accounts of low-cost hepatitis vaccine development, the Children's Vaccine Initiative and Global Alliance for Vaccines and Immunization, loosely resembles oral history. While anecdotes about corporations and individuals associated with corporations feature in these works, they are not the primary focus. Moreover, Muraskin does not self-identify as an oral historian, and it is unclear whether he recorded or transcribed his interviews for they are not publicly accessible.

There are opportunities to apply oral history to study the inner workings of corporations impacting on GHG. As noted earlier, much of the existing corporation-focused oral histories has been commissioned by the companies themselves. As noted by Perks (2010a), the rationale for oral history projects by corporations is that narrators are more likely to be candid, if they are familiar with their interviewers, and their testimonies will not be subject to public scrutiny in the short- to medium term while housed in company archives or other repositories with prearranged conditions on access (Perks 2010a). However, these accounts face criticism from the oral history community for being insufficiently willing to pose challenging questions, and overly laudatory if not hagiographic, in their intent and content (Frisch 1979). The end products of commissioned oral histories, or those conducted by organisations themselves, can shape historical accounts by being unwilling or unable to ask challenging questions regarding specific events or practices that may cast the corporation in poor light (Hordes 1986; Walkowitz 1986; Perks 2010a), or, worse, purposely obscure facts in order to prevent reputational harm (Gourvish 2006; Perks 2010a). To reduce the chances of self-censure, and to increase the likelihood that difficult questions will be addressed and historians are sufficiently critical in their analyses, the history of any institution is likely to be best told by independent (i.e. external) experts (Morrissey 1978). Indeed, there is a need for greater application of oral history to the study of corporations. Limited examples of published oral history collections focused on corporations include the Smithsonian National Museum of History's assemblage of large American advertising campaigns, which include material related to PepsiCo and Marlboro; a collection on the Federated Department Stores (the original name of Macy's Inc.) housed at the Columbia Oral History Research Office; and interviews with notable American entrepreneurs housed at the University of California, Los Angeles (Ryant 1988).

While narratives were initially viewed as passive, first-hand accounts that could then be subject to interpretation over time, oral historians have come to see their relationship with narrators, and their role in the interview process, as shaping both what is said or what is not said in the interview (Summerfield 2005). From the perspective of oral history pioneer Ronald Grele (1998), former director of the Columbia Oral Research Office, it is impossible to separate the final 'conversational narratives' from the circumstances within which they are created. Moreover, because the process of transcribing audio recordings may involve minor edits, or inadvertently fail to capture emotive aspects of the original conversation, transcription itself is viewed as adding another layer of interpretation to the end product (Di Leonardo 1987).

THE STRENGTHS AND WEAKNESSES OF ORAL HISTORY AS A METHOD

The strengths of oral history arise from its role in affirming the importance of the lived experience of narrators. Oral history collects and preserves for perpetuity subjective self-assessments of individuals' contributions to particular events or organisations. As Portelli (1998) notes, oral history is special for never being the same twice. Moreover, because recordings provide the opportunity to revisit accounts and are thus open to reinterpretation, the greatest contribution of oral historians is not how they themselves use interviews but the act of collecting and preserving material for long-term use (Samuel 1998; Keulen and Kroeze 2012).

Oral history also provides a unique opportunity for narrators to speak honestly about, or reflect upon, important periods of their careers, if needed providing clarification on issues where they feel misunderstood or insights into decisions not be captured in official documents (Keulen and Kroeze 2012). Given the often powerful emotions and memories generated, through the very process of conveying personal stories, the method can create a degree of trust between the researcher and narrator, which can help generate deeper understanding than other methodologies. This, in turn, can improve access to other potential narrators.

Unlike semi-structured interviews (Chapter 11), which begin with the needs of the researcher, oral history can give the narrator considerable control over the subject, focus, or topic spoken about (Field 2007). This creates latitude to explain actions in their own words and reflect on the significance of their lived experience. This, in turn, may create opportunities for bringing untold stories to light that had previously been excluded from the public record (Welch et al. 2002). Moreover, multiple oral histories of linked individuals provide an opportunity to 'connect the dots' and to tease out contestation and complexity surrounding an issue.

While there is scope for oral history to fill gaps in knowledge, due to lack of access to or incomplete formal documentation (Ryant 1988), the method has four main challenges. First, because narrators may draw from distant memories, and sometimes be advanced in age, there is a potential for recall bias. This concern, while valid, has nonetheless lessened among oral historians over time as how and why narrators reconstruct their memories in certain ways (i.e. 'mediated memory') has become part of the analytical process (Summerfield 2005). Second, the need for interviewers to be empathetic to narrators, while not synonymous with agreement, nonetheless means attempting to see the world through their eyes. This is needed during both interviewing and analysis. As noted by Blight and Lang (2005), an unwillingness or inability to empathise is a key driver of misinterpretation. While oral history recognises that all researchers come to research with a particular theoretical lens, it is essential for researchers to be critically reflexive of their own perspectives, while seeking to understand those of narrators.

A third potential challenge is that the process of securing, conducting and processing interviews can be labour-intensive and time-consuming. Accessing some individuals as narrators can be simple and straightforward. When seeking to study corporations, others such as senior executives can be difficult to locate, communicate with and secure access to. As private institutions, there is nothing to compel corporate actors to cooperate with researchers, especially those intent on asking difficult questions. There is likely to be reluctance if there is a risk of reputational harm to narrators, their friends and colleagues or affiliated firms. Confidentiality agreements might also restrict participation. How then might existing or former employees be given the opportunity to speak? Perks (2010a) writes that researchers may need to provide anonymity to narrators, despite the importance of identity in oral history, as well as agreement on the specific use of, and public access to, recordings (Perks 2010a).

Finally, when using oral history to study corporations, there may be a need to operate according to rules determined largely by the research subject (Gardner 1992). This is particularly pertinent if the research is funded by the corporation under scrutiny. If researchers are unable to determine who is interviewed, what they are asked or not asked; lack control over the interview or transcription process; or are forced to work with imposed conditions related to the access to or use of materials (Ryant 1988), then the oral history method may not meet their critical research needs.

CONCLUSION

Oral history as a research method is highly relevant to the study of corporations and GHG. It can provide credible, empirically rich and supplemental accounts from document sources. More specifically, oral history can be used as a means for engaging with, and finding value in, a broader range of individuals associated with health-relevant corporations. This might be individuals who are members of populations whose health and well-being are affected by corporate activity. Or this may be the many individuals who were, or are still, employed by corporations that shape their strategies and activities. To date, oral history has been used to study 'ordinary people' and public figures. Individuals within corporations have been studied as part of company histories. There is thus a major gap, and much scope, for oral history to contribute to new insights on the corporation as an increasingly dominant form of economic organisation, including its impacts on GHG.

FURTHER READING

Keulen, Sjoerd and Ronald Kroeze. 2012. 'Back to Business: A Next Step in the Field of Oral History – The Usefulness of Oral History for Leadership and Organizational Research'. *Oral History Review* 39(1): 15–36.

Perks, Rob. 2010. '"Corporations Are People Too!": Business and Corporate Oral History in Britain'. *Oral History* 38(1): 36–54.

Perks, Robert and Alistair, Thompson, ed. 2006. *The Oral History Reader*, 2nd edition. London: Routledge.

REFERENCES

Abrams, Lynn. 2010. *Oral History Theory*. London: Routledge.

Blight, James G. 2010. 'When Empathy Failed: Using Critical Oral History to Reassess the Collapse of US-Soviet Détente in the Carter-Brezhnev Years'. *Journal of Cold War Studies* 12(2): 29–74.

Blight, James G. and Janet M. Lang. 2005. *The Fog of War: Lessons from the Life of Robert S. McNamara*. Lanham, MA: Rowman & Littlefield.

Brown, Garrett D. 2002. 'The Global Threats to Workers' Health and Safety on the Job'. *Social Justice* 29(3): 12–25.

Crane, Susan A. 1996. '(Not) Writing History: Rethinking the Intersections of Personal History and Collective Memory with Hans von Aufsess'. *History and Memory* 8(1): 5–29.

Di Leonardo, Micaela. 1987. 'Oral History as Ethnographic Encounter'. *Oral History Review* 15(1): 1–20.

Errante, Antoinette. 2000. 'But Sometimes You're Not Part of the Story: Oral Histories and Ways of Remembering and Telling'. *Educational Researcher* 29(2): 16–27.

Evans, George Ewart. 1956. *Ask the Fellows Who Cut the Hay*. London: Faber & Faber.

Field, Sean. 2007. *Oral History Methodology*. South-South Exchange Programme for Research on the History of Development.

Frisch, Michael. 1979. 'Oral History and Hard Times: A Review Essay'. *Oral History Reader* 7(1): 70–79.

Gardner, Joel R. 1992. 'Oral History and Philanthropy: Private Foundations'. *Journal of American History* 79(2): 601–5.

Gluck, Sherna. 1977. 'What's So Special about Women? Women's Oral History'. *Frontiers: A Journal of Women Studies* 2(2): 3–17.

Gourvish, Terry. 2006. 'What Can Business History Tell Us about Business Performance?' *Competition & Change* 10(4): 375–92.

Grele, Ronald J. 1998. 'Movement without Aim: Methodological and Theoretical Problems in Oral History'. In *The Oral History Reader*, 1st edition, edited by Robert Perks and Alistair Thomson, 38–52. London: Routledge.

Hordes, Stanley M. 1986. 'Does He Who Pays the Piper Call the Tune? Historians, Ethics, and the Community'. *The Public Historian* 8(1): 53–56.

Keulen, Sjoerd and Ronald Kroeze. 2012. 'Back to Business: A Next Step in the Field of Oral History – The Usefulness of Oral History for Leadership and Organizational Research'. *Oral History Review* 39(1): 15–36.

Margai, Florence M. and Fatoumata B. Barry. 2011. 'Global Geographies of Environmental Injustice and Health: A Case Study of Illegal Hazardous Waste Dumping in Cote d'Ivoire'. In *Geospatial Analysis of Environmental Health*, edited by Juliana A. Maantay and Sara McLafferty, 257–81. New York: Springer.

Morrissey, Charles T. 1978. 'Rhetoric and Role in Philanthropy: Oral History and the Grant-Making Foundations'. *Oral History Review* 6(1): 5–19.

Muraskin, William A. 1995. *The War against Hepatitis B: A History of the International Task Force on Hepatitis B Immunization*. Philadelphia: University of Pennsylvania Press.

Muraskin, William A. 1998. *The Politics of International Health: The Children's Vaccine Initiative and the Struggle to Develop Vaccines for the Third World*. Albany: State University of New York Press.

Muraskin, William A. 2005. *Crusade to Immunize the World's Children: The Origins of the Bill and Melinda Gates Children's Vaccine Program and the Birth of the Global Alliance for Vaccines and Immunizations*. Los Angeles, CA: USC Marshall BioBusiness Initiative.

Oral History Association. 2009. 'Principles and Best Practices: Principles for Oral History and Best Practices for Oral History'. Accessed September 19, 2016. http://www.oralhistory.org/about/principles-and-practices/.

Perks, Rob. 2010a. '"Corporations Are People Too!": Business and Corporate Oral History in Britain'. *Oral History* 38(1): 36–54.

Perks, Rob. 2010b. 'The Roots of Oral History: Exploring Contrasting Attitudes to Elite, Corporate, and Business Oral History in Britain and the US'. *Oral History Review* 37(2): 215–24.

Portelli, Alessandro. 1998. 'What Makes Oral History Different'. In *The Oral History Reader*, 1st edition, edited by Robert Perks and Alistair Thomson, 63–74. London: Routledge.

Postel, Danny. 2002. 'Revisiting the Brink: The Architect of "Critical Oral History" Sheds New Light on the Cold War'. *Chronicle of Higher Education* 49(8): A16.

Ryant, Carl. 1988. 'Oral History and Business History'. *Journal of American History* 75(2): 560–66.

Samuel, Raphael. 1998. 'Perils of the Transcript'. *Oral History Reader* 1(2): 389–92.

Summerfield, Penny. 2005. 'Oral History as a Research Method'. In *Research Methods for English Studies*, edited by Gabrielle Griffin, 47–66. Edinburgh, UK: Edinburgh University Press.

Thompson, Paul. 2000. *Voice of the Past: Oral History*. Oxford, UK: Oxford University Press.

Thomson, Alistair. 2007. 'Four Paradigm Transformations in Oral History'. *Oral History Review* 34(1): 49–70.

Walkowitz, Daniel J. 1986. 'Corporate History, or Giving History the Business'. In *Presenting the Past: Essays on History and the Public*, edited by Susan Porter Benson and Roy Rosenzweig, 225–36. Philadelphia, PA: Temple University Press.

Welch, Catherine, Rebecca Marschan-Piekkari, Heli Penttinen and Marja Tahvanainen. 2002. 'Corporate Elites as Informants in Qualitative International Business Research'. *International Business Review* 11(5): 611–28.

World Health Organization. 2004. 'Global Health Histories Initiative'. Accessed September 19, 2016. http://www.who.int/global_health_histories/en/.

World Health Organization. 2007. 'WHO's 60 Years and the Global Health Histories Initiative'. *Bulletin of the World Health Organization* 85(4): 254–55.

Yow, Valerie. 1997. '"Do I Like Them Too Much?": Effects of the Oral History Interview on the Interviewer and Vice-Versa'. *Oral History Review* 24(1): 55–79.

Chapter 14

Participation of Corporations in International Organisations

Brandon Barclay Derman

Corporations can exert influence over global health governance (GHG) by participating in the work of a wide range of international organisations (IOs). This includes those dedicated explicitly to health, such as the World Health Organization (WHO), and those whose work is more indirect but nonetheless holds significant implications for GHG like the World Bank (WB). Individual IOs differ markedly, with each representing a complex, multidimensional subject of investigation. This poses significant challenges for policy analysts. IOs are institutions structured by formal rules, but also 'social settings' (Lofland et al. 2005) where informal practices, relationships and 'cultural' factors shape governance practices and the conduct of policy actors within them. Furthermore, they are 'event spaces', where the business of governance occurs, shaped by the interaction of key participants during major meetings (Little 1995).

This complexity poses significant substantive and methodological demands of researchers seeking to understand corporations and GHG. On the one hand, researchers must develop a nuanced understanding of the rules, structures and processes associated with each IO examined. On the other hand, their analyses of corporate influence within those structures and processes must also account for the less formalised practices and fleeting interactions of individual organisational cultures and meetings. A variety of methods and data sources can be deployed for this purpose.

This chapter sets out an analytical framework for researchers, which addresses these challenges, by drawing on different approaches to the study of IOs and their integration. In so doing, it will identify different data sources and methods which researchers might use to undertake comprehensive, critical analyses of the influence corporations can exert through participation in IOs. The chapter discusses studies which employ each method and data source, from the field of GHG and other IO settings. Examples and data sources specific to WHO are given particular focus.

METHODS AND DATA SOURCES FOR TRACKING CORPORATE PARTICIPATION IN IOS

The multidimensional nature of IOs suggests that any one research method or data source can offer only limited understanding of participation by corporations within them. Each available method and associated data type constitutes a different, and necessarily partial, 'window' into the workings of a given organisation, revealing some, but not all, dimensions of corporate participation. Existing sources, such as the official records and publications of IOs, corporate actors and observers, for instance, help the researcher to understand the IO as an institution with formal rules, which participates in the wider aims, relations and processes of governance. Researchers may need to generate their own data, however, through interviews, focus groups, surveys and participant observation to understand crucial aspects of the social settings and events that also constitute IO governance (Van Der Heijden 2006; Mahoney 2008). Many of these methods are discussed elsewhere in this volume. This section discusses benefits and considerations associated with each of these 'windows'. Combining the views they each offer creates potential for more complete analysis of a wide range of research questions. At the same time, such combinations pose epistemological challenges worthy of careful consideration.

Existing sources

Each IO has specific histories, mandates, structures, functions and policies, and it is imperative that researchers first gain familiarity with these particulars in order to identify and characterise corporate actors' participation in them. An obvious starting point is the records of the IO itself, available on-site or, increasingly, online. IOs may maintain a variety of records on the organisation itself, its initiatives and its relationships with other organisations, which are relevant to research on corporate participation. Organisational records can, in particular, provide information on entry points for corporations into the work and proceedings of IOs, which then inform research questions and the design of the researcher's inquiry. These can include the following:

- Lists of participants, members and holders of observer status in governing bodies, meetings and committees
- Lists of members of industry-level lobbying groups

- Briefs, oral testimony and other evidence submitted by corporate representatives as public comment on the organisation's initiatives
- Records of corporate representatives' presence and contributions as technical advisers and expert witnesses, for example to informational meetings, seminars, training events, hearings and other decision-making processes
- Financial records of corporate donations and sponsorship of organisations, subsidiary bodies and supported initiatives

WHO's website, for instance, provides links to numerous sources within these categories, a subset of which is listed in Table 14.1.

As the categories enumerated suggest, the types of data available from organisational records vary widely, from numerical tabulations to lists of individuals and organisations to textual, audio and video documents (e.g. footage of hearings). Importantly, data from organisational records must often be processed before it can be analysed in a manner that will further the researcher's enquiry. This may include standardising quantities, developing categories, cross-referencing or coding the organisation's lists using additional sources (e.g. corporate board memberships), or developing transcripts from recordings. Suitable analytical methods can then vary correspondingly and in conjunction with research questions and paradigms (e.g. Guba and

Table 14.1. Online resources on World Health Organization governance

Resource	*Website address*
Constitution and basic documents	http://www.who.int/about/mission/en/
Portal on governance	http://www.who.int/governance/en/
World Health Assembly Rules of Procedure	http://www.who.int/governance/WHA_Rules_of_Procedure-en.pdf?ua=1
Executive Board Rules of Procedure	http://www.who.int/governance/EB_Rules_of_Procedure-en.pdf?ua=1
Official Records of Governance (resolutions, decisions and annexes; summaries and verbatim records)	http://apps.who.int/gb/or/
Governing Body Documentation (World Health Assembly and Executive Board documents and webcasts)	http://apps.who.int/gb/
Statement and documentation on engagement with non-state actors	http://www.who.int/about/collaborations/non-state-actors/en/
Statement and documentation on partnerships	http://www.who.int/about/collaborations/partnerships/en/
Statement on funding and related portals	http://www.who.int/about/finances-accountability/funding/en/
Application for observer status	http://www.who.int/fctc/cop/ngo_application/en/

Lincoln 1994; Babbie 2015). Participant lists, for instance, can be used to track networks of overlapping or shifting membership (and even influence) among individuals and across organisations. For example, Weishaar, Amos and Collin (2015) used quantitative social network analysis of publicly available comments, submitted during European Union smokefree policy debates, to explain the success of tobacco control advocates in terms of network properties of relatedness and polarisation.

The documents of other organisations can also be useful for understanding a specific IO and corporate participation. Many civil society organisations (CSOs), for example, follow the specific activities of certain IOs, evaluate their performance and produce summaries or reports on their activities that can serve as useful background, as well as provide valuable secondary data. A 2015 statement by CSOs to WHO's World Health Assembly, for instance, summarises the relevance of two items put before the assembly on the issue of corporate influence within WHO (People's Health Movement 2015). Such statements are usually timed to correspond with specific events of internal IO governance, but they can also help researchers identify the framing of longer-standing social and academic concerns within the IO's institutional structures and processes.

The statements of corporate actors and industry associations (e.g. annual reports, marketing campaigns, submissions, press releases) can be useful sources of information on IOs. They can provide valuable insights into the policy positions adopted by corporate actors, their influencing strategy regarding a particular issue or IO and their attempts to frame or set the terms of a particular debate. Clapp and Fuchs (2009) consider the framing deployed in corporations' statements as levers of the considerable 'discursive power' they wield in governance. They highlight the influence corporate lobbying groups exerted over the Rio Earth Summit and Johannesburg World Summit on Sustainable Development, for instance, through discursive tropes that cast voluntary corporate measures as more effective, efficient and 'user friendly' than regulation (see Finger and Kilcoyne 1997; Clapp 2005).

Finally, the existing scholarly and other secondary literature can serve a variety of purposes. As well as providing important background information and essential data, this literature can help identify and locate further records, assess the content of those records in relation to the stated priorities of IOs and corporate actors and identify opportunities and directions for further investigation.

Overall, existing sources offer researchers important orienting information and data as a starting point. The official records and publications of IOs, CSOs and corporate actors are particularly valuable for understanding the formal institutional dimensions of corporate participation in IOs. As researchers explore the less formal, and often more difficult to observe, social dimension of IOs, or track the involvement of corporate actors over time (including real time), existing sources are likely to need supplementing with data collected using other methods.

Interviews

Interviews allow the researcher to access participants' views and experiences of governance, which may help to clarify, or contrast with, information found in institutionally sanctioned sources. Moreover, through interviews the researcher can approach issues left unaddressed in available organisational records or the existing scholarly literature (Rubin and Rubin 2005; Seidman 2013). Sandberg, Andresen and Bjune (2010) use interview data to study interests in the formation of the Global Alliance for Vaccines and Immunization (GAVI), a public–private partnership involving the Gates Foundation, WHO, United Nations Children's Fund, WB, national governments, civil society, industry and research groups. The authors conduct interviews with key actors to explain the construction of GAVI, which, they argue, 'ushered in a new era of global health institutions' (Sandberg, Andresen and Bjune 2010, 1355), by reinvigorating the work of older IOs, while enrolling private sector partners in programmatically influential capacities.

More generally, interview data can complement existing sources in at least two important ways. First, through interviews, observers and participants in IOs can explicate 'unwritten rules', common practices and other aspects of organisational culture, which are seldom detailed or even mentioned in official publications but are nonetheless highly consequential (Mahoney 2008). Second, key informants may provide nuanced, or critical, analyses of organisational proceedings, which are largely absent from official accounts. While individuals external to an IO, such as civil society representatives, are more likely to offer such critiques, guarantees of confidentiality or anonymity to 'insiders' can create opportunities to capture departures from official accounts.

The individual characteristics of interviewees are relevant to the data they are likely to provide. On the one hand, researchers may seek out individuals with longer experience of an IO as more likely to provide useful insights into changes over time. On the other hand, long-serving officials may be so deeply embedded within the culture of an IO that they may be less able to be reflexive about organisational issues. Interviews with differently positioned individuals are likely to allow multiple and distinct views on a given topic to emerge. Such distinctions can illuminate contrasting interests, and levels of power within the organisation, which are important aspects of governance arrangements. Moreover, some individuals move between different roles within an IO setting, adding to their knowledge and social networks. Interviews with such individuals can help the researcher understand the social world of the IO as composed of specific roles and relationships.

Focus groups – which are effectively surveys conducted through interviews with multiple respondents simultaneously – give researchers the opportunity to learn from a larger number of participants and their interactions. Focus groups provide an opportunity for participants to voice their views interactively with each other (Morgan 1998; Berg and Lune 2014, chapter 5). Participants can thus build on the responses of others, potentially generating richer data than if individuals were interviewed separately. Importantly, however, researchers must remain wary of biases and vested interest–informing statements by participants. Focus groups may also not be representative of the larger population, which the researcher may be interested in studying.

The fact that the experiences and affiliations, of interview and focus group participants, affect the data generated underscores the importance of sampling. A variety of approaches exist to sampling in general and interviewee selection in particular (Rubin and Rubin 2005; Babbie 2015). In interviews with actors concerned with global climate governance, Derman (2014, 2015) employed two types of sampling methods. Conversations with actors in different institutional roles (purposive sampling) helped to clarify organisational relationships and provide a rounded picture of events. Drawing on interviewees' networks to identify subsequent respondents (snowball sampling) then helped to fill specific gaps in understanding and facilitate contact with highly placed, and highly knowledgeable but less visible, respondents.

The value of the data collected will depend, in part, on the researcher's skill, knowledge, positionality vis-à-vis interviewees, social setting and practice of interviewing itself. A specific pitfall of research on IOs is the propensity of many participants to deliver the 'party line' associated with their role in governance. The researcher must remain aware of this tendency, working to recognise and, when possible, discourage it. Assurances of anonymity, demonstrable familiarity with nuances of organisational culture and professional or personal rapport may help.

Deriving research findings from interviews and focus groups requires rigorous data preparation and analytical practices (Cope 2003; Charmaz 2004; Rubin and Rubin 2005; Richards 2009). Audio recordings are typically made, whenever possible, along with notes jotted down in the course of the conversation. Recordings (or key segments thereof) can then be transcribed. Two orientations to analysing notes and transcripts present themselves. In the first, researchers can take an 'etic' or deductive approach to textual data, seeking to understand them from a set of pre-defined concepts derived from the literature and/or research questions. In the second, the salient concepts and relations are derived from the statements of respondents themselves (an 'emic', or inductive, approach) (Cook and Crang 1995). In either case, the primary means of summarising data involves coding wherein the researcher selects and tags sections of the text, using a finite set of labels or 'codes'. Coding allows the researcher to track key concepts and themes across the full set of transcripts (and other textual materials). In this way, contextual knowledge and experiences of carefully chosen respondents can be mobilised, to understand dimensions of GHG in IO settings that go unaddressed or under-addressed by more widely available, existing sources. The use of interviews as a method for studying corporations and global health is discussed in more detail in Chapter 12 in this volume.

Surveys

Survey methods enable researchers to produce their own data, hear directly from GHG actors and address questions that may be difficult or impossible to answer through existing sources alone. Survey data differ, though, in important ways from those produced by interviews. Surveys tend towards larger sample sizes and more traditional sampling designs, that is those which strive for wide representation rather than elucidation (Babbie 2015). Accordingly, survey data facilitate the robust generalisation, comparison and ready summary offered by quantitative analysis. A good example is a survey conducted by Cetindamar and Husoy (2007) among corporate participants in the UN Global Compact to understand why they adopt environmentally responsible behaviour.

Once again, opportunities and compromises attend each method. On the one hand, the quantitative summaries enabled by survey methods travel easily, retaining greater currency in policy circles, for instance, than interpretive results from qualitative analysis. On the other hand, because surveys usually include few open-ended questions and elicit shorter responses, the latter are more often framed in researchers' (rather than participants') terms. Survey findings are commonly more etic and deductive, therefore capturing details of pattern more readily than those of process or explanation.

(Participant) Observation

A researcher may generate unique data on corporate involvement in the governance activities of IOs as a direct observer or even participant. Observational data is particularly useful for capturing the interactional dimension of governance during meetings and larger gatherings (Little 1995). As an observer, the researcher can identify and observe key actors, processes, practices and relationships which emerge in real time. The researcher can also document the facets of corporate and industry representatives' participation within, and immediately outside, the spaces of IO formal proceedings that leave little or no impression in official records. This might take place in the corridors outside of meetings and at parallel events (e.g. briefings, fairs, displays, fringe meetings). Researchers can observe, for example, informal interactions, such as who is speaking to whom, the content of displays, pamphlets and gifts for attendees, unpublicised gatherings, routine interactions and offsite events. In this way, observational data and methods offer a distinct window on the participation of corporate actors in the activities of IOs.

Observation can complement the methods and data sources discussed earlier. At exploratory stages of a study, observation can help the investigator hone research questions and design; generate specific prompts for interviews, focus groups and surveys; and identify relevant respondents or documents. Later, the researcher's presence allows comparative accounts of events from interviews, focus groups and official sources, alongside his or her own impressions. Finally, 'being there' affords unique opportunities to conduct informal interviews and convene focus groups with rarely assembled collections of participants in GHG.

Generating usable data from observation requires the researcher's physical presence and therefore securing access. A researcher's access to an IO's proceedings may require accreditation, membership in an observer or participant organisation or some other status or affiliation. Data quality also depends on the disciplined practice of faithfully recording experiences and reflections before they fade from memory (Lofland et al. 2005). The assiduous practice of writing field notes (see Emerson, Fretz and Shaw 2011) is therefore essential, along with whatever audio, photographic and/or video documentation can be captured in the course of events. Analysing notes and transcripts typically entails repeated review, thematic 'memo-ing' (Emerson, Fretz and Shaw 2011) and coding methods as described earlier. There are also ethical considerations about data collection without subject consent, which need to be considered beforehand (see Chapter 21).

Many aspects of observation in IOs, in this sense, are common to ethnographic research (see Chapter 14; Herbert 2000). However, the multiple, simultaneous processes and distinct spaces of large international events can pose special challenges, especially to the solo researcher who can attend to only one setting at a time. Collaborative approaches to 'event ethnography' offer a means of resolving this dilemma, albeit at the cost of additional coordination (see e.g. Brosius et al. 2010; Campbell et al. 2014).

Merry's study of the construction of women's rights through the UN Convention on the Eradication of Discrimination Against Women (CEDAW, see Merry 2006) offers an example of research in an IO (and beyond), combining extensive participant observation with documentary and interview methods. Merry's presence at UN negotiations enabled her to demonstrate how institutional culture and practice shaped the meanings of women's empowerment under CEDAW, with implications for practice around the globe. As mentioned earlier, participant observation is widely used in the discipline of anthropology as part of an ethnographic research methodology, which is discussed at greater length in Chapters 7 and 12 of this volume, respectively.

Analysing and combining multiple data sources and methods

Multiple data sources and methods are likely to be required in the study of corporations and their participation in IOs, including GHG arrangements. This is because IOs are complex empirical subjects. Each category of data and method discussed earlier offers a distinct, and inherently limited, perspective on the nature of organisations and their relationships with corporate actors. Combining different methods, and types of data, holds the greatest promise for understanding organisations and the ways in which they produce GHG.

However, the mixing of methods also demands considerable care, since the validity of any study depends on the methodological correspondence between research practices (or methods) and specific philosophical commitments about the construction and character of knowledge (see Elwood 2009). Official sources and most surveys, for instance, mobilise established theoretical categories and discourses of governance, while the validity of quantitative survey results depends on the comparability of individuals within respondent groups. By contrast, qualitative interviewing and participant observation often valorise the unique insights of particularly placed individuals and facilitate the inductive discovery of meaningful concepts and relations. Thus, while combined approaches can support rigorous and critical findings, researchers must develop suitable research methods for answering specific research questions and ensure that the combination of different approaches in multi-method results is consistent and coherent.

CONCLUSION

Despite the significant, and possibly increasing, participation of corporate actors in GHG through their participation in IOs, this subject remains under-analysed. Studying the involvement of corporations in IOs relevant to GHG poses methodological challenges. Nevertheless, there are opportunities to draw on multiple data sources and methods to document, and more fully analyse, this key means of corporate influence. Further research will improve understanding of the formal and informal ways in which corporations can influence the very institutions that create and maintain GHG. Case studies of specific institutional arrangements, for instance, can tell us about the means by which particular corporate actors have, and could continue, to shape GHG through particular IOs. Comparative and longitudinal analyses, in turn, can illuminate the extent to which corporations exert such influence over time. Findings would demonstrate that institutional design matters – in an era of proliferating global governance, corporate power and health inequality – for structuring and mediating corporate influence.

FURTHER READING

Campbell, Lisa M., Catherine Corson, Noella J. Gray, Kenneth I. MacDonald and J. Peter Brosius. 2014. 'Studying Global Environmental Meetings to Understand Global Environmental Governance: Collaborative Event Ethnography at the Tenth Conference of the Parties to the Convention on Biological Diversity'. *Global Environmental Politics* 14(3): 1–20.

Clapp, Jennifer and Doris A. Fuchs. 2009. *Corporate Power in Global Agrifood Governance*. Cambridge, MA: MIT Press.

Sandberg, Kristin Ingstad, Steinar Andresen and Gunnar Bjune. 2010. 'A New Approach to Global Health Institutions? A Case Study of New Vaccine Introduction and the Formation of the GAVI Alliance'. *Social Science & Medicine* 71(7): 1349–56.

REFERENCES

Babbie, Earl. 2015. *The Practice of Social Research*. Canada: Cengage Learning.

Berg, Bruce Lawrence and Howard Lune. 2014. *Qualitative Research Methods for the Social Sciences*. Essex, UK: Pearson Education.

Brosius, J. Peter, Lisa M. Campbell and others. 2010. 'Collaborative Event Ethnography: Conservation and Development Trade-Offs at the Fourth World Conservation Congress'. *Conservation and Society* 8(4): 245–55.

Campbell, Lisa M., Catherine Corson, Noella J. Gray, Kenneth I. MacDonald and J. Peter Brosius. 2014. 'Studying Global Environmental Meetings to Understand Global Environmental Governance: Collaborative Event Ethnography at the Tenth Conference of the Parties to the Convention on Biological Diversity'. *Global Environmental Politics* 14(3): 1–20.

Cetindamar, Dilek and Kristoffer Husoy. 2007. 'Corporate Social Responsibility Practices and Environmentally Responsible Behaviour: The Case of the United Nations Global Compact'. *Journal of Business Ethics* 76(2): 163–76.

Charmaz, Kathy. 2004. 'Grounded Theory'. In *Approaches to Qualitative Research: A Reader on Theory and Practice*, edited by Sharlene Nagy Hesse-Biber and Patricia Leavy. Oxford, UK: Oxford University Press.

Clapp, Jennifer. 2005. 'Global Environmental Governance for Corporate Responsibility and Accountability'. *Global Environmental Politics* 5(3): 23–34.
Clapp, Jennifer and Doris A. Fuchs. 2009. *Corporate Power in Global Agrifood Governance*. Cambridge, MA: MIT Press.
Cook, Ian and Mike Crang. 1995. *Doing Ethnographies*. Norwich, UK: Geobooks.
Cope, Megan. 2003. 'Coding Transcripts and Diaries'. In *Key Methods in Geography*, edited by Nicholas Clifford, Shaun French and Gill Valentine, 445–59. Thousand Oaks, CA: Sage.
Derman, Brandon. 2014. 'Climate Governance, Justice, and Transnational Civil Society'. *Climate Policy* 14(1): 23–41.
Derman, Brandon. 2015. 'Making Climate Justice: Social Natures and Political Spaces of the Anthropocene'. Unpublished Dissertation, University of Washington.
Elwood, Sarah. 2009. 'Mixed Methods: Thinking, Doing, and Asking in Multiple Ways'. In *The SAGE Handbook of Qualitative Geography*, edited by Dyda DeLyser, Steve Herbert, Stuart Aitken, Mike Crang and Linda McDowell, 94–114. London: Sage.
Emerson, Robert M., Rachel Fretz and Linda Shaw. 2011. *Writing Ethnographic Fieldnotes*, 2nd edition. Chicago, IL: University of Chicago Press.
Finger, Matthias and James Kilcoyne. 1997. 'Why Transnational Corporations Are Organizing to Save the Global Environment'. *Ecologist* 27(4): 138–42.
Guba, Egon G. and Yvonna S. Lincoln. 1994. 'Competing Paradigms in Qualitative Research'. In *Handbook of Qualitative Research*, edited by Norman K. Denzin and Yvonna S. Lincoln, 105–88. Thousand Oaks, CA: Sage.
Herbert, Steve. 2000. 'For Ethnography'. *Progress in Human Geography* 24(4): 550–68.
Little, Paul E. 1995. 'Ritual, Power and Ethnography at the Rio Earth Summit'. *Critique of Anthropology* 15(3): 265–88.
Lofland, John, David A. Snow, Leon Anderson and Lyn H. Lofland. 2005. *Analyzing Social Settings: A Guide to Qualitative Observation and Analysis*, 4th edition. Belmont, CA: Wadsworth Publishing.
Mahoney, Christine. 2008. *Brussels versus the Beltway: Advocacy in the United States and the European Union*. Washington, DC: Georgetown University Press.
Merry, Sally Engle. 2006. *Human Rights and Gender Violence: Translating International Law into Local Justice*. Chicago, IL: University of Chicago Press.
Morgan, David L. 1998. *The Focus Group Guidebook*. Thousand Oaks, CA: Sage.
People's Health Movement. 2015. 'Civil Society Organisations Call for Delegates to World Health Assembly to Defend the Integrity and Independence of the WHO'. 18 May. http://www.phmovement.org/en/node/9980.
Richards, Lyn. 2009. *Handling Qualitative Data: A Practical Guide*. Thousand Oaks, CA: Sage.
Rubin, Herbert J. and Irene Rubin. 2005. *Qualitative Interviewing: The Art of Hearing Data*. Thousand Oaks, CA: Sage.
Sandberg, Kristin Ingstad, Steinar Andresen and Gunnar Bjune. 2010. 'A New Approach to Global Health Institutions? A Case Study of New Vaccine Introduction and the Formation of the GAVI Alliance'. *Social Science & Medicine* 71(7): 1349–56.

Seidman, Irving. 2013. *Interviewing as Qualitative Research: A Guide for Researchers in Education and the Social Sciences*, 4th edition. New York: Teachers College Press.

Van Der Heijden, Hein-Anton. 2006. 'Globalization, Environmental Movements, and International Political Opportunity Structures'. *Organization & Environment* 19(1): 28–45.

Weishlaar, Heide, Amanda Amos and Jeff Collin. 2015. 'Best of Enemies: Using Social Network Analysis to Explore a Policy Network in European Smoke-Free Policy'. *Social Science & Medicine* 133: 85–92.

Chapter 15

Studying the Influence of Corporations on Democratic Processes

William H. Wiist

Corporations seek to influence governments to lower their costs, expand markets, gain competitive advantage or obtain subsidies. The ability of corporations to systemically dominate government and the policy agenda is termed *corporate capture* (Mindel et al. 2012) and *legal corruption* (Kaufmann and Vicente 2011), which results in policies that favour corporate over public interests. Given the significant impact of corporations on health (Wiist 2010), their ability to influence democratic processes is of concern to research on global health governance (GHG).

This chapter introduces public health researchers to a range of online data sources to study how corporations influence health laws, policies and regulations, provides examples of existing scholarship on corporate influence on democratic processes and identifies potential areas for further research. Given the volume of information available about the extent and scope of corporate-influencing activities in the United States resulting from federal and state laws and court rulings, this chapter focuses on the United States as a case study of how to study corporate influence on democracy. However, the approach described here, research questions proposed and types of data sources identified are applicable to other contexts.

RESEARCH ON CORPORATE INFLUENCE ON DEMOCRACY

Social scientists have developed theoretical approaches and empirical methods to study corporate influence on democratic processes, which could be usefully applied to GHG research (Stratman 2005; Ciepley 2013). The following are selected examples of research about the four principal methods corporations use to influence democratic processes and from which corporations benefit (Alexander, Mazza and Scholz 2009; Hill and Painter 2011; Akey 2015).

Corporation donations to political campaigns

During the 2014 US congressional election, more than 75% of the US$266 million contributed by the top 50 campaign donors came from corporations or business groups (Zubak-Skees and Whyte 2015). The money raised and spent during the 2012 state legislative elections totalled more than US$1 billion, and the gubernatorial and lower state-wide elections exceeded US$300 million (Nichols and McChesney 2013, 53). Corporations vary as to which political party they donate to (Gimpel, Lee and Parrott 2014). About one-third of congressional roll-call votes reflect the campaign contributions to members (Roscoe and Jenkins 2005), but the effect can occur earlier in the legislative process (Powell 2014).

Research suggests that corporate donations can influence the behaviour of government officials. More than 90% of the judicial business in the United States is conducted by state courts, in which 89% of judges are elected. The more contributions judges receive from business, the more likely they are to rule in favour of business interests (Shepherd 2013). Congressional members who rely most on donations from business Political Action Committees (PACs) for their campaigns are more likely to support pro-business spending programmes (Fellowes and Wolf 2004). PACs are more likely to donate to members of committees with industry-relevant policy expertise who are on committees with jurisdiction relevant to their industry (Bonica 2013).

The more campaign contributions Congress members receive from the tobacco industry, the more likely they are to vote pro-tobacco on related bills (Luke and Krauss 2004). Corporate contributions also reduce citations for corporate health and safety violations from the Occupational Safety and Health Administration (Witko 2013). Environmental groups' PAC donations promote members of Congress to advocate for an environmental issue (Riddel 2003). Neurobiological and psychological research shows that favours (e.g. corporate contributions to medical research) from others influence a recipient's decisions, outside of his or her own awareness, to act favourably towards the donor ('influence reciprocity') (Friedlander 2007).

Corporate influence through lobbying

In 2014, US$2.2 billion was spent on lobbying Congress and government agencies by 11,781 registered and active lobbyists (Center for Responsive Politics 2015). The US Chamber of Commerce, a corporate membership group, spent US$124 million on lobbying in 2014, more than any other association (Center for Responsive Politics n.d.a). The pharmaceutical and health products industry spent US$229 million on lobbying, more than any other industry sector (Center for Responsive Politics n.d.b). In some instances, lobbying provided a 20,000% return on expenditure (Alexander, Mazza and Scholz 2009).

Lobbyists meet with congressional members and committee staff and members of the executive branch, provide testimony during hearings, may write bills for legislators, may help select legislators' staff (Chang 2013; Palmer and Sherman 2014) and serve on advisory boards (Davis 2014). They lobby the staff of government agencies that recognise that politicians and appointees, to whom they are responsible, may favour certain corporations and that unfavourable agency decisions can incur strong congressional opposition, including budgetary threats.

Most lobbying is done by a few highly connected lobbyists whose influence depends on their prior experience as a congressional staff member (LaPira and Thomas 2014). The largest numbers of revolving door lobbyists are former congressional staff, but when their former employer exits Congress, they lose income and leave lobbying (Vidal, Draca and Fons-Rosen 2012).

Tobacco industry lobbying influences state legislatures and marketing regulations (Givel and Glantz 2001; Savell et al. 2014), and wields its political power globally (Holden and Lee 2009). Lobbying influences health care expenditures and policy (Landers and Sehgal 2004), alcohol problems (McCambridge, Hawkins and Holden 2014) and environmental policy (Johal and Ulph 2002).

The 'revolving door' between business and government

After the 2014 congressional election, 75 members either left or were defeated. Of the 42 who found new employment, 45% (n = 19) went to work for lobbying firms and 19% (n = 8) for their lobbying clients (Center for Responsive Politics n.d.c). About half of former senators and state governors serve on corporate boards after leaving office for which they are highly compensated (Palmer and Schneer 2015, Table 1), a prospect that may unduly influence their actions while in office (Drutman and Fornas 2014).

This revolving door also rotates in the other direction. Key US congressional committees, where policy is written, are predominantly staffed by former lobbyists (Bryner 2011). The perceived value of having insiders in key governmental positions leads corporations to pay bonuses to senior executives who enter government (Fang 2013).

The conflicts of interest created by political appointees to positions in the US Department of Defense, for example, have abnormally favourable effects on the appointee's former corporate employer's stock prices, profits and government contract procurement (Luechinger and Moser 2014); have corrupting effects; and divert public resources (Brezis 2014). Agencies often provide corporations with favourable regulation to obtain political support in Congress, and for employment after leaving government (Livermore and Revesz 2013).

A search of the health literature found no empirical studies of the revolving door. However, examples are numerous (Jasso-Aguilar and Waitzkin 2011), including officials of the US Centers for Disease Control and Prevention (Cragle and Keller 2014), the National Institutes of Health (Herper 2010), the Office of the US Trade Representative (Lee 2013), Medicare and Medicaid Services (Potter 2015), the Department of Agriculture (Brasher 2015), the Environmental Protection Agency (Harkinson 2009) and the Food and Drug Administration (Carome 2014).

Corporations and tax avoidance

Some corporations pay no income tax (MacIntyre, Gardner and Phillips 2014), pay less than the statutory rate or receive a refund cheque (US Government Accountability Office 2013a), resulting in US$2.8 billion lost to government health functions alone (US Government Accountability Office 2013b). Profit shifting costs US$10–$90 billion annually (Gravelle 2013). Tax avoidance limits governments' ability to fulfil their obligations to provide food, water and shelter; alleviate poverty (Lipsett 2013); and provide programmes and institutions for economic, social, cultural and political rights (Organisation for Economic Co-operation and Development 2013), and it gives corporations a free ride on public services paid for by others, along with after-tax profits that can be translated into increased political and economic power (Tax Justice Network 2015). Government subsidies to corporations ('corporate welfare') can have effects similar to tax avoidance and warrant further research (Farnsworth 2013).

There appears to be no empirical health research examining the effects of corporate tax avoidance on health status, public health infrastructure, programmes, research or monitoring and enforcement of health regulations.

DATA SOURCES FOR STUDYING CORPORATE INFLUENCE ON DEMOCRACY

There are a variety of US data sources (Table 15.1) for researchers to study corporate influence on democracy and that illustrate the possibilities for research in other countries (Ohman 2012). When such data is not available,

Table 15.1. Resources for studying the influence of corporations on democratic processes

World Wide Web information resources	*Election campaign donations*	*Lobbying*	*Revolving door*	*Tax avoidance*	*Type of information available*
Center for Responsive Politics	*	*	*		Data and reports
Sunlight Foundation	*	*	*		Reports
Center for Political Accountability		*			Reports
Political MoneyLine	*	*	*		Reports
National Institute on Money in State Politics	*				Data
Transparency International	*				Reports
Campaign Finance Center	*				Data and reports
MapLight			*		Social networks
TheyRule.net			*		Social networks
Powerbase			*		Social networks
Little Sis			*		Social networks
NNDB Mapper			*		Social networks
Influence Explorer			*		Social networks
Integrity in Science Database			*		Social networks
Revolving Door Watch			*		Data
Institute on Taxation and Economic Policy				*	Data and reports
Citizens for Tax Justice				*	Reports
Tax Justice Network				*	Reports
Center for Research on Multinational Corporations				*	Reports

(Continued)

Table 15.1. Continued

World Wide Web information resources	*Election campaign donations*	*Lobbying*	*Revolving door*	*Tax avoidance*	*Type of information available*
CrocTail				*	Reports
Tax Justice Corporate Tax Explorer				*	Data
Center for Effective Government				*	Reports
Good Jobs First Subsidy Tracker				*	Data
Federal Elections Commission	*				Data
Internal Revenue Service	*			*	Data
Securities and Exchange Commission				*	Data
Office of the Clerk of the US House of Representatives		*			Data
US Senate Office of Public Records		*			Data

Note: 'Reports' for all sources indicate availability of tabulated data and/or reports with data. 'Data' indicates availability of data for analysis.

researchers may need to advocate for laws requiring transparency and reporting, or use other methods to collect data about corporate influence (Mialon, Swinburn and Sacks 2015).

Data sources on election campaign donations

US election campaign finance laws require that information be available from the Federal Election Commission (FEC) about individual contributions to candidates, parties and PACs. Internal Revenue Service (IRS) tax regulations also make campaign contribution information available for some tax-exempt organisations. Some FEC and IRS information about contributions and expenditures can be obtained from various organisations (Table 15.1), including groups such as ProPublica, the World Economic Forum's Survey of Global Competitiveness Report and the International Institute for Democracy and Electoral Assistance.

Data sources on lobbying

US lobbyists are required by law to register and to report quarterly on who their clients are, the issues on which they lobby and their political contributions (US Senate 1995; Office of the Clerk, U.S. House of Representatives 2013; Federal Election Commission 2015), but there are also many unregistered lobbyists (Auble 2014; LaPira 2014). Lobbying information is available at the Lobbying Disclosure web page of the Office of the Clerk of the U.S. House of Representatives, and the US Senate's Office of Public Records. Organisations such as the Center for Responsive Politics and LobbyWatch publish reports from that data, including lobbyists' profiles. Some researchers make their data about lobbying available for free (Drutman and Furnas 2014). Data and reports are also available from fee-based services such as Quorum Analytics, CQ Roll Call, Popvox, FiscalNote, Lobbydata.com and Ipsos.

Data sources about the revolving door

The developments in social network analysis (Sandström and Carlsson 2008; Christakis and Fowler 2009), including free programmes on social network analysis websites (see Table 15.1) and reports (e.g. SourceWatch), have facilitated research on individuals' connections to and movements between corporations, government agencies, academia, foundations and elected office. The Revolving Door Index, a measure of the concentration of revolving door regulators in a business sector, can also be useful (Brezis 2014).

Information from business publications, corporate websites and required reports from corporations to the Securities and Exchange Commission (SEC) can be useful in identifying corporate officials. Political appointments to government agencies may be available from the agency (e.g. Department of Defense), *The Plum Book* from the U.S. Government Publishing Office, Congress.Gov (until recently known as THOMAS) or TheyRule.net. PowerBase can be used to monitor networks (Miller and Ahmad 2010). The US Office of Government Ethics specifies public reports that senior officials in the executive, legislative and judicial branches must file about their finances and interests outside the government. Some federal agencies require public reporting by employees and advisory committee members (e.g. rosters are public information).

Data sources on tax avoidance

Some corporate tax information is available in corporate reports to the IRS (e.g. based on Forms 1120 and M3) and to the SEC (e.g. 10-K reports and exhibits). Some organisations (see Table 15.1) publish reports based on IRS and SEC data. The Organisation for Economic Co-operation and Development (OECD) makes available national tax receipt data (and a list of tax havens). The OECD iLibrary ORBIS database has corporate financial and ownership information. The International Center for Tax and Development's Government Revenue Dataset, World Bank and International Monetary Fund also make tax receipt data available. Information from sources such as the International Consortium of Investigative Journalists (e.g. Panama Papers) and WikiLeaks may also be relevant.

Sources of information about congressional activities

Although legislators' votes on bills are often a measured outcome of research, other actions taken in committee, caucus membership, funds budgeted for specific programmes and so on can also be important. Congress.Gov and websites of the House of Representatives and the Senate are the primary sources of information about legislation, members, committees, calendars, votes, caucuses, nomination hearings, bills and the Congressional Record. Budget information is published by the Office of Management and Budget.

Other sources of information about government activities include LexisNexis (e.g. testimony given before Congress), govtrack.us, Sunlight Foundation's Open Congress website, Measuring American Legislatures (roll-call estimates of state legislators' ideological positions) and Inter-University

Consortium for Political and Social Research (researchers' data). Ballotpedia and Github are user-driven resources about Congress. Many political scientists use a spatial model of congressional and parliamentary roll-call votes, decisions and ideology named DW-Nominate (Poole and Rosenthal 2007); data is available at voteview.com. Some organisations (e.g. American Public Health Association) publish tallies of congressional votes on key issues. Fee-based subscription services (e.g. Legistorm, CQPress and Lobbyists.info) provide databases and reports about Congress. Information in the World Bank's Database of Political Institutions is also relevant.

Limitations of data sources

The complexity and intricacy of the legislative process makes drawing causal inferences difficult. Not all actions of legislators are recorded or reported, nor is all information about campaign donations or lobbying activity. It is also difficult to separate the influence of campaign donations from that of lobbying. Information about the revolving door may require combining information from several sources. Access to corporate tax information is limited because its tax filing documents are usually not made public. Social network analysis software can be expensive, and the validity of the underlying statistical methods of some programmes is questionable. The size, terminology and complexity of some government websites, reports and databases make analysis challenging. An alternative to using existing data, conducting primary data collection, is expensive and time consuming.

CONCLUSIONS

Theories, methods and data resources used to study the corporate influence on democracy can be applied to understand corporations and GHG. Despite some of the limitations of these data sources, the topics open to global health research about corporate influence on democracy are vast because the laws and policies established by elected officials are the paramount determinants of corporate actions that affect a society's health and welfare. The extent of that influence holds true at the national, regional and global levels of public policy making.

Thus, the major focus of future GHG research should be on corporate influence through financial contributions to political campaigns. Longitudinal studies are needed about donations from specific health-related industries (e.g. pharmaceuticals) to members of legislative bodies with oversight of relevant health issues. Studies are also needed on corporate donations influencing judicial appointments, dispute settlement bodies and the patterns of their rulings on health issues.

Social network research is needed about the conflicts of interest posed by individuals from corporations appointed to government positions as employees or volunteers who make recommendations on health research proposals, contracts and medical devices and drugs. This type of research can usefully include interviews with agency employees, former employees and whistle-blowers. Longitudinal research is needed to compare health industrial sectors' (e.g. pharmaceutical) income tax and other taxes with government budgets for related health regulatory agencies, and health services, programmes and research. Similar research is needed about government subsidies to corporations whose products and services affect health. Research to evaluate the effectiveness of law, policy, regulations and advocacy interventions is also needed.

The types of research described in this chapter are needed at many different jurisdictional levels (i.e. state, county and city), and within and across different countries, particularly those such as member-states of the European Union that have transparency and reporting regulations about lobbying, election campaign donations and the revolving door (Greenwood and Dreger 2013). Some research (e.g. revolving door, lobbying) is also relevant to studying corporate influence on multilateral institutions such as the World Health Organization, World Bank, International Monetary Fund and the World Trade Organization.

Finally, global health researchers need to effectively and expeditiously convey their research results to support advocacy by practitioners, not-for-profit organisations and public interest groups. Despite the limitations of existing data sources, and the novelty of this type of research to public health researchers, a deeper understanding of the systemic influence of corporations on democracy is critically important to building effective forms of GHG to limit corporations' influence that threatens human and planetary health.

FURTHER READING

Gilens, Martin. 2012. *Affluence & Influence: Economic Inequality and Political Power in America*. New York: Russell Sage Foundation.

Sklair, Leslie. 2001. *The Transnational Capitalist Class*. Malden, MA: Blackwell Publishing.

Wilks, Stephen. 2013. *The Political Power of the Business Corporation*. Cheltenham, UK: Edward Elgar.

REFERENCES

Alexander, Raquel, Stephen W. Mazza and Susan Scholz. 2009. 'Measuring Rates of Return on Lobbying Expenditures: An Empirical Case Study of Tax Breaks for Multinational Corporations'. *Journal of Law & Politics* 25(4): 401–57.

Akey, Pat. 2015. 'Valuing Changes in Political Networks: Evidence from Campaign Contributions to Close Congressional Elections'. *Review of Financial Studies* 28(11): 3188–223.

Auble, Dan. 2014. 'Waning Influence? Part 1: Tracking the "Unlobbyist"'. Washington, DC: Centre for Responsive Politics. http://www.opensecrets.org/news/2014/03/waning-influence-part-1-tracking-the-unlobbyist/.

Bonica, Adam. 2013. 'Ideology and Interests in the Political Marketplace'. *American Journal of Political Science* 57(2): 294–311.

Brasher, Philip. 2015. 'Lobbyist Picked to Lead Senate Ag Committee as It Rewrites Nutrition Programs'. *Agri-Pulse*, 9 January. http://www.agri-pulse.com/Pepsico-lobbyist-to-lead-Senate-Agriculture-staff-01092015.asp.

Brezis, Elise S. 2014. 'The Revolving Door Indicator: Estimating the Distortionary Power of the Revolving Door'. U4 Brief No. 10. Clermont-Ferrand, France: Foundation for Research and Studies on International Development. http://www.u4.no/publications/the-revolving-door-indicator-estimating-the-distortionary-power-of-the-revolving-door/.

Bryner, Sarah McKinnon. 2011. 'From Hired Guns to Hired Hands: "Reverse Revolvers" in the 111th and 112th Congresses'. Washington, DC: Center for Responsive Politics.

Carome, Michael. 2014. 'Outrage of the Month: Revolving Door at FDA Undermines Public Confidence'. Public Citizen, May. http://www.citizen.org/Page.aspx?pid=6298.

Center for Responsive Politics. 2015. 'Lobbying Database: Total Lobbying Spending and Number of Lobbyists'. Accessed September 19, 2016. http://www.opensecrets.org/lobby/.

Center for Responsive Politics. n.d.a. 'Top Industries 2014'. Accessed September 19, 2016. http://www.opensecrets.org/lobby/top.php?indexType=i&showYear=2014.

Center for Responsive Politics. n.d.b. 'Top Spenders 2014'. Accessed September 19, 2016. http://www.opensecrets.org/lobby/top.php?indexType=s&showYear=2014.

Center for Responsive Politics. n.d.c. 'Revolving Door: Former Members of the 113th Congress'. Accessed September 19, 2016. https://www.opensecrets.org/revolving/departing.php?cong=113.

Chang, Ailsa. 2013. 'When Lobbyists Literally Write the Bill'. National Public Radio, 11 November. http://www.npr.org/blogs/itsallpolitics/2013/11/11/243973620/when-lobbyists-literally-write-the-bill?sc=tw&cc=share.

Christakis, Nicholas A. and James H. Fowler. 2009. 'Social Network Visualization in Epidemiology'. *Norsk Epidemiologi* 19(1): 5–16.

Ciepley, David. 2013. 'Beyond Public and Private: Toward a Political Theory of the Corporation'. *American Political Science Review* 107(1): 139–58.

Cragle, Steven and Lainie Keller. 2014. 'Merck Announces Appointment of Dr. Julie Gerberding as Executive Vice President for Strategic Communications, Global Public Policy and Population Health'. Kenilworth, NJ: Merck Sharp & Dohme. http://www.mercknewsroom.com/news-release/corporate-news/merck-announces-appointment-dr-julie-gerberding-executive-vice-president.

Davis, Julie Hirschfeld. 2014. 'Obama Administration Loosens Ban on Lobbyists in Government'. *The New York Times*, 12 August. http://www.nytimes.com/.

Drutman, Lee and Alexander Furnas. 2014. 'K Street Pays Top Dollar for Revolving Door Talent'. Accessed September 19, 2016. https://sunlightfoundation.com/blog/2014/01/21/revolving-door-lobbyists-government-experience/.

Fang, Lee. 2013. 'The Reverse Revolving Door: How Corporate Insiders Are Rewarded Upon Leaving Firms for Congress'. *The Nation*, 4 May. http://www.thenation.com/article/reverse-revolving-door-how-corporate-insiders-are-rewarded-upon-leaving-firms-congres/.

Farnsworth, Kevin. 2013. 'Bringing Corporate Welfare'. *Journal of Social Policy* 42(1): 1–22.

Federal Election Commission. 2015. 'Honest Leadership and Open Government Act of 2007'. Accessed September 19, 2016. http://www.fec.gov/law/feca/s1legislation.pdf.

Fellowes, Matthew C. and Patrick J. Wolf. 2004. 'Funding Mechanisms and Policy Instruments: How Business Campaign Contributions Influence Congressional Votes'. *Political Research Quarterly* 57(2): 315–24.

Friedlander, Michael. 2007. 'Scientific Background and Introduction of Speakers'. Paper presented at the Scientific Basis of Influence and Reciprocity: A Symposium, Association of American Medical Colleges and Baylor College of Medicine, Department of Neuroscience and Computational Psychiatry Unit, Washington, DC, 12 June.

Gimpel, James G., Frances E. Lee and Michael Parrott. 2014. 'Business Interests and the Party Coalitions: Industry Sector Contributions to U.S. Congressional Campaigns'. *American Politics Research* 42(6): 1034–76.

Givel, Michael and Stanton Glantz. 2001. 'Tobacco Lobby Political Influence on US State Legislatures in the 1990s'. *Tobacco Control* 10: 124–34.

Gravelle, Jane. 2013. 'Tax Havens: International Tax Avoidance and Evasion'. 7-5700, R40623. Washington, DC: Congressional Research Service. https://www.fas.org/sgp/crs/misc/R40623.pdf.

Greenwood, Justin and Joanna Dreger. 2013. 'The Transparency Register: A European Vanguard of Strong Lobby Regulation?' *Interest Groups & Advocacy* 2(2): 139–62.

Harkinson, Josh. 2009. 'Revolving Door: Climate Edition'. *Mother Jones*, 14 December. http://motherjones.com/blue-marble/2009/12/how-bush-insiders-are-influencing-climate-debate.

Herper, Mathew. 2010. 'Former NIH Director to Lead Sanofi's Labs'. *Forbes*, 14 December. http://www.forbes.com/sites/matthewherper/2010/12/14/former-nih-director-to-lead-sanofis-labs/.

Hill, Claire and Richard Painter. 2011. 'Compromised Fiduciaries: Conflicts of Interest in Government and Business'. *Minnesota Law Review* 95: 1637–91.

Holden, Chris and Kelley Lee. 2009. 'Corporate Power and Social Policy: The Political Economy of the Transnational Tobacco Companies'. *Global Social Policy* 9(3): 328–54.

Jasso-Aguilar, Rebeca and Howard Waitzkin. 2011. 'Multinational Corporations, the State, and Contemporary Medicine'. *Health Sociology Review* 20(3): 245–57.

Johal, Surjinder and Alistair Ulph. 2002. 'Globalization, Lobbying, and International Environmental Governance'. *Review of International Economics* 10(3): 387–403.

Kaufmann, Daniel and Pedro C. Vicente. 2011. 'Legal Corruption'. *Economics & Politics* 23(2): 195–219.

Landers, Steven H. and Ashwini R. Sehgal. 2004. 'Health Care Lobbying in the United States'. *American Journal of Medicine* 116(7): 474–77.

LaPira, Timothy. 2014. 'Lobbying in the Shadows: How Private Interests Hide from Public Scrutiny, and Why That Matters'. Accessed September 19, 2016. http://papers.ssrn.com/sol3/papers.cfm?abstract_id=2507300.

LaPira, Timothy and Herschel Thomas. 2014. 'Revolving Door Lobbyists and Interest Representation'. *Interest Groups & Advocacy* 3(1): 4–29.

Lee, Timothy. 2013. 'Here's Why Obama Trade Negotiators Push the Interests of Hollywood and Drug Companies'. *Washington Post*, 26 November. http://www.washingtonpost.com/.

Lipsett, Lloyd. 2013. 'Tax Abuses, Poverty and Human Rights'. London: International Bar Association. http://www.ibanet.org/Article/Detail.aspx?ArticleUid=4A0CF930-A0D1-4784-8D09-F588DCDDFEA4.

Livermore, Michael and Richard Revesz. 2013. 'Regulatory Review, Capture, and Agency Inaction'. *Georgetown Law Journal* 101(5): 1337–98.

Luechinger, Simon and Christoph Moser. 2014. 'The Value of the Revolving Door: Political Appointees and the Stock Market'. *Journal of Public Economics* 119: 93–107.

Luke, Douglas and Melissa Krauss. 2004. 'Tobacco Industry Campaign Contributions and U.S. Congressional Voting'. *American Journal of Preventive Medicine* 27(5): 363–72.

MacIntyre, Robert, Matthew Gardner and Richard Phillips. 2014. *The Sorry State of Corporate Taxes: What Fortune 500 Firms Pay (or Don't Pay) in the USA and What They Pay Abroad – 2008 to 2012*. Washington, DC: Citizens for Tax Justice and the Institute on Taxation and Economic Policy. http://www.ctj.org/corporatetaxdodgers/sorrystateofcorptaxes.pdf.

McCambridge, Jim, Benjamin Hawkins and Chris Holden. 2014. 'Vested Interests in Addiction Research and Policy. The Challenge Corporate Lobbying Poses to Reducing Society's Alcohol Problems: Insights from UK Evidence on Minimum Unit Pricing'. *Addiction* 109(2): 199–205.

Mialon, Melissa, Boyd Swinburn and Gary Sacks. 2015. 'A Proposed Approach to Systematically Identify and Monitor the Corporate Political Activity of the Food Industry with Respect to Public Health Using Publicly Available Information'. *Obesity Reviews* 16(7): 519–30.

Miller, David and Idrees Ahmad. 2010. 'Powerbase: A Collaborative Resource for Monitoring Power Networks'. *Radical Statistics* 102: 4–16.

Mindel, Jennifer, Lucy Reynolds, David Cohen and Martin McKee. 2012. 'All in This Together: The Corporate Capture of Public Health'. *BMJ* 345: e8082. doi:10.1136/bmj.e8082.

Nichols, John and Robert W. McChesney. 2013. *Dollarocracy: How the Money-and-Media Complex Is Destroying America*. New York: Nation Books.

Office of the Clerk, U.S. House of Representatives. 2013. 'Lobbying Disclosure Act Guidance Section 4 – Lobbying Registration'. Accessed September 19, 2016. http://lobbyingdisclosure.house.gov/amended_lda_guide.html#section4.

Ohman, Magnus. 2012. *Political Finance Regulations around the World: An Overview of the International IDEA Database*. Stockholm, Sweden: International Institute for Democracy and Electoral Assistance.

Organisation for Economic Cooperation and Development. 2013. 'Addressing Base Erosion and Profit Shifting'. OECD Publishing. doi:10.1787/9789264192744-en.

Palmer, Anna and Jake Sherman. 2014. 'To Pick Staff, Scalise Turns to Lobbyist'. Accessed September 19, 2016. http://www.politico.com/story/2014/08/steve-scalise-staff-john-feehery-109739.html.

Palmer, Maxwell and Benjamin Schneer. 2015. 'Capitol Gains: The Returns to Elected Office from Corporate Board Directorships'. *Journal of Politics* 78(1): 181–96.

Poole, Keith and Howard Rosenthal. 2007. *Ideology and Congress*. New Brunswick, NJ: Transaction Publishers.

Potter, Wendell. 2015. 'Latest Swing of Revolving Door Puts Former Medicare Czar in Charge of Health Insurance Lobby'. Accessed September 19, 2016. https://www.publicintegrity.org/2015/07/20/17689/latest-swing-revolving-door-puts-former-medicare-czar-charge-health-insurance-lobby.

Powell, Lynda. 2014. 'The Influence of Campaign Contributions on the Legislative Process'. *Duke Journal of Constitutional Law & Public Policy* 9(1): 75–101.

Riddel, Mary. 2003. 'Candidate Eco-Labelling and Senate Campaign Contributions'. *Journal of Environmental Economics and Management* 45(2): 177–94.

Roscoe, Douglas and Shannon Jenkins. 2005. 'A Meta-Analysis of Campaign Contributions' Impact on Roll Call Voting'. *Social Science Quarterly* 86(1): 52–68.

Sandström, Annica and Lars Carlsson. 2008. 'The Performance of Policy Networks: The Relation between Network Structure and Network Performance'. *The Policy Studies Journal* 36(4): 497–524.

Savell, Emily, Anna Gilmore and Gary Fooks. 2014. 'How Does the Tobacco Industry Attempt to Influence Marketing Regulations? A Systematic Review'. *PLoS ONE* 9(2): e87389. doi:10.1371/journal.pone.0087389.

Shepherd, Joanna. 2013. *Justice at Risk: An Empirical Analysis of Campaign Contributions and Judicial Decisions*. Washington, DC: American Constitution Society for Law and Policy. http://www.acslaw.org/ACS%20Justice%20at%20Risk%20(FINAL)%206_10_13.pdf.

Stratman, Thomas. 2005. 'Some Talk: Money in Politics. A (Partial) Review of the Literature'. *Public Choice* 124: 135–56.

Tax Justice Network. 2015. *Ten Reasons to Defend the Corporation Tax: How the Corporate Income Tax Protects Democracy and Curbs Inequality*. Bucks, UK: Tax Justice Network Limited. http://www.taxjustice.net/wp-content/uploads/2013/04/Ten_Reasons_Full_Report.pdf.

US Government Accountability Office. 2013a. *Corporate Income Tax: Effective Tax Rates Can Differ Significantly from the Statutory Rate*. GAO-13-520. Washington, DC: U.S. Government Accountability Office. http://www.gao.gov/assets/660/654957.pdf.

US Government Accountability Office. 2013b. *Corporate Tax Expenditures: Information on Estimated Revenue Losses and Related Federal Spending Programs*. GAO-13-339. Washington, DC: US Government Accountability Office. http://www.gao.gov/assets/660/653120.pdf.

US Senate. Lobbying Disclosure Act of 1995. Accessed 18 March 2015. http://www.senate.gov/legislative/Lobbying/Lobby_Disclosure_Act/TOC.htm.

Vidal, Jordi Blanes i, Mirko Draca and Christian Fons-Rosen. 2012. 'Revolving Door Lobbyists'. *American Economic Review* 102(7): 3731–48.

Wiist, William H. ed. 2010. *The Bottom Line or Public Health: Tactics Corporations Use to Influence Health and Health Policy, and What We Can Do to Counter Them*. New York: Oxford University Press.

Witko, Christopher. 2013. 'Party Government and Variation in Corporate Influence on Agency Decision Making: OSHA Regulation, 1981–2006'. *Social Science Quarterly* 94(4): 894–911.

Zubak-Skees, Chris and Liz Essley Whyte. 2015. 'Who Tried to Buy the 2014 Ballot Measures?' Accessed September 19, 2016. http://www.publicintegrity.org/2015/02/05/16678/who-tried-buy-2014-ballot-measures#donor/monsanto-co.

Chapter 16

Analysing Corporate Documents

Ross MacKenzie and Chris Holden

Almost all organisations, from small businesses to transnational corporations, government departments and non-governmental organisations, are 'routinely, often extensively, involved in the production and consumption of paperwork' (Atkinson and Coffey 2004). Such paperwork can include reports and communications, meeting agendas and minutes, business plans, budgets and diaries that provide potentially important primary source material for researchers from history, sociology, public health, education, political science and other fields seeking to understand those organisations (Forster 1994; Bero 2003; Abbott, Shaw and Elston 2004; Jupp 2006; Bowen 2009). Corporate document collections, however, have limitations. They are unavoidably incomplete and provide only a partial account and are *not*, as Atkinson and Coffey (2004) caution, transparent representations of organisational routines or decision-making processes.

This chapter focuses on documents produced by corporations and how they can be used by researchers. Two document collections are used as examples of how they can be used in researching corporate activities. The provenance and value of the previously confidential tobacco industry documents, made public from the 1990s, are described, as is the development of analytical approaches to their analysis. The second document set comprises corporate submissions to a public consultation on alcohol policy, and two approaches to analysis are considered. First, these submissions were combined with other public company documents and qualitative interviews, to understand how the industry sought to frame public debate on alcohol policy. Second, evidence claims within companies' submissions were compared and contrasted with independent scientific evidence. We emphasise throughout the need to understand the reasons for documents' production and retention when using them for research purposes.

INTERNAL CORPORATE DOCUMENTS

Internal document collections made public voluntarily, generally through company-operated depositories or public archives, are subject to a range of procedures and protocols. Some documents may not be released or may be heavily redacted, because their content is deemed sensitive or privileged. Similarly, documents may be produced or filed by 'information gate-keepers with ulterior motives' (Forster 1994). Document owners, company lawyers and the archival sorting and classification process of a company will combine to filter document collections before they reach the public domain (Hill 1993). Internal document collections made public as the result of legal proceedings undergo a lesser degree of filtration but, as described later, remain partial in their contents and scope.

The public release of previously confidential tobacco industry documents, described later, has been critical to the understanding of tobacco corporations' strategies and opposition to effective public health policy. Similar publicly accessible documents of other health-relevant corporations do not currently exist on a comparable scale, but smaller collections from other industries, disclosed via legal proceedings, have yielded important findings. One relatively large collection is the University of California, San Francisco (UCSF), Library's Drug Industry Documents, which contains some 3,800 documents that provide insights into pharmaceutical industry advertising, manufacturing, marketing, sales and scientific research. It houses documents that demonstrate how the pharmaceutical industry, regulatory/funding agencies and other organisations 'operate in ways that are detrimental to public health' (UCSF 2016a). Analysis of the internal documents of the US lead and vinyl industries demonstrated that corporate officials were aware of the associated dangers of their products and endeavoured to keep information from the public to prevent regulation of products they knew to be dangerous (Markowitz and Rosner 2002), while documents of leading asbestos corporations suggest formulation of similar strategies (Environmental Working Group 2016).

Corporate documents can also be found within collections of personal papers. The plans and communications of the World Sugar Research Organization were found, for example, in the personal papers of a University of Illinois emeritus professor. Analysis of these documents uncovered industry knowledge, as early as the 1950s, that sugar causes tooth decay, and strategies to deflect attention from oral health by funding research on ineffective interventions (Kearns, Glantz and Schmidt 2015).

Tobacco industry document collections

Available tobacco industry documents are remarkably diverse in content and format, comprising inter alia, correspondence; reports on advertising, marketing and promotional strategies; corporate structure; and country, regional and international business plans and strategies. Much of this material is the stuff of day-to-day operations of any large corporation. However, given the nature of the tobacco industry's business, and the decades-long battle to regulate its deadly products, the documents reveal what has been described as 'the dishonest and starkly cynical nature' of transnational tobacco companies (Blanke 2002).

The value of the tobacco industry documents was first demonstrated in 1994 when a legal clerk at Brown & Williamson, a US-based company, leaked around 4,000 pages of company files to Professor Stanton Glantz at UCSF and prominent journalists (Glantz et al. 1996). Analysis of these documents revealed industry 'strategies to avoid product liability litigation, understand nicotine addiction, and manipulate both internal and external scientific research on the effects of both active and passive smoking' (Glantz et al. 1995, 219). The same year, the US states of Minnesota and Mississippi sued seven leading cigarette manufacturers and two industry organisations[1] to recover treatment costs of smoking-related illness.[2] The initial claimants were subsequently joined by 46 other states and two Minnesota-based private health insurers (Blanke 2002). The legal settlements reached in 1998 between claimant states and the industry resulted in the release of around 40 million pages of industry documents under the terms of two related agreements (Walburn 2000). The Minnesota Consent Agreement (between the state of Minnesota and Minnesota Blue Cross, Blue Shield and tobacco industry defendants) compelled tobacco companies to make millions of pages of internal documents accessible in hardcopy form at depositories in Minneapolis, Minnesota, where documents of US-based companies are held, and at Guildford, England, which housed those of UK-based British American Tobacco (BAT) until the company repository was closed in 2015. The Master Settlement Agreement (between the attorneys general of 46 US states and four largest US tobacco companies) required companies to post those documents on publicly accessible websites until 2010, a requirement that did not extend to UK-based BAT. The agreement further stipulated that documents filed in discovery in future US lawsuits were to be added to these websites. Temporary online availability, combined with unreliability of collections maintained by tobacco corporations, made posting the industry documents on permanent websites administered by the tobacco control community essential. Concerted international efforts by public health academics and advocates, supported by a range of funders, led to the launch of the Legacy Tobacco Documents Library (renamed the Truth Tobacco Industry Documents in 2015) by the UCSF Library and Center for Knowledge Management (2016) in 2002. By 2016, approximately 88 million pages in 14.6 million documents were available online (UCSF 2016b).

Significance and limitations

The significance of the release of tobacco industry documents has been compared to the human genome project, in that the documents have provided the public health community with its 'first clear understanding of how the tobacco contagion works' (Glantz 2000). Former US surgeon general C. Everett Koop cites the release of the documents as among the most important public health achievements of the twentieth century (Blanke and Humphrey 2006). This is demonstrated by their transformation of litigation, in the US and other countries, by making cases against the industry more affordable for potential plaintiffs, and official recognition of the legal team behind the initial disclosures by a World Health Organization's Tobacco Free World Award (Blanke and Humphrey 2006).

It is important to recognise that, as with all internal corporate materials, there are limitations to tobacco industry documents as a data source. Documents made available are only from those companies and organisations that were party to the two 1998 legal settlements. The documents are also limited to those documents identified during the legal discovery process, which are an unknown proportion of the total held by a given company. It has also been established that tens of thousands of pages of documents have been withheld on contested claims of legal privilege, confidentiality and trade secrets (US Department of Justice 2006; LeGresley and Lee 2016), and an unknown number is unavailable as the result of tobacco industry strategies to store documents offshore, destroy those considered potentially incriminating and dilute the court-ordered release of internal records since the 1990s (Diethelm, Rielle and McKee 2004; Hammond et al. 2009).

Finally, documents released via court decisions do not extend past the date of the relevant legal proceeding, and most documents currently available date to no later than the mid-2000s. Charges of obsolescence can be answered, however, by the prospective nature of many documents which contain, for example, corporate strategies for periods extending past the date of their original circulation, and by contemporary documents leaked to the media (Doward 2013) or available via more recent legal proceedings. The most significant release of internal documents since the 1998 settlement agreements has been the approximately one million pages produced in the US Department of Justice case against the tobacco industry from 1999 to 2006. Under the Racketeer Influenced and Corrupt Organizations Act, tobacco companies and industry organisations[3] were found guilty and ordered to make future documents under legal discovery processes publicly available (Guardino, Banthin and Daynard 2007). It is reasonable to assume that increased vigilance, in committing potentially sensitive or incriminating information to paper, now exists. Such limitations notwithstanding, the value of research based on the tobacco industry internal documents to strengthening global tobacco governance, and public health more broadly, is well established (Hurt et al. 2009).

Evolving approaches to industry document analysis

The urgency felt by researchers to make their findings public during initial excavations of tobacco industry documents outpaced deeper reflections on methodology. As the value of the documents became more widely appreciated, greater attention was paid to methodological development (Malone and Balbach 2000; Bero 2003; Carter 2005). Analytical approaches have evolved, from a largely 'descriptive mainstream' of chronological narratives into more systematic and more deeply theorised studies based on 'iteratively reviewing data to construct an account that is coherent, supported by the evidence, and deeply contextualized' (Bero 2003). Forster's (1994) hermeneutic model of document research, which describes the central role of iterative search techniques, interpretation, contextualisation and validation, provides a useful template that can be applied to tobacco industry document research (Box 16.1).

Box 16.1 Stages of the hermeneutic process

(i) Understanding meanings of individual texts

The focus is on reading and re-reading documents to gain understanding of the content, and identifying and recording key bibliographic information: type (correspondence, report, prospective plan), author, recipient, date, countries/regions named, broad topics/themes and brief summary of content. New terms arising from this initial scrutiny are recorded in a separate file for subsequent searches.

(ii) Identifying themes and sub-themes

Disparate findings identified in stage i are categorised into central themes and sub-themes; this leads to stage iii.

(iii) Identifying thematic clusters

Researchers consider intertextuality or how documents relate to one another. Groupings of text emerge with clear cohesion and unity, and these can be compared with others. Correspondence produced by a company subsidiary office, for instance, on a given topic can be compared with correspondence from head office to determine organisational structure and lines of communication within a company.

(iv) Contextualising documentary data

Research findings are contextualised within their geographical, temporal and corporate settings to minimise misinterpretation, and reassessed in the light of new material consulted and growing comprehension of the issues under examination.

(v) Triangulating documentary data

The focus is on efforts to determine whether strategies or tactics outlined in documents were carried out. The fragmented nature of documents means that it is not always clear when, or if, mooted strategies are translated into action and, if so, to what degree of success. Information taken from document analysis is compared to other data resources to establish outcomes of plans described. These may include

- relevant documents produced by other tobacco companies that include discussion of a particular plan or strategy, or its impact;
- media accounts;
- civil society reports;
- published articles; and
- interviews with key informants.

(vi) Reliability and validity checks

Findings and interpretations are discussed at length with co-authors and colleagues.

(vii) Presenting representative case material

Findings are published and/or publicly presented.

Source: Adapted from Forster (1994).

One example is a study of tobacco industry complicity in cigarette smuggling in Thailand in the 1980s and 1990s (MacKenzie, Lee and LeGresley 2016). The authors searched the Truth Tobacco Documents Library using broad initial search terms, including industry euphemisms for smuggling,[4] that were generated from a review of scholarly works, non-governmental reports and the media. The snowball technique, by which initial searches generate additional search terms including names of individuals, associated organisations, projects and products (Malone and Balbach 2000; Bero 2003), was then applied. The resulting 74 industry documents were iteratively reviewed, and triangulated with other sources, to build a narrative related to tobacco industry strategies in Thailand during the late 1980s. This narrative revealed the role of smuggling in BAT's global business strategy, as well as its manipulation of the relative supply and pricing of both legal and illegal products. These findings emphasised the need to address the mixing of legal and illegal trade by the tobacco industry in order to implement the Protocol to Eliminate Illicit Trade in Tobacco Products.

PUBLIC CORPORATE DOCUMENTS

For research purposes, industry documents produced with the objective of communication with the public, government or another external entity must be distinguished from those intended for internal use. Communications intended for an external audience cannot be used alone, and uncritically, to construct an objective account of corporate activity over time. However, such materials are amenable to other types of analysis and can be triangulated with documents of other organisations and with other data sources to gain insights into corporate behaviour. For example, the Centre for International Environmental Law (CEIL) analysed documents that suggest that the oil industry had been aware of carbon-based climate change for decades and acted so as to not only conceal this knowledge but also discredit unfavourable independent scientific findings. Through detailed analysis of statements made by US government officials, reports both issued by and submitted to government agencies and reports funded by the industry itself, CEIL researchers uncovered evidence that the oil industry was explicitly warned of climate risks as early as the 1960s and that it funded research aimed at creating public scepticism of independent science and environmental regulation (CEIL 2016).

Miller and Harkins (2010, 566) argue that external communication strategies are a fundamental aspect of corporate efforts to influence public opinion and policy, as part of an attempt to 'dominate the information environment'. Analysing corporate communications of various kinds can, therefore, help understanding of how industry actors attempt to influence public debate and the views of policymakers as part of their lobbying efforts. Documents made available on company websites or in response to public consultations, academic papers written by corporate employees, company annual reports, media releases, investment prospectuses, industry journals and oral histories are all potential sources of valuable research data (Fridenson 2009). In addition, the tobacco document collections discussed earlier include materials intended for public communications. These can often be particularly useful when different iterations of a draft public communications document are available. This allows analysis of how a public message has been crafted within a company, prior to a final version being released for public consumption.

Submissions to public consultations by corporations are a particular form of external communication that requires specific analytic approaches. Researchers have analysed documents of this kind in a number of ways, including using quantitative content analysis (Costa et al. 2014) and qualitative thematic analysis (Miller et al. 2011; see Bryman 2012 for an introduction to content analysis and the use of documents in research more generally). Here, we review two examples of qualitative analyses of submissions to a public consultation on alcohol policy.

Frame analysis

In 2008, the Scottish Government (2008) conducted a public consultation on its plans to change alcohol policy, publishing consultation submissions on its website. These plans marked a decisive break with previous policy in Scotland, and elsewhere in the United Kingdom, by adopting a 'whole-population' approach to alcohol-related harm including minimum unit pricing (MUP), which was widely opposed by the alcohol industry.

A 'frame analysis' of company submissions to this consultation was used to understand how industry actors attempted to influence policy by promoting a particular set of ideas. Frames are 'underlying structures of belief, perception and appreciation' upon which particular policy positions rest (Schön and Rein 1994, 23). The way an issue is framed points towards certain kinds of policy responses and precludes others (Hawkins and Holden 2013). Frame analysis can be used to understand the ways that actors seek to advance their political agendas by defining the nature of a policy problem and the requisite solutions. Political actors, including corporations, thus attempt to frame debates in ways that are amenable to their interests and objectives (Snow and Benford 1992; Rein and Schön 1996). Using this approach, Hawkins and Holden (2013) analysed alcohol industry submissions to the consultation, triangulating submissions with documents culled from company websites and interviews with industry actors. Documents were analysed and coded manually, and then cross-referenced with interview transcripts that had been coded using Nvivo software. The aim was to map the frames used by companies and the role these frames played in the policy debate. It was found that the dominant industry frames conflicted substantially with those prevalent in the public health community. While corporations tended to individualise both problems and solutions, seeing the causes of alcohol-related harm as lying primarily with a small minority of 'problem drinkers' who require targeted interventions, public health professionals advocated whole-population approaches to reduce the overall consumption of alcohol via measures such as MUP.

Analysing evidence claims

The differences between industry and public health frames raise the important question of the evidence base supporting these contrasting policy approaches. To examine industry evidence claims, McCambridge, Hawkins and Holden (2013) identified and extracted the main evidential claims made by industry consultation submissions and evaluated these against the most authoritative and up-to-date review of alcohol policy effectiveness (Babor et al. 2010). By examining the frequency and prominence of evidence claims across these submissions, they were able to identify the main methods used by alcohol companies to attempt to link evidence to policy: the misrepresentation of strong evidence, the promotion of weak evidence, the making of unsubstantiated claims about the adverse effects of policy proposals and the promotion of alternatives without any evidence for their efficacy. Analysis of this kind has the potential to be applied to various policy consultations and public proceedings relevant to global health governance.

CONCLUSION

Bowen's (2009, 27) observation that 'document analysis requires that data be examined and interpreted in order to elicit meaning, gain understanding, and develop empirical knowledge' holds true for documents originally produced for both internal and external communication. In analysing document collections, whether intended for internal or public use, it is crucial to understand their provenance, notably who produced them and for what purpose, before attempting to interpret their meaning. The potential value of corporate documents to researchers is made clear by the extensive scholarly literature that has emerged from their analysis.

FURTHER READING

Atkinson, Paul and Amanda Coffey. 2004. 'Analysing Documentary Realities'. In *Qualitative Research: Theory, Method and Practice*, 2nd edition, edited by David Silverman, 56–74. London: Sage.

Carter, Stacy. 2005. 'Tobacco Document Research Reporting'. *Tobacco Control* 14(6): 368–76.
Forster, Nick. 1994. 'The Analysis of Company Documentation'. In *Qualitative Methods in Organizational Research*, edited by Catherine Cassell and Gillian Symon, 147–66. London: Sage.

NOTES

1. Philip Morris Incorporated, R.J. Reynolds Tobacco Company, Brown & Williamson Tobacco Corporation, BAT Industries Plc, Lorillard Tobacco Company, American Tobacco Company, Liggett Group and two industry organisations (Council for Tobacco Research and the Tobacco Institute). The Council for Tobacco Research was founded by the industry to fund ostensibly independent research on tobacco and health. The Tobacco Institute oversaw public relations and lobbying duties. Both were shut down under the terms of the 1998 Master Settlement Agreement.

2. Details of the 1998 legal proceedings and settlement are available in Ciresi (1999) and Ciresi, Walburn and Sutton (1999).

3. Philip Morris (now Philip Morris USA), Philip Morris companies (now Altria), R.J. Reynolds Tobacco (now Reynolds American), Brown & Williamson Tobacco (now part of Reynolds American), Lorillard Tobacco Company, Liggett Group, American Tobacco (merged with Brown & Williamson and now part of Reynolds American), BATCo, Council for Tobacco Research and Tobacco Institute.

4. Industry code and euphemisms for smuggling include transit, general trade and duty not paid (see Collin et al. 2004).

REFERENCES

Abbott, Stephen, Sara Shaw and Julian Elston. 2004. 'Comparative Analysis of Health Policy Implementation: The Use of Documentary Analysis'. *Policy Studies* 25(4): 259–66.
Atkinson, Paul and Amanda Coffey. 2004. 'Analysing Documentary Realities'. In *Qualitative Research: Theory, Method and Practice*, 2nd edition, edited by David Silverman, 56–74. London: Sage.
Babor, Thomas, Raul Caetano, Sally Casswell, Griffith Edwards, Norman Giesbrecht, Kathryn Graham, Joel W. Grube, Linda Hill, Harold Holder, Ross Homel, Michael Livingston, Esa Österberg, Jürgen Rehm, Robin Room and Ingeborg Rossow. 2010. *Alcohol, No Ordinary Commodity: Research & Public Policy*. Oxford, UK: Oxford University Press.
Bero, Lisa. 2003. 'Implications of the Tobacco Industry Documents for Public Health and Policy'. *Annual Review of Public Health* 24: 267–88.
Blanke, Douglas. 2002. *Towards Health with Justice: Litigation and Public Inquiries as Tools for Tobacco Control*. Geneva: World Health Organization.
Blanke, Douglas and Hubert Humphrey III. 2006. 'Putting Truth into Action: Using the Evidence for Justice'. *Tobacco Control* 15(Supp IV): v1–iv3.

Bowen, Glenn. 2009. 'Document Analysis as a Qualitative Research Method'. *Qualitative Research Journal* 9(2): 22–40.

Bryman, Alan. 2012. *Social Research Methods*. Oxford, UK: Oxford University Press.

Carter, Stacy. 2005. 'Tobacco Document Research Reporting'. *Tobacco Control* 14(6): 368–76.

Centre for International Environmental Law. 2016. 'How We Learned "What They Knew"'. Accessed September 19, 2016. http://www.ciel.org/how-we-learned-what-they-knew/.

Ciresi, Michael. 1999. 'An Account of the Legal Strategies That Ended an Era of Tobacco Industry Immunity'. *William Mitchell Law Review* 25(2): 439–46.

Ciresi, Michael, Roberta Walburn and Tara Sutton. 1999. 'Decades of Deceit: Document Discovery in the Minnesota Tobacco Litigation'. *William Mitchell Law Review* 25(2): 477–566.

Collin, Jeff, Eric LeGresley, Ross MacKenzie, Sue Lawrence and Kelley Lee. 2004. 'Complicity in Contraband: British American Tobacco and Cigarette Smuggling in Asia'. *Tobacco Control* 13(Supplement 2): ii104–ii111.

Costa, Hélia, Anna Gilmore, Sylvie Peeters, Martin McKee and David Stuckler. 2014. 'Quantifying the Influence of the Tobacco Industry on EU Governance: Automated Content Analysis of the EU Tobacco Products Directive'. *Tobacco Control* 23(6): 473–78.

Diethelm, Pascal, Jean-Charles Rielle and Martin McKee. 2004. 'The Whole Truth and Nothing but the Truth? The Research that Philip Morris Did Not Want You to Wee'. *Lancet* 364(9479): 86–92.

Doward, Jamie. 2013. 'Tobacco Giant Philip Morris "Spent Millions in Bid to Delay EU Legislation"'. *The Guardian*, 7 September. http://www.theguardian.com/business/2013/sep/07/tobacco-philip-morris-millions-delay-eu-legislation.

Environmental Working Group. 2016. 'Understanding Asbestos'. Accessed September 19, 2016. http://www.ewg.org/asbestos/facts/.

Forster, Nick. 1994. 'The Analysis of Company Documentation'. In *Qualitative Methods in Organizational Research*, edited by Catherine Cassell and Gillian Symon, 147–66. London: Sage.

Fridenson, Patrick. 2009. 'Business History and History'. In *The Oxford Handbook of Business History*, edited by Geoffrey Jones and Jonathan Zeitlin, 9–36. Oxford, UK: Oxford University Press.

Glantz, Stanton. 2000. 'The Truth about Big Tobacco in Its Own Words'. *British Medical Journal* 321(8257): 313–14.

Glantz, Stanton, Deborah Barnes, Lisa Bero, Peter Hanauer and John Slade. 1995. 'Looking through a Keyhole at the Tobacco Industry: The Brown and Williamson Documents'. *Journal of the American Medical Association* 274(3): 219–24.

Glantz, Stanton, John Slade, Lisa Bero, Peter Hanauer and Deborah Barnes. 1996. *The Cigarette Papers*. Berkeley, CA: University of California Press.

Guardino, Sara, Christopher Banthin and Richard Daynard. 2007. *USA v. Philip Morris USA, Inc., et al.: Analysis of Judge Kessler's Final Opinion and Order*. Boston, MA: Tobacco Control Resource Centre. http://www.tobacco.neu.edu/litigation/cases/DOJ/doj_opinion_summary.pdf.

Hammond, David, Michael Chaiton, Alex Lee and Neil Collishaw. 2009. 'Destroyed Documents: Uncovering the Science That Imperial Tobacco Canada Sought to Conceal'. *Canadian Medical Association Journal* 181(10): 691–97.

Hawkins, Benjamin and Chris Holden. 2013. 'Framing the Alcohol Policy Debate: Industry Actors and the Regulation of the UK Beverage Alcohol Market'. *Critical Policy Studies* 7(1): 53–71.

Hill, Michael R. 1993. *Archival Strategies and Techniques*. Newbury Park, CA: Sage.

Hurt, Richard, Jon Ebbert, Monique Muggli, Nikki Lockhart and Channing Robertson. 2009. 'Open Doorway to Truth: Legacy of the Minnesota Tobacco Trial'. Mayo Clinic Proceedings 84(5): 446–56.

Jupp, Victor. 2006. 'Documents and Critical Research'. In *Data Collection and Analysis*, 2nd edition, edited by Roger Sapsford and Victor Jupp, 298–316. London: Sage.

Kearns, Cristin, Stanton Glantz and Laura Schmidt. 2015. 'Sugar Industry Influence on the Scientific Agenda of the National Institute of Dental Research's 1971 National Caries Program: A Historical Analysis of Internal Documents'. *PLOS Medicine* 12(3): e1001798. doi:10.1371/journal.pmed.1001798.

LeGresley, Eric and Kelley Lee. 2016. 'An Analysis of British American Tobacco's Questionable Use of Privilege and Protected Document Claims at the Guildford Depository'. *Tobacco Control*. doi:10.1136/tobaccocontrol-2016-052955.

MacKenzie, Ross, Kelley Lee and Eric LeGresley. 2016. 'To "Enable Our Legal Product to Compete Effectively with the Transit Market": British American Tobacco's Strategies in Thailand Following the 1990 GATT Dispute'. *Global Public Health* 11(3): 1–15.

Malone, Ruth and Edith Balbach. 2000. 'Tobacco Industry Documents: Treasure Trove or Quagmire?' *Tobacco Control* 9(3): 334–38.

Markowitz, Gerald and Rosner David. 2002. *Deceit and Denial: The Deadly Politics of Industrial Pollution*. Berkeley, CA: University of California Press.

McCambridge, Jim, Ben Hawkins and Chris Holden. 2013. 'Industry Use of Evidence to Influence Alcohol Policy: A Case Study of Submissions to the 2008 Scottish Government Consultation'. *PLoS Medicine* 10(4): e1001431. doi:10.1371/journal.pmed.1001431.

Miller, David and Claire Harkins. 2010. 'Corporate Strategy, Corporate Capture: Food and Alcohol Industry Lobbying and Public Health'. *Critical Social Policy* 30(4): 564–89.

Miller, Peter, Florentine de Groot, Stephen McKenzie and Nicolas Droste. 2011. 'Vested Interests in Addiction Research and Policy. Alcohol Industry Use of Social Aspect Public Relations Organizations against Preventative Health Measures'. *Addiction* 106(9): 1560–67.

Rein, Martin and Donald Schön. 1996. 'Frame-Critical Policy Analysis and Frame-Reflective Policy Practice'. *Knowledge and Policy* 9(1): 85–103.

Schön, Donald and Martin Rein. 1994. *Frame Reflection*. New York: Basic Books.

Scottish Government. 2008. *Changing Scotland's Relationship with Alcohol: A Discussion Paper on Our Strategic Approach*. Edinburgh: Scottish Government.

Snow, David and Robert Benford. 1992. 'Master Frames and Cycles of Protest'. In *Frontiers in Social Movement Theory*, edited by Aldon Morris, 133–55. New Haven, CT: Yale University Press.

UCSF Library. 2016a. 'Drug Industry Documents'. Accessed September 19, 2016. https://industrydocuments.library.ucsf.edu/drug/.

UCSF Library. 2016b. 'Truth Tobacco Industry Documents'. Accessed September 19, 2016. https://industrydocuments.library.ucsf.edu/tobacco/.

Walburn, Roberta. 2000. 'The Role of the Once-Confidential Tobacco Industry Documents'. *William Mitchell Law Review* 25(2): 431–38.

US Department of Justice. 2006. 'United States v. Philip Morris et al.' Civil Action No. 1999–2496 [GK]. Final Opinion issued 17 August 2006. http://www.tobaccofreekids.org/reports/doj/FinalOpinion.pdf.

Chapter 17

Social Media Research Methods

Becky Freeman

Social media are Internet-based applications that allow the creation and exchange of user-generated content. Social media platforms are no longer simply ways for consumers to communicate with each other but for corporations to engage with both consumers and key decision makers.

This chapter describes how social media and other digital sources, such as blogs, apps and podcasts, can provide rich data sources for research on corporations and global health governance (GHG). The examples and research studies cited are primarily drawn from tobacco control and obesity prevention, the two fields where much of the health-related research has been undertaken. Corporations may use social media to undermine health policies that run counter to their commercial interests and negatively influence consumer health behaviours. Monitoring and tracking social media content is essential in analysing the influence of corporations on global health. While there are tools and applications available to systematically collect this type of data, there is also a need for researchers to test data collection and management methods to determine if they yield relevant content. While much of this data is freely available, the costs in undertaking this kind of research lie in the need to invest significant human resources in the collection, recording and analysis of that data.

PUBLIC HEALTH AND SOCIAL MEDIA

The influence of media on attitudes, beliefs and behaviours is an established field of public health research and practice (Strasburger, Jordan and Donnerstein 2012). The rise of new media, and its emphasis on consumer-generated content, presents unique challenges to researchers, programme planners and regulators. Three primary difficulties created by these participatory platforms are (1) the sheer volume of content, (2) the borderless nature of the Internet and (3) consumer willingness to engage with corporations on social media. In addition, much of the research into corporate use of social media, as it impacts on public health, has been case studies. While case studies illustrate specific examples, and highlight how corporations are using these platforms, they do not systematically monitor or present a complete picture of activities. Case studies in isolation do not allow generalisations to be drawn and theories to be developed.

Nevertheless, there is a burgeoning field of research assessing how social media tools can assist public health researchers in tracking and countering corporate behaviour and activity. There is a growing body of research on how social media impacts on public health. Industries that heavily influence health and lifestyle behaviours, such as tobacco, alcohol and food, are the most studied in the literature. The tobacco control field has a long history of actively monitoring the industry as a means for developing and improving regulations and policies to reduce use (Cruz 2009). Tobacco industry monitoring has traditionally included an array of techniques, such as analysis of internal documents (see Chapter 16), collation and scrutiny of marketing campaigns (Toll and Ling 2005), critiques of corporate social responsibility efforts (Hirschhorn 2004) and appraisal of tobacco industry influence on legislative reform (Savell, Gilmore and Fooks 2014). With the advent of new media, this monitoring has extended to tobacco industry activity on social media platforms.

Unlike tobacco products, for which stringent marketing restrictions are commonplace in many countries, food and beverage, and alcohol, marketing is far less regulated (Hawkins et al. 2016). The obesity prevention and alcohol control fields have recognised that, despite limited regulation of marketing of these products in traditional media, social media platforms cannot be ignored. Social media has been embraced by tobacco, food and beverage and alcohol industries (Nicholls 2012) as an effective tool for corporate communication and product promotion. Social media must not then be considered a poor substitute to traditional mass media channels and may well prove to be a more effective means of reaching and influencing younger consumers (Boelsen-Robinson, Backholer and Peeters 2015). The proliferation of harmful products advertising on social media has occurred alongside these same corporations using social media to advance corporate social responsibility campaigns to undermine proposed legislation to reduce consumption (McCambridge et al. 2014). Monitoring the use of social media by industries with such a direct impact on public health is an essential first step in curtailing this powerful influence.

Box 17.1. Key terms and definitions

Mass media – Traditional media channels (television, newspaper, radio), which can be thought of as 'one-to-many communication' platforms. In contrast, new media democratise mass media and create 'many-to-many communication' possibilities (Tambini 1999).

New media – The combination and convergence of computing and information technology, communications networks and digitised media and information content. The interlinking of these three key pillars is due to the development and popularisation of the Internet coupled with the accessibility of activities, products and services within the digital media sphere (Flew 2008).

Web 2.0 – The evolution of the Internet, from an expert-driven information source to an interactive, participatory and consumer-driven medium (O'Reilly 2005).

Social media – A group of Internet-based applications (e.g. Facebook, YouTube, Twitter, Instagram, Snapchat) that build on the ideological and technological foundations of Web 2.0 and that allow the creation and exchange of user-generated content (Kaplan and Haenlein 2010).

User-generated content – Digital media (e.g. photographs, videos, songs) created by social media users.

Post – A message (can be text, photo, video, graphic, etc.) published in an online forum/social media page.

Apps – An abbreviation for *application*. An app is a piece of software. It can run on the Internet, a computer or smartphone or other electronic devices (Karch 2014).

Sources: Tambini (1999), Flew (2008), Kaplan and Haenlein (2010), Karch (2014) and O'Reilly (2005).

KEY QUESTIONS POSED BY SOCIAL MEDIA MONITORING RESEARCH OF CORPORATIONS THAT IMPACT PUBLIC HEALTH

To date, social media monitoring has been more extensively and effectively used as a method for tracking corporate communications and marketing strategies. There are a variety of platforms to consider, from image-based sharing services such as Instagram to services with a greater focus on text and web link sharing such as Twitter. These platforms require different approaches to data collection and analysis. The primary questions that public health researchers, using social media for corporate monitoring, seek to answer fall into the following broad themes:

- What are the key marketing strategies, techniques and messages being used on social media channels to promote products that impact on public health?
- What key messages and themes are disseminated through social media in response to health issues and/or proposed policy reforms that impact these corporations?
- What is the level of public engagement and reach with these corporations on social media? And how is the public engaging with these corporations on social media?
- Where regulations apply to corporate activity on traditional media platforms, are there loopholes/gaps in regulating this same activity on social media?
- Which corporations and associated partners are most influential in the social media space?

The open and highly public nature of social media and their associated content means that accessing data to help answer these questions is generally not difficult. A bigger challenge lies in identifying parties that may appear to be independent voices but are, in fact, acting in the interests of corporations. While it is becoming increasingly risky for organisations not to declare their funding sources, in an era that demands transparency, corporate documents reveal that significant conflicts of interest are still often undeclared. It is essential for researchers to carefully investigate the provenance and connections of all online sources.

Social media platforms also collect extensive analytics and insight data on page administrators and users, and their associated activities. Some of this basic data can be accessed freely, with more detailed information available for purchase either directly from social media providers or through third parties (Socialbakers 2016). For example, all YouTube videos have a number of views, comments, thumbs-up and thumbs-down ratings, posting date, posting account and length of video. Third-party platforms also rank YouTube channel popularity and videos by sector and/or topic, allowing researchers to track corporations of interest. This makes estimates of reach possible and assists researchers in assessing which companies/brands are cutting through the vast amount of online content. This can also help focus monitoring efforts only on those corporations that have a significant social media presence. One limitation of this approach, however, is that popularity of content does not necessarily mean it is the most influential. Corporations may employ methods to artificially inflate their reach in an effort to appear more influential or popular.

However, popularity is not the sole criterion that makes social media content worthy of examination. For example, the British American Tobacco (BAT) YouTube channel has very few subscribers or viewers (BAT n.d.), but the high-production value videos posted give clear insights into how the company frames opposition to tobacco control reforms, and the key messages it may be using to influence policymakers. This information is highly valuable in assisting public health advocacy organisations in preparing to counter these messages and in disassembling tobacco industry arguments. Again, the limitations of this approach must be acknowledged. Messages conveyed on social media are for public consumption and are designed to convey a positive image of the company or serve their commercial interests. They are unlikely to represent the corporate strategy fully. The messages relayed by corporations to politicians through lobbying activities may be shaped quite differently to the publicly available content on social media. There are parallels to the discussion of public versus private corporate communications, and the types of research questions that they can answer (see Chapter 16).

METHODS

Three common methods employed to investigate and monitor corporations on social media include (1) content analysis, (2) reporting of key case studies and (3) network analysis. Social media *content analysis* entails selecting a topic and systematically assessing the characteristics of posts and/or accounts associated with that topic, usually over a set period of time. For example, a content analysis of the marketing techniques employed by energy-dense and nutrient-poor food and beverage brands involved categorising the posts from 27 Facebook pages across 19 marketing categories (Freeman et al. 2014). The study showed that these pages widely used marketing features that increase consumer interaction and engagement, such as competitions based on user-generated content, interactive games and apps.

Undertaking *case studies* of high-profile corporate campaigns or illustrative examples is one of the useful ways of documenting the emerging use of social media for promotional opportunities. A case study of BAT employee activity on Facebook found that some employees were energetically promoting the company and its brands by 'liking', joining and administering groups, and then posting images of BAT events, products and promotional items (Freeman and Chapman 2010). On publication of this research in the journal *Tobacco Control*, BAT submitted a letter to the editor stating that the employees in question violated company policy and would be reminded that posting advertising content on social media is not permitted. Had there been evidence of BAT being aware of these actions, this could be in violation of existing tobacco advertising laws.

Network analysis is a third method that could be used in social media research. Many of the illnesses associated with the consumption of tobacco, alcohol and energy-dense, nutrient-poor food and drink, are traditionally described as non-communicable diseases (NCD). However, the norms and behaviours associated with NCD progression are increasingly recognised as being spread through social networks. Simply put, network analysis shows that if our close social connections are obese, we are more likely to be obese ourselves (Coiera 2013). While there is a body of work using network analysis to track the spread of infectious diseases (Christakis and Fowler 2010), little research has been done to assess how corporations may be exploiting online social networks to normalise the consumption of harmful products. For example, corporations can make use of friend networks on social media platforms to promote products. If a person 'likes' a product on his or her Facebook page, such as Coca-Cola, then promotions for Coca-Cola are more likely to appear on the page newsfeeds of his or her Facebook friends. Equally, the images that friends share on social media may be considered a form of word-of-mouth advertising. Corporations can foster this sharing by encouraging users to post images of themselves consuming products or by paying highly influential social media users to use and promote their products (London 2015).

CONTRIBUTION TO THE STUDY OF CORPORATIONS AND GHG

The most significant contribution made by social media research is exposing how inadequately advertising is regulated on new media channels, even for highly controlled industries like tobacco (Freeman 2012) and alcohol (Brodmerkel and Carah 2013). This research can assist in developing appropriate legislation to fill this policy gap. The borderless nature of the Internet, however, presents a serious challenge to the effectiveness and enforceability of such laws unless there is collective action. The World Health Organization Framework Convention for Tobacco Control is an example of how an international treaty can improve regulation of an industry that operates globally (Roemer, Taylor and Lariviere 2005).

Social media research is also useful for understanding how corporations attempt to reframe criticisms of their products and practices. For example, the comments sections of online news articles are a form of social media, allowing users to interact and engage with other readers, and the authors, of news articles they read. There is evidence that comments are often skewed towards negative remarks and can be overly critical (Wolchover 2012). These comments are an opportunity to analyse what arguments industry may be perpetrating to stall and prevent health policy reforms. Content analysis of the comments posted on online news stories about tobacco plain packaging reforms in Australia, for example, revealed the most common arguments against such laws (Freeman 2011). These comments reflected similar arguments the tobacco industry and its third-party allies were touting through news reports and websites, with the most common argument being plain packaging would not work to reduce smoking rates.

Corporations may also use social media to promote what appear to be public health–focused messages but are, in fact, promotional corporate communications. For example, the Coca-Cola Company responded to increasing public pressure, that sugar-sweetened beverages are a key driver of obesity, by reframing obesity as a consequence of inactivity, not dietary consumption (O'Connor 2015a). The company funded research that claimed to show that physical activity is more important to health than what consumers eat and drink (O'Connor 2015a). Coca-Cola then strategically used social media channels to reinforce this message, reassuring consumers that a little exercise can offset massive sugar consumption. For example, a video with a catchy soundtrack and images of young fit people from the Coca-Cola YouTube channel claimed that 'a 12oz can of Coke = 140 calories. There are many ways to burn those calories through EXTRA physical activity and have fun while doing so. Balance your lifestyle. Be OK. Open happiness' (Coca-Cola Co 2013). Coca-Cola reassured consumers that their products are harmless. Researchers can systematically monitor social media communications and make these activities transparent to the public.

One benefit of social media research is that it allows for tracking of trends in real time. Corporations can be monitored to assess how they immediately respond, when facing criticism, when policy changes are announced or when research is published that may impact on profitability. When high-profile nutrition researcher Marion Nestle was about to publish her book, *Soda Politics*, the International Food Information Council Foundation (IFICF), an organisation funded by food and beverage manufacturers, paid for the placement of social media posts critiquing her book (Freeman 2015). These posts directed readers to an article written by researchers and nutritionists, and funded by the IFICF. Identifying the links among researchers, third-party groups and corporations has, in some ways, been made easier as the Internet has shifted to an interactive, participatory and consumer-driven medium.

Given that consumers can quickly contribute to, and dominate, online campaigns, social media is not a risk-free medium for corporations. Corporations with controversial reputations, like those that harm health, have experimented and failed to improve their corporate reputations through social media. Again, these incidents represent opportunities for researchers to learn what messages resonate most with consumers and how social media users may effectively push back against corporate communications. When the fast-food chain McDonald's took to the social media site Twitter, highlighting how the company works with local farmers worldwide, the campaign quickly turned negative when users were asked to share their own feel-good McDonald's stories. Instead of positive examples, Twitter posts that included #McDStories were overwhelmingly critical of McDonald's, particularly regarding food quality and animal welfare (Lubin 2012).

CONCLUSION

Systematic monitoring and analysis of the social media activities of corporations relevant to global health is an increasingly important field of research. Monitoring can be readily achieved through joining online social networks and groups, following key individuals and companies, and reading blogs and websites that have connections to these corporations. It is not necessary to do this in a surreptitious way, as much of this type of information is publicly available and easily captured and analysed. Indeed, publicly available content is often well-crafted public relations and product advertising that is readily available as artefacts of corporate strategy.

Social media can be used to apply pressure on corporations to disclose information that reveals strategies to undermine the scientific process. In 2015, when the North American arm of the Coca-Cola Company was pressed to publish a complete list of researchers it had funded, to advance the notion the exercise is more important to health than the food and drinks we consume, it triggered intense media and public scrutiny. This resulted in universities and individual researchers returning Coca-Cola funding, and declaring their conflicts of interest in undertaking such work (O'Connor 2015b). The openness and transparency espoused by social media platforms and users may allow the public not only to demand corporations behave similarly but also to act to limit these same corporations from unduly influencing independent research.

Finally, social media can serve as a simple and efficient way to disseminate research on corporations and GHG. Sharing research findings beyond traditional academic journals is deemed essential to translating evidence into policy change (Cherney et al. 2012). However, given that many corporations and their third-party allies are active on social media, it should be assumed that research disseminated in this way will be closely monitored. Any content shared on new media, including any urge to goad or publicly shame corporations, should then be well considered as it is likely to provoke some of the tactics described in this chapter (Bunyan 2014). This does not mean that researchers should not be active social media users. This means simply that the same care and attention put into producing traditional peer-reviewed scholarly papers should also underpin social media posts.

FURTHER READING

Huang, Jidong, Rachel Kornfield, Glen Szczypka and Sherry L. Emery. 2014. 'A Cross-Sectional Examination of Marketing of Electronic Cigarettes on Twitter'. *Tobacco Control* 23(Supplement 3): iii26–iii30.

Kelly, Bridget, Stefanie Vandevijvere, Becky Freeman and Gabrielle Jenkin. 2015. 'New Media but Same Old Tricks: Food Marketing to Children in the Digital Age'. *Current Obesity Reports* 4(1): 37–45.

Wang, Fan, Pinpin Zheng, Dongyun Yang, Becky Freeman, Hua Fu and Simon Chapman. 2014. 'Chinese Tobacco Industry Promotional Activity on the Microblog Weibo'. *PLoS ONE* 9(6): e99336.

REFERENCES

BAT. n.d. 'Welcome to BAT'. Accessed September 19, 2016. https://www.youtube.com/user/WelcomeToBAT.

Boelsen-Robinson, Tara, Kathryn Backholer and Anna Peeters. 2016. 'Digital Marketing of Unhealthy Foods to Australian Children and Adolescents'. *Health Promotion International* 31(3): 523–33.

Brodmerkel Sven and Nicholas Carah. 2013. 'Alcohol Brands on Facebook: The Challenges of Regulating Brands on Social Media'. *Journal of Public Affairs* 13(3): 272–81.

Bunyan, Nigel. 2014. 'Health Chief Steps Down after Crude "e-cig" Rant on Twitter: Professor Stands Aside after Online Attack on Supporter of Quitting Aide'. *Daily Mail Australia*, 13 September. http://www.dailymail.co.uk/news/article-2754917/Health-chief-steps-crude-e-cig-rant-Twitter-Professor-leaves-post-online-attack-supporter-quitting-aide.html.

Cherney, Adrian, Brian Head, Paul Boreham, Jenny Povey and Michele Ferguson. 2012. 'Perspectives of Academic Social Scientists on Knowledge Transfer and Research Collaboration: A Cross-Sectional Survey of Australian Academics'. *Evidence & Policy: A Journal of Research, Debate and Practice* 8(4): 433–53.

Christakis, Nicholas A. and James H. Fowler. 2010. 'Social Network Sensors for Early Detection of Contagious Outbreaks'. *PLoS ONE* 5(9): e12948.

Coca-Cola Co. 2013. 'Be OK'. Accessed September 19, 2016. https://youtu.be/yfh0BeNMxGY?list=UU5JBB_E5mzPEbDupD-6fA4A.

Coiera, Enrico. 2013. 'Social Networks, Social Media, and Social Diseases'. *BMJ* 346: f3007.

Cruz, Tess Boley. 2009. 'Monitoring the Tobacco Use Epidemic IV. The Vector: Tobacco Industry Data Sources and Recommendations for Research and Evaluation'. *Preventive Medicine* 48(1): S24–34.

Flew, Terry. 2008. *New Media: An Introduction*, 3rd edition. Melbourne: Oxford University Press.

Freeman, Becky. 2011. 'Tobacco Plain Packaging Legislation: A Content Analysis of Commentary Posted on Australian Online News'. *Tobacco Control* 20(5): 361–66.

Freeman, Becky. 2012. 'New Media and Tobacco Control'. *Tobacco Control* 21(2): 139–44.

Freeman, Becky. 2015. 'Sweet Tweets: How Big Soda Uses Social Media to Dilute Critique'. *PLoS Blogs, Transnational Global Health*, 23 October. http://blogs.plos.org/globalhealth/2015/10/sweet-tweets-how-big-soda-uses-social-media-to-dilute-critiques/.

Freeman, Becky and Simon Chapman. 2010. 'British American Tobacco on Facebook: Undermining Article 13 of the Global World Health Organization Framework Convention on Tobacco Control'. *Tobacco Control* 19(3): e1–e9.

Freeman, Becky, B. Kelley, L. Baur, K. Chapman, Simon Chapman, T. Gill and L. King. 2014. 'Digital Junk: Food and Beverage Marketing on Facebook'. *American Journal of Public Health* 104(2): 356–64.

Hawkins, Benjamin, Chris Holden, Jappe Eckhardt and Kelley Lee. 2016. 'Reassessing Policy Paradigms: A Comparison of the Global Tobacco and Alcohol Industries'. *Global Public Health* (epub): 1–19.

Hirschhorn, Norbert. 2004. 'Corporate Social Responsibility and the Tobacco Industry: Hope or Hype?' *Tobacco Control* 13(4): 447–53.

Kaplan, Andreas M. and Michael Haenlein. 2010. 'Users of the World, Unite! The Challenges and Opportunities of Social Media'. *Business Horizons* 53(1): 59–68.

Karch, Marziah. 2014. 'Apps'. About Tech, Google. http://google.about.com/od/a/g/apps_def.htm.

London, Bianca. 2015. 'How Much Are YOUR Instagram Posts Worth? Users with 1,000 Followers Could Net £4,160 a Year by Promoting Brands (and Anyone with 100,000 Can Earn More Than a Lawyer)'. *Daily Mail Online*. http://www.dailymail.co.uk/femail/article-3313864/How-Instagram-posts-worth-Users-1-000-followers-net-4-160-year-promoting-brands-100-000-earn-lawyer.html.

Lubin, Gus. 2012. 'McDonald's Twitter Campaign Goes Horribly Wrong #McDStroies'. *Business Insider Australia*, 24 January. http://www.businessinsider.com.au/mcdonalds-twitter-campaign-goes-horribly-wrong-mcdstories-2012-1.

McCambridge, Jim, Kypros Kypri, Peter Miller, Benjamin Hawkins and Gerard Hastings. 'Be Aware of Drinkaware'. *Addiction* 109(4): 519–24.

Nicholls, James. 2012. 'Everyday, Everywhere: Alcohol Marketing and Social Media – Current Trends'. *Alcohol and Alcoholism* 47(4): 468–93.

O'Connor, Anahad. 2015a. 'Coca-Cola Funds Scientists Who Shift Blame for Obesity Away from Bad Diets'. *The New York Times*, 9 August. http://well.blogs.nytimes.com/2015/08/09/coca-cola-funds-scientists-who-shift-blame-for-obesity-away-from-bad-diets/?_r=0.

O'Connor, Anahad. 2015b. 'Coca-Cola's Top Obesity Scientist Departs amid Murky Research Claims'. *The Sydney Morning Herald*, 25 November. http://www.smh.com.au/business/cocacolas-top-obesity-scientist-departs-amid-murky-research-claims-20151125-gl7gvl.html.

O'Reilly, Tim. 2005. 'What's Web 2.0?' Accessed September 19, 2016. http://www.oreilly.com/pub/a//web2/archive/what-is-web-20.html.

Roemer, Ruth, Allyn Taylor and Jean Lariviere. 2005. 'Origins of the WHO Framework Convention on Tobacco Control'. *American Journal of Public Health* 95(6): 936–38.

Savell, Emily, Anna B. Gilmore and Gary Fooks. 2014. 'How Does the Tobacco Industry Attempt to Influence Marketing Regulations? A Systematic Review'. *PloS ONE* 9(2): e87389.

Socialbakers. 2016. 'About Socialbakers'. Accessed September 19, 2016. http://www.socialbakers.com/.

Strasburger, Victor C., Amy B. Jordan and Ed Donnerstein. 2012. 'Children, Adolescents, and the Media: Health Effects'. *Pediatric Clinics of North America* 59(3): 533–87.

Tambini, Damian. 1999. 'New Media and Democracy: The Civic Networking Movement'. *New Media & Society* 1(3): 305–29.

Toll, Benjamin A. and Pamela M. Ling. 2005. 'The Virginia Slims Identity Crisis: An Inside Look at Tobacco Industry Marketing to Women'. *Tobacco Control* 14(3): 172–80.

Wolchover, Natalie. 2012. 'Why Is Everyone on the Internet So Angry?' Accessed September 19, 2016. http://www.scientificamerican.com/article/why-is-everyone-on-the-internet-so-angry/.

Chapter 18

Making Use of Business and Financial Data

Kelley Lee

Corporations collect a range of data to support their commercial operations, including information about customers, products, suppliers, sales, markets, finances, human resources and regulatory obligations. Business and financial data is used internally to analyse a corporation's operations and environment, and to make decisions about strategy and planning. This data is also required for external reporting to shareholders, regulators and prospective investors. Rapid changes in information technologies have expanded the capacity for global data gathering and analysis, known as 'business data analytics', which is seen as 'the next frontier for business productivity and competition' (*Financial Times* 2013).

The business and financial data produced by a corporation describes what activities are carried out, how they are undertaken, what strategies drive operations and how successfully corporate goals are achieved over time. While much of this data is for internal use, and thus confidential, certain types of data from publicly traded companies are available to researchers. In addition, there is a wealth of information on specific corporations, industries, sectors and markets, within and across countries, produced by governments, business research firms, financial analysts, business media, academics and civil society organisations. These are potentially rich data sources which are currently underused by global health researchers.

This chapter describes the types of business and financial data publicly available to researchers seeking to analyse corporations and global health governance (GHG), and selected sources for obtaining this data. While this chapter is focused on selected English-language sources, primarily from the United States and the United Kingdom, it should be seen as a guide to the type of information which may be available elsewhere and a starting point for locating comparable data in other languages and settings. The chapter then discusses four types of research questions, relevant to corporations and GHG, which might be advanced through these data sources. A brief review of how such data has been used to date for research is provided. The strengths and weaknesses of using business and financial data are then presented.

TYPES AND SOURCES OF BUSINESS AND FINANCIAL DATA

An important source of business and financial data issued by corporations is the annual report to shareholders, prospective investors, regulators and the general public about business operations over the previous year. The specific content required in an annual report varies depending on the financial regulatory authority of the country where the company is formally registered (e.g. US Securities and Exchange Commission [SEC], and the Securities and Exchange Board of India). Most annual reports, however, contain four main sub-reports. First, the *directors' report* provides information to enable shareholders to make an informed assessment of the operations of the company, its financial position, business strategies and prospects for future financial years. This includes information on

- significant changes in the company's state of affairs;
- principal activities and any significant changes;
- matters since the previous year that may significantly affect the company's future operations, results or state of affairs;
- likely developments in the company's future operations and expected results of those operations (unless their inclusion would be unreasonably prejudicial);
- performance in relation to any particular and significant environmental regulation; and
- directors and officers of the company, and how they are remunerated (CPA Australia 2014).

Second, the *corporate governance report* is a statement of compliance with principles under a given jurisdiction concerning such matters as management and oversight, election of directors, remuneration, reporting and disclosure, risk management and decision making. For example, the Nestlé Corporate Governance Report 2015 states that the global food corporation 'follows the SIX Swiss Exchange Directive on Information relating to Corporate Governance . . . [and] complies with the recommendations of the Swiss Code of Best Practice for Corporate Governance' (Nestlé 2015, 3). Corporate governance reports provide information on its management and decision-making structure, and thus how a company makes decisions, manages risk and abides by certain legal and ethical standards.

Third, the *financial report* provides audited statements on the financial performance and position of a corporation commensurate with prevailing legal requirements. The financial report usually consists of the following:

(a) *Income statement*: This is a statement of profit and loss based on a report of revenues and expense generated and incurred by the corporation over a specified period of time. It shows the net gain or loss from the company's equity position during the stated accounting period.
(b) *Balance sheet*: This is a report, for a given date, of the accounting value of all of the corporation's assets, liabilities and shareholder's equity.
(c) *Cash flow statement*: This report is an analysis of all activities during the accounting period that affected cash, impacted primarily by operations, financing and investments.

Financial reports can serve as a gauge for overall financial health, as well as the direction of specific operations, of a company. For example, in 2015 PepsiCo reported that restructuring charges of US$450 million were incurred during 2012–2014 which enhanced the company's 'cost-competitiveness and . . . funding for future brand-building and innovation initiatives' (Pepsico 2015, 143). A global health researcher might seek to understand how this impacted on the type of food products produced by PepsiCo and where in the world they are marketed successfully in terms of profits.

Fourth, annual reports usually contain a two-part *auditor's report* prepared by independent accountants (appointed by shareholders) on whether the corporation's financial report complies with relevant legislation, national accounting practices and international financial reporting standards. The purpose of this sub-report is to give 'a true and fair view of the reported financial performance, financial position and cash flows of the company' (CPA Australia 2014, 11). An auditor's report should also state whether 'all information, explanations and assistance necessary for the audit has been given, whether sufficient financial records have been kept to enable the financial report to be prepared and audited, and whether other records and registers as required' (CPA Australia 2015, 11). A modified or qualified opinion is given if the auditor does not have access to sufficient or relevant information.

A good starting point, for obtaining current and previous annual reports, is corporate websites. Many companies, whether publicly- or privately owned, use websites for public communication purposes. Information made available may also include non-compulsory reports such as on corporate social responsibility (CSR) initiatives, company histories, organisational charts, senior executive or director biographies, speeches, policy statements, product information and supply chains.

Beyond information issued by corporations, other types of data sources are assembled and analysed by third-parties for regulatory, advisory, monitoring and educational purposes. These data concern the finances, assets, holdings, markets and products of a specific company, industry, sector or market. Company filings (e.g. annual reports, registration statements, stock acquisitions, share issues) to regulatory authorities may be searchable to track a corporation's acquisitions. Financial data vendors provide market data to financial firms, traders and investors to inform their decision making. Industry associations may conduct and disseminate information to support their members. For example, the industry-funded International Tobacco Growers Association (ITGA) 'publicises and disseminates a range of specialised materials that include . . . [a] quarterly newsletter, The Tobacco Courier, reports, research and issues papers' (ITGA n.d.). Table 18.1 sets out these additional types of data.

Table 18.1. Additional types of data on transnational corporations

Type of data	*Description*
Company profiles and registers	Financial and operational profiles of publicly traded companies, including history, business descriptions, annual sales, financial statistics, analyst ratings, valuations, stock symbols, stock price quotes, company news, competitor information, investor and industry reports, employees and the names of senior executives and company officers
Directory of company directors	Names and profiles of board of director members and executives of companies, including directorships and offices held, education and professional associations
Dividends data	Records of payments to shareholders from company profits or holdings, reinvestment plans, rights offerings (shareholders to buy further shares), foreign currency dividends and history of dividend payments
Financial performance data	Company performance data compared to competitors based on benchmarks such as number of businesses in industry, profitability (including net profits/losses), revenues and expenses, assets/liabilities and financial ratios.
Fixed income data	Data on bonds and preferred stocks, which pay fixed returns, issued by corporations to raise financing for ongoing operations, M&A, or to expand business; levels and outstanding corporate debt; yields and maturity dates

Type of data	*Description*
Fund reports	Mutual fund profiles that include an overview of each fund, holdings, comparison of the fund's performance with the market and its competitors, risk and return information, a current quote, charts and statistics
Industry and sector surveys	Business and financial analysis by industry and sector, including trends and forecasts over time and market
Market share research	Rankings of top companies in a given industry or sector by share of revenues in a given market
Mergers and acquisitions	Mergers, acquisitions and divestitures including transaction values, buyers and sellers, resultant industry concentration ratios
New issues data	New stock and bond offerings by publicly traded companies, governments and agencies by security type, market, currency and other features
Predecessor and defunct companies	Record of company name, incorporation changes, amalgamations, takeovers, acquisitions and dissolutions
Stock reports	Equity evaluations of public companies, quantitative and technical analysis and analyst recommendations for stocks listed on industry, national and regional stock exchanges
Trade data	International shipment of goods; profiles of suppliers including data on their shipments

These types of data, which are particularly relevant to transnational corporations, can be obtained from four main sources (Table 18.2). The first is *search engines* (e.g. Google Finance, Yahoo Finance), which provide financial data, notably stock prices, in real time and over time so that investors can track the performance of specific listed companies. The second is *research or consultancy firms* (e.g. Euromonitor, Economist Intelligence Unit, McKinsey), which undertake paid analysis of companies, industries or markets. The third is *specialist media* (e.g. *Financial Times*, Bloomberg, Reuters), which provide news and information to the business community, and produce company, industry and market profiles. The fourth is *business information service providers* (e.g. Business Insights: Global, Factiva, LexisNexis Academic), which bring together other sources in searchable databases. In practice, these four types of data sources are increasingly converging, with providers supplying many types of data and analytical services. When deciding which sources to use, the main factors to consider are the companies, industries, sectors and markets covered; historical range of data; types of data (i.e. annual reports, stock prices, news); independence from conflicts of interest; searchability; and affordability.

Table 18.2. Selected sources of business and financial data on transnational corporations

Source	*Information available*	*Terms of access*
Google Finance	• Financial information in real time, stock quotes and charts, news and currency conversions • Summary, news, related companies, historical prices and financial data on major publicly listed companies worldwide	Free
Yahoo Finance	• Financial information in real time on stock prices and trends, stock markets, bonds, commodities, indices, currencies, business news, videos	Free
StockCharts.com	• Technical charts for US and Canadian stocks, funds and indices	Free and fee
Hoover's Online	• Detailed company profiles for 28 million international companies • In-depth coverage of >40,000 leading companies by revenue, market share, technology and industry • Company histories, strategies, market positions, major events, links to news and financial analyses	Free and fee
Thompson ONE	• Financial data on public companies, as well as merger and acquisition information and industry and market data	Subscription
Economist Intelligence Unit	• Free reports, webinars and podcasts on current issues affecting specific countries, regions and industries • Analyses of countries, risk and industries	Free, subscription and fee
Euromonitor International	• Market research on every key trend and driver produced by analysts in over 80 countries • Business intelligence reports and data to industry • Historic trends and forecasts by region, country, category, channel and consumer	Free and fee
Bloomberg	• Data on markets, commodities, stocks, currencies and futures in the Americas, Europe, Asia and Middle East • Company profiles • Business news and analysis	Free
Financial Times Companies	• Data on markets, commodities, stocks, currencies and futures • Company profiles • Business news and analysis by sector and region	Subscription

Source	*Information available*	*Terms of access*
Fortune Global 500	• Rankings of world's largest corporations by sector, revenue, profits, assets, employees and home country	Free and subscription
Business Insights: Global (Gale Cengage Learning)	• Economic and business indicators to analyse economies, companies and industries • Global company, industry and country overviews and interactive rankings and statistics, with quick links to associated news, case studies and academic journal articles • Global industry research reports for specific industries within specific countries • Articles from academic journals, periodicals and news media • Topic overviews on major areas of international business • Company histories and market share data	Individual or institutional subscription
Factiva	• International news and business information drawn from more than 28,000 sources in 23 languages in more than 150 countries • Full-text coverage of hundreds of business magazines	Subscription
LexisNexis Academic	• Full text resources on business and financial information, news media (including transcripts), company reports, regulation	Subscription

WHAT TYPE OF QUESTIONS CAN BUSINESS AND FINANCIAL DATA ANSWER?

There are four main types of questions relevant to corporations and GHG that business and financial data can help to address. First, effective GHG seeks to prevent or mitigate adverse impacts on population health. Business and financial data can help identify and document what Freudenberg and Galea (2008, 87) call 'corporate practices', that is 'decisions about production, pricing, distribution and promotion of their products' as social determinants of health. This data can help understand what health-related goods and services are produced, how many are sold and in which markets and what production and employment practices are used. For instance, a study of 43 countries by Goran, Ulijaszek and Ventura (2013) found that type 2 diabetes rates are 20% higher where high-fructose corn syrup (HFCS) is used. To develop appropriate regulatory measures, business and financial data can be used to analyse changes in global patterns of HFCS production and consumption. Researchers may, for instance, identify trends in the size and structure of producers and industry, concentration of industry ownership, production methods, revenues and costs and use of HFCS along a global value chain (IbisWorld 2016).

Second, effective GHG requires understanding of the reasons why corporations behave as they do. Business and financial data can be used to more fully explain *corporate business strategies and tactics*. For example, through annual report statements by senior executives of past decisions and future plans, a researcher can determine why a company operates in one jurisdiction over another (e.g. tax liability, regulatory environment). The reports can also provide trend data on profits and losses for specific goods and services, and shifts in targeted markets. For example, the Annual Report of Diageo (2015), the transnational alcoholic beverages company, describes 'acquisitions to broaden our geographical footprint and our category depth and range', including the brand's acquisitions in Nigeria, India and Mexico. Company statements can be triangulated with reports by business analysts on shifts in global production and consumption worldwide. While these reports are intended to support the business community, available data can help global health researchers understand the rationale behind new products and brands, anticipate populations at growing risk of alcohol-related diseases and evaluate marketing strategies in emerging markets. The public health community, in turn, can develop appropriate policy responses, including regulatory frameworks.

Third, effective GHG requires a better understanding of how corporations increasingly operate across and beyond national jurisdictions. Business and financial data can be used to identify affiliated companies of a corporation, including those operating in different countries or sectors. This can help researchers understand a corporation's economic reach and potential political influence. Data can also be used to analyse the globalisation strategies of firms and the extent to which they are achieved. This can be measured, for example, by a shift from the *multinational corporation*, whereby domestic operations of a firm are replicated in foreign operations through a parent company-subsidiary structure, to the *transnational corporation* where a more decentralised and globally distributed organisational structure is adopted, divided by function, production or service, customer or location (Dicken 2015). This restructuring of a corporation, in turn, suggests the potential need for coordinated adoption and implementation of regulatory measures. Lee, Eckhardt and Holden (2016, 2), for example, argue that 'collective action to stem the tobacco pandemic requires fuller understanding of the nature and dynamics of tobacco industry globalization'. The authors set out an interdisciplinary research agenda, including clearer definition and measurement, which draws on many of the data sources described in this chapter.

Finally, business and financial data offers a fuller understanding of the varied *external relations of corporations*. The political influence of corporations, for instance, can be facilitated by a so-called revolving door between the business and policy worlds (see Chapter 15). Annual reports (notably corporate governance and remuneration reports) list company directors and senior executives (Mattera 2014). Additional roles and affiliations held by such individuals, in other companies, charities or public bodies, may be found in directories of directors. Filings to regulatory bodies detail share issues to company directors, which can help identify potential conflicts of interest when analysing policy influence. For instance, in the searchable online US SEC database of filings, there are documents pertaining to the issuing of shares to seven individually named non-executive directors by UK pharmaceutical company GlaxoSmithKline (US SEC 2016). These interpersonal relationships can, in turn, be mapped using network analysis to illuminate the political economy of corporate–state relations (Mizruchi 2007).

External relations extend to CSR initiatives which many corporations describe in non-compulsory reports on social and environmental sustainability. For global health researchers, such reports can be used to inform the conduct of *social accounting* (or non-financial reporting) defined as 'an approach to reporting a firm's activities which stresses the need for the identification of socially relevant behaviour, the determination of those to whom the company is accountable for its social performance and the development of appropriate measures and reporting techniques' (Crowther 2000, 20). For example, Moerman and van der Laan (2013) undertook a social accounting of corporate disclosures relating to the uncertainty arising from long-term ('long-tail') liabilities of the Australian asbestos industry. The study found 'significant gaps between what companies disclose in relation to asbestos, and what is reported in the media. These findings reinforce the widely held belief that mandatory corporate disclosures or "accounts" suffer from inherent limitations, providing no more than a partial picture of an entity's impact on society' (Moerman and van der Laan 2013, 5). Civil society organisations provide useful summaries of the financial records of large companies for social accounting purposes. For instance, the Transnationale Project compiles data on operating results, ownership structures, shareholders, investments, litigation and fines on thousands of companies worldwide, which is accessible via a searchable online database. *Corporate Watch*, CorporateRegister.com and the Dutch organisation SOMO, for example, compile data on the charitable contributions of corporations. In the United States, the Corporate Giving Directory publishes profiles of major American corporate foundations and corporate giving programmes. The Foundation Center is an online source of information on US corporate and other foundations, and publishes the National Directory of Corporate Giving. All are useful sources for improving the transparency of CSR activities and their potential use in furthering the policy influence of corporations.

HOW HAS THIS DATA BEEN USED TO STUDY CORPORATE ACTORS AND GHG?

There are limited examples to date of the application of business and financial data in global health research to study corporations. Gilmore (2012) draws on annual reports, investor relations materials, financial analyst reports and market research to analyse how the world tobacco market is changing, adaptation by transnational tobacco companies (TTCs) and the implications for tobacco control. There is much potential to increase the use of this type of data by drawing on currently available internal tobacco industry documents (see Chapter 16). In a study of direct-to-consumer drug advertising, Liang and Mackey (2011) identify the ten largest pharmaceutical companies and top ten grossing medicines worldwide using IMS Health sales data (revenue by company and product). The authors then use this data as a starting point for a detailed analysis of the companies' use of social media.

There has been extensive use of business and financial data in the study of corporations in other disciplines, most notably political science, international political economy and business studies. Magnan (2015, 1) examines new patterns of financial investment in farmland and agricultural production, as part of the 'financialization of the global agri-food sector, a process through which finance capital and financial logics exercise increasing influence over food production and distribution'. Research on corporations forms a core focus in business studies, with the analysis of CSR activities providing a useful model for applying business and financial data. Using the *Business Week* ranking of corporations (average of eight publicly reported measures of historical financial performance), for example, Verschoor (1998) finds an association between overall financial performance and an emphasis on ethics as an aspect of corporate governance.

STRENGTHS AND WEAKNESSES OF BUSINESS AND FINANCIAL DATA

Global health research has focused, to date, on documenting the health impacts of particular products produced by corporations such as alcoholic beverages, asbestos or highly processed foods. Additionally, global health researchers have examined industry or market-level trends, and the increased production and consumption of health-harming products and practices. Business and financial data can offer a fuller, and more nuanced, account of why and how specific products are produced, where they fit within corporate and industry strategy and the prospects for improving corporate practices through GHG. Analysis addressing the entire global supply chain, for example, enables researchers to pinpoint where there are needs and opportunities for strengthening regulation. For example, Maloni and Brown (2006, 35) develop 'a comprehensive tool to support food industry practitioners and researchers in the assessment of strategic and operational supply chain CSR practices'.

One weakness of this type of data is the need for specialist knowledge of core concepts and terms from the business and finance worlds before the meaning and significance of these data sources can be derived. There are several helpful introductory guides to interpreting annual reports and other data sources available which researchers can draw upon. Another weakness is the need to critically analyse data originating from corporate actors because it is carefully generated and presented to put the corporation or industry in a positive light. In many cases, third-party news and analyses draw directly from corporate sources. Even where public relations are not the primary purpose, business and financial data is collected to serve commercial rather than social purposes. Using such data, to address global health research questions, must take account of the purpose and methodology of the data. Data provided by consultancy firms, such as KPMG, must be contextualised with knowledge of their financial relationships with specific industries. There may also be concerns about the reliability of data reported by some companies to third parties. Financial reporting standards and audits can improve reliability, but implementation of such requirements varies across jurisdictions. Moreover, business and financial data produced by some sources, such as financial data analysts, is sold commercially and may be unaffordable to global health researchers. For all the aforementioned reasons, where possible, researchers need to triangulate business and financial data with other sources such as interviews, surveys and focus groups.

CONCLUSION

There is an opportunity for global health researchers to substantially expand their repertoire of information sources through the use of business and financial data. To date, there has been limited application of these data sources despite their growth in scope, abundance and accessibility. Indeed, the sheer scale of data available, alongside the need for specialist knowledge, has hindered their application to analyse corporations and GHG. This introduction to business and finance data is intended to encourage researchers to explore this rich resource, develop methods relevant to global health and undertake analyses complementing other efforts to achieve more effective GHG.

FURTHER READING

CPA Australia. 2014. 'A Guide to Understanding Annual Reports'. Sydney. https://www.cpaaustralia.com.au/~/media/corporate/allfiles/document/professional-resources/reporting/guide-to-understanding-annual-reporting.pdf?la=en.

Global Corporate Governance Forum and the International Center for Journalists. 2012. *Whose Running the Company? A Guide to Reporting on Corporate Governance*. Washington, DC. http://www.ifc.org/wps/wcm/connect/aa93d6804d394d5eabc8eff81ee631cc/Whos+Running+the+Company+Rev+-+Lo+Res.pdf?MOD=AJPERES.

Mattera, Philip. 2014. *Dirt Diggers Guide to Strategic Corporate Research*. Washington, DC: Corporate Research Project. September. http://corp-research.org/dddresearchguide.

US Securities and Exchange Commission. 'Beginners Guide to Financial Statements'. Accessed September 19, 2016. http://www.sec.gov/investor/pubs/begfinstmtguide.htm.

REFERENCES

CPA Australia. 2014. 'A Guide to Understanding Annual Reports'. Sydney. https://www.cpaaustralia.com.au/~/media/corporate/allfiles/document/professional-resources/reporting/guide-to-understanding-annual-reporting.pdf?la=en.

Crowther, David. 2000. *Social and Environmental Accounting*. London: *Financial Times*/Prentice Hall.

Diageo. 2015. 'Annual Report'. file:///C:/Users/Kelley%20Lee/Downloads/Diageo_AR15%20Strategic%20Report.pdf. Accessed September 19, 2016. https://www.diageo.com/Lists/Resources/.../Diageo%20Interactive%20AR2015.pdf.

Dicken, Peter. 2015. *Global Shift, Mapping the Changing Contours of the World Economy*, 7th edition. New York: Guilford Press.

Financial Times. 2013. 'The Future of Business Data'. 22 May. http://databoard.ft.com/.

Freudenberg, Nicholas and Sandro Galea. 2008. 'The Impact of Corporate Practices on Health: Implications for Health Policy'. *Journal of Public Health Policy* 29(1): 86–104.

Gilmore, Anna. 2012. 'Understanding the Vector in Order to Plan Effective Tobacco Control Policies: An Analysis of Contemporary Tobacco Industry Materials'. *Tobacco Control* 21(2): 119–26.

Goran, Michael, Stanley J. Ulijaszek and Emily E. Ventura. 2013. 'High Fructose Corn Syrup and Diabetes Prevalence: A Global Perspective'. *Global Public Health* 8(1): 55–64.

IbisWorld. 2016. 'High Fructose Corn Syrup Production Market Research Report'. June. Accessed September 19, 2016. http://clients1.ibisworld.com/reports/us/industry/default.aspx?entid=5945.

ITGA. n.d. *Who We Are and What We Do*. Castelo Branco, Portugal: International Tobacco Growers Association. http://www.tobaccoleaf.org/conteudos/default.asp?ID=7&IDP=2&P=2.

Lee, Kelley, Jappe Eckhardt and Christopher Holden, C. 2016. 'Tobacco Industry Globalization and Global Health Governance: Towards an Interdisciplinary Research Agenda'. *Palgrave Communications* 2: 16037. doi:10.1057/palcomms.2016.37.

Liang, Bryan A. and Timothy K. Mackey. 2011. 'Prevalence and Global Health Implications of Social Media in Direct-to-Consumer Drug Advertising'. *Journal of Medical Internet Research* 3(3): e64.

Magnan, André. 2015. 'The Financialization of Agri-Food in Canada and Australia: Corporate Farmland and Farm Ownership in the Grains and Oilseed Sector'. *Journal of Rural Studies* 41: 1–12.

Maloni, Michael J. and Michael E. Brown. 2006. 'Corporate Social Responsibility in the Supply Chain: An Application in the Food Industry'. *Journal of Business Ethics* 68(1): 35–52.

Mattera, Philip. 2014. *Dirt Diggers Guide to Strategic Corporate Research*. Washington, DC: Corporate Research Project. September. http://corp-research.org/dddresearchguide.

Mizruchi, Mark. 2007. 'Political Economy and Network Analysis: An Untapped Convergence'. *Sociologica* 2. doi:10.2383/24765.

Moerman, Lee and Sandra van der Laan. 2013. *Accounting and Long-Tail Liabilities: The Case of Asbestos*. London: Certified Accountants Educational Trust.

Nestlé. 2015. 'Corporate Governance Report 2015'. Geneva. http://www.nestle.com/asset-library/documents/library/documents/corporate_governance/corp_governance_report_2015_en.pdf.

Pepsico. 2015. 'Annual Report'. New York. http://pepsico.ca/en/downloads/pepsico-2015-annual-report_final_s57dqszgmy22ggn.pdf.

US SEC. 2016. 'GlaxoSmithKline plc, Notification of Transactions of Directors, Persons Discharging Managerial Responsibilities or Connected Persons'. Washington, DC. 1 July. https://www.sec.gov/Archives/edgar/data/1131399/000119163816002259/gsk201607016k2.htm.

Verschoor, Curtis. 1998. 'A Study of the Link between a Corporation's Financial Performance and Its Commitment to Ethics'. *Journal of Business Ethics* 7(3): 1509–16.

Chapter 19

Using Freedom of Information Requests

Becky Freeman

Freedom of Information (FOI) legislation is neither new nor novel, with Sweden adopting the first FOI law in 1766. A wave of FOI laws have been adopted worldwide since the late 1990s (Ackerman and Sandoval-Ballesteros 2006). FOI laws recognise that citizen participation in government cannot be considered complete without mechanisms for ensuring access to government information. Access to information, in turn, enhances accountability and promotes more effective decision making and greater trust in the policies implemented.

Many countries have long-standing laws based on similar principles of transparency, accountability and openness. As Ackerman and Sandoval-Ballesteros (2006) write:

> FOI law gives citizens, other residents, and interested parties the right to access documents held by the government without being obliged to demonstrate any legal interest or 'standing'. Under a FOI law, government documents are assumed to be public unless specifically exempt by the law itself, and individuals can access them without explaining why or for what purpose they need them. In short, FOI laws imply a change in the principle of the provision of government information from a 'need to know' basis to a 'right to know' basis.

At the same time, FOI laws vary across different countries in terms of their operational effectiveness in four primary areas (Ackerman and Sandoval-Ballesteros 2006):

- Coverage, the extent to which FOI laws apply to all aspects of government and publicly funded initiatives
- Exemptions, how readily government can withhold information even when covered by the law

- Enforcement, including compliance monitoring
- Ease of access, whether information can be retrieved efficiently and at low cost

This chapter discusses the scope for using FOI requests as a source of data for research on corporations and global health governance (GHG). After describing what FOI requests are and how they are made, the research questions that can be pursued through such requests are considered. Possibilities and examples of using FOI requests to study corporations and GHG are also presented. Finally, the chapter concludes with a discussion on how corporations can themselves use FOI requests to thwart research that challenges their interests.

WHAT CAN YOU REQUEST UNDER FOI?

Individuals can make FOI requests to access documents held by government institutions that are otherwise not exempt from FOI laws. These include, but are not limited to, reports, correspondence, meeting minutes, electronic files, maps, photographs, plans and financial information. Applicants may also find out what personal information is being held about them or others. FOI processes may be used to obtain submissions to government policy consultation processes that have otherwise not been published.

FOI laws present researchers with an opportunity to access documentation of relevance to the research questions they are investigating. This is especially useful for researchers working in the areas of controversy or political sensitivity, where relevant data sources may be limited or difficult to identify. An example is an FOI submission made to the Treasury Department of the Australian government for data on total cigarettes entering the country after payment of taxes and duties. The Treasury does not routinely publish this data, but it is an excellent means to assess trends in population-level consumption and tax revenue from tobacco over time. It is also a method for estimating sales volumes, which are not publicly accessible from tobacco companies operating in Australia. After receiving this request, the Treasury published its response, including the requested information, on its FOI Disclosure Log website (Australian Government and the Treasury 2015). This means that not only does the original applicant receive the information, but it also becomes available to the public, other researchers and the media.

HOW FOI REQUESTS ARE MADE

The discussion of FOI requests in this section focuses on the Australian system of FOI requests, with which the author is most familiar. However, the principles identified are widely applicable and serve to highlight the types of issues which may arise when making FOI requests elsewhere. The FOI laws of each country have their own particular processes and procedures, and researchers should familiarise themselves with them prior to making a request to ensure they are successful and to avoid unnecessary delays and impediments to data access.

Generally, requests are made, either directly through the government department concerned (often online) or through an officer/commissioner of information. While there is usually no fee to place an FOI request, there are often processing charges (for staff time, photocopying) if an applicant decides to proceed after a request has been evaluated. There may be limits to the range and volume of documents which can be requested. Or requests may need to be highly specific. FOI requests may be returned to an applicant, and an additional request necessary, if insufficient detail is provided to allow the identification of relevant documents within a specific timeframe. A sample of this step-by-step process, and associated fees, from the Australian National Health and Medical Research Council is provided in Box 19.1.

Box 19.1. Sample FOI request process, from the Australian National Health and Medical Research Council

The application must:
- be made in writing;
- state that it is an application for the purposes of the FOI Act;
- provide enough information about the documents for a responsible officer of the agency to identify them; and
- specify how notices and documents can be sent to you (for example an email address).

Fees and charges

There is no application fee for an FOI application (including an interview review application). There are no costs where you request access to documents containing only your personal information. However, processing charges may apply to other requests. The most common charges are:

Search and retrieval: time we spend searching for or retrieving a document	$15.00 per hour
Decision making: time we spend in deciding to grant or refuse a request, including examining documents, consulting with other parties, and making deletions.	First five hours: nil. Subsequent hours: $20 per hour
Transcript: preparing a transcript from a sound recording, shorthand or similar medium	$4.40 per page of transcript

(*Continued*)

Box 19.1. Continued

Photocopy	$0.10 per page
Inspection: supervision by an NHMRC officer of your inspection of documents or hearing or viewing an audio or visual recordings at our premises.	$6.25 per half hour (or part thereof)
Delivery: posting or delivering a copy of a document at your request.	Cost of postage or delivery

What you can expect from us:
Once you have made an FOI application, we will tell you within 5 working days that we have received your application. We will also give you an estimate of the charges that apply to your application. We will give you our decision within 30 calendar days unless that time has been extended. If a document contains information about a third party, we will need to consult them and may need to extend the time to give you our decision by another 30 calendar days. We may also seek your agreement to extend the time by up to 30 calendar days if your application is complex.

Source: Australian National Health and Medical Research Council (2012).

Some scholars have pointed out that FOI requests are not as well used by researchers as they could be and that some researchers may avoid using such processes for fear they may appear confrontational or difficult (Brown 2009). Researchers may avoid unnecessary confrontation by first directly requesting documents of interest from a relevant government body. If this proves unsuccessful, a formal FOI request could then be submitted. In addition, journalists can be helpful in lodging FOI requests. Working collaboratively with media, to request and analyse information procured through FOI processes, can be a powerful way of ensuring public dissemination of findings.

FOI REQUESTS AND RESEARCH ON CORPORATIONS

FOI laws are built on the principle of a citizen's right to transparent government. Given that public bodies, which corporations seek to influence, are subject to FOI laws in many countries, requests can be used to gain important insights into corporate interaction with government. Requests can thus be used to expose concealed conflict of interests or undue influence by corporations on public policy. Key research questions that may be answered using information obtained from FOI requests include the following:

- How corporations influence or block policy reforms?
- How closely do government agencies, and corporations with vested interests, work together?
- What influences and pressures might corporations put on government agencies, including both financial and political, to further their interests?

FOI requests can also be used to find out if public statements are obscuring uncomfortable truths about government–corporate relations. In 2014, the Australian government launched a website that provided consumers with information about the nutritional value of packaged foods. The website used a voluntary star-rating system to rank the relative healthiness of food products. It was then suddenly shut down, without clear explanation, on the insistence of the chief of staff to the assistant health minister. Media subsequently reported on the conflict of interest by the chief of staff, who was also a co-owner of a lobbying business, Australian Public Affairs, which had a number of food companies as clients. The minister insisted that the chief of staff had outlined in a letter 'how he would ensure his co-ownership of the lobbying company . . . would not interfere with his role in creating healthy food policy' (Corderoy 2014). Journalists filed FOI requests to obtain a copy of this supposed letter and were told that such a document could not be shared as 'it did not exist' (Corderoy 2014). The minister was subsequently censured for her actions, and the website was relaunched several months later.

FOI processes can also be used to obtain submissions to government policy consultation processes that have otherwise not been published. The submissions can then be analysed to give clues as to which think tank and front group organisations are being paid by corporations to try and influence policy debates. These sorts of lobby groups are notoriously silent on their membership and financial donors (Sourcewatch 2009), but assessing their arguments and message framing gives clues as to which corporate interests they are likely representing.

Finally, there is substantial literature on the positive features, and limitations, of specific FOI laws (see Further Reading). One important imbalance of existing FOI laws is that they only apply to certain government-funded entities and do not apply at all to the private sector. For example, while the tobacco industry may demand transparency from government departments, and other publicly funded institutions, about the process of formulating and adopting tobacco control policies, this same level of transparency is not required of the tobacco industry's own efforts to influence policy making (Dimopoulos, Mitchell and Voon 2015). As shown later, this imbalance is currently exploited by the tobacco industry to prevent, stall and discredit tobacco control.

USING FOI REQUESTS TO RESEARCH CORPORATIONS AND GHG

While FOI law has largely been adopted by national governments, there are opportunities for them to be used to obtain information on the transnational activities of corporations, including their efforts to influence GHG. One approach is to employ FOI requests to obtain information that can be triangulated with what is available in the public domain. For example, a study of the scale and nature of lobbying by transnational tobacco companies against the European Union Tobacco Products Directive included analysis of 581 documents obtained through FOI requests. The documents were used to identify industry lobbying positions and strategies to delay and prevent certain regulations, and the extensive use of third parties. The authors deductively analysed the documents by applying an understanding of a document's content in a wider policy context, while identifying conceptual themes that were then tested as data collection progressed. This study revealed the true extent of tobacco industry lobbying, with one company employing over 160 lobbyists. It also showed repeated and undisclosed contact between senior EU officials and the tobacco industry, resulting in successful delay and amendments to the Tobacco Products Directive (Peters et al. 2016).

Another example is the use of FOI requests to document the full extent of partnership between leading obesity scientists and the North American arm of Coca-Cola, the world's largest producer of sugary drinks. In a 2015 article published in *The New York Times*, it was revealed that

> the beverage giant has teamed up with influential scientists who are advancing this message in medical journals, at conferences and through social media. To help the scientists get the word out, Coke has provided financial and logistical support to a new non-profit organization called the Global Energy Balance Network (GEBN), which promotes the argument that weight-conscious Americans are overly fixated on how much they eat and drink while not paying enough attention to exercise. (O'Connor 2015)

While the researchers in question had disclosed that they had received an unrestricted educational gift from Coca-Cola, in an editorial published in the *British Journal of Sports Medicine* (Blair, Hand and Hill 2015), the degree of influence this carried over the conduct of the research was not made clear. FOI requests to the University of South Carolina showed that the lead investigator of the GEBN had received more than US$3.5 million from Coca-Cola since 2008. The GEBN team, which included researchers from the University of Colorado, West Virginia University and University of South Carolina, denied that Coca-Cola had any influence on the research design or publication of results. However, FOI requests for correspondence between GEBN researchers and Coca-Cola executives revealed that Coca-Cola helped choose the GEBN leaders, create its mission statement and design the promotional website. The researchers, in return, expressed their intentions to be supportive of Coca-Cola's corporate agenda, stating in one email: 'I want to help your company avoid the image of being a problem in people's lives and back to being a company that brings important and fun things to them' (The Associated Press 2015). Following these revelations, the University of Colorado returned all funds to Coca-Cola, and the GEBN was shut down.

EXPOSING CORPORATE ABUSE OF FOI LAWS

Mitchell and Voon (2014) outline how the Australian tobacco industry used FOI requests to divert, frustrate and intimidate Department of Health officials in an effort to derail plain packaging. British American Tobacco Australasia (BATA) and Philip Morris (PM) both filed numerous, high-volume and vague FOI requests that required months of processing time and hundreds of thousands of dollars to prepare. For example, a 2010 BATA FOI request resulted in a final charge to BATA of more than US$100,000, but the actual cost to the Australian Department of Health for dealing with the request over 18 months was estimated at over US$600,000. Similarly, abuse of the FOI process is illustrated in PM's actions. A PM FOI request took months to prepare and release. Following actual receipt of documents requested, PM requested an internal review. PM then appealed the internal review findings. Health officials undertook significant work to prepare for the appeal, which was then abruptly withdrawn by PM a week before the actual hearing. Despite these industry make-work tactics, plain packaging was enacted in Australia in December 2012 and is being adopted in many other countries.

It is clear that corporations may seek to use FOI requests to intimidate, stall and deflect attention from their own agendas. This misuse of FOI processes is not limited to corporations but also includes the think tanks and lobbyists they employ. In Australia, the Institute of Public Affairs (IPA) submitted hundreds of FOI requests for documents on climate change, prompting a government warning that the volume of requests was unreasonable and vexatious (Ries 2015). The IPA is not required, in turn, to make public its donors or members, although tellingly, the think tank focuses its work on challenging 'bad' climate change policies, the Nanny State, high taxes and excess regulation (Hamilton 2012).

Researchers in some jurisdictions may also be subject to corporate-motivated FOI requests, including to confidentially collected data. Researchers at the University of Stierling were subjected to an FOI request concerning a study of teen smoking from PM. The request was sent under the guise of an international law firm, demanding full access to information on the study, including primary data files. The research team prepared a 60-page response, outlining why ethical principles did not allow them to share data that participants had been promised would be kept secure and confidential. A two-year legal battle ensued between PM and the university, which was eventually dropped by PM following scathing media attention. However, this was not before many months of precious time and substantial university resources had been wasted. As the lead researcher for the project Gerard Hastings (2015) observed, 'The identity of the applicant is irrelevant in FOI. The fact that this was not a request from "the people of the United Kingdom" but a powerful multinational producing an addictive and lethal carcinogen, mattered not a whit.'

CONCLUSION

FOI requests can be usefully applied by researchers seeking to study corporations and GHG, including their undue influence of public institutions at the national, regional and global levels. Much of the knowledge we have about the tobacco industry results from the release of internal documents following US litigation (Hurt et al. 2009). Lack of access to comparable documents from other industries means much less is known about the global health impacts of their products and their attempts to shape GHG. There is need to seek alternative sources of such data, and FOI requests offer a potentially effective means of doing so, even despite their current limitations. Such requests can expose corporate influence on policy making, research and funding.

There are growing calls to hold corporations to the same FOI standards as government agencies (Monbiot 2012). The lack of corporate accountability and transparency, for example, was a significant contributory factor to the global financial crisis beginning in the mid-2000s (Crotty 2009). Furthermore, revelations about the widespread use of phone hacking, and a wider culture of unethical practices within the UK media (UK Government 2015), have provided compelling evidence of the need for fuller transparency and accountability to protect public interest (Dorfman et al. 2012). It bears repeating that the tobacco industry, which successfully hid knowledge of the true nature of its highly addictive and deadly products for decades (Bero 2003), strategically uses FOI laws to prevent effective public health regulations. Yet documents about its tactics and products have been released only when required by legal action or for carefully crafted public relations purposes (Cummings, Morley and Hyland 2002). Extending FOI laws to the private sector is not without precedence. South Africa has implemented an access to information law that includes the private sector, although there is limited evidence it has been operationalised to its full potential (Adeleke 2011). The Promotion of Access to Information Act states that individuals and government may access records held by private bodies when the record is deemed 'necessary for the exercise or protection' of human rights (Banisar 2006).

Meanwhile, there is much potential for researchers to make fuller use of current FOI requests, learning from the ways that investigative journalists and civil society organisations have done so. FOI laws can provide essential information on the inner workings of government and make them more subject to critical scrutiny. In this way, researchers can make corporate efforts to influence GHG more transparent and curb corporate abuse of FOI laws.

FURTHER READING

Berger, Mitchell. 2011. 'The Freedom of Information Act: Implications for Public Health Policy and Practice'. *Public Health Reports* 126(3): 428–32.

Dimopoulos, Georgina, Andrew D. Mitchell and Tania S.L. Voon. 2015. 'The Tobacco Industry's Strategic Use of Freedom of Information Laws: A Comparative Analysis'. *Oxford University Comparative Law Forum* (forthcoming). http://ssrn.com/abstract=2725638.

Rutgers University. 2015. '1st Global Conference on Transparency Research'. Rutgers University, Newark, 19–20 May. https://spaa.newark.rutgers.edu/1stGCTR.

REFERENCES

Ackerman, John M. and Irma E. Sandoval-Ballesteros. 2006. 'The Global Explosion of Freedom of Information Laws'. *Administrative Law Reviews* 58(1): 85–130.

Adeleke, F. 2011. 'The Case for Corporate Transparency in Africa'. Paper presented at the First Global Conference on Transparency Research, Rutgers University, Newark, 19–20 May. https://spaa.newark.rutgers.edu/sites/default/files/files/Transparency_Research_Conference/Papers/Adeleke_Fola.pdf.

The Associated Press. 2015. 'Excerpts from Emails between Coke, Anti-Obesity Group'. *The Associated Press*, 24 November. http://bigstory.ap.org/article/eac573c073b6429bb302d94acc787c2b/excerpts-emails-between-coke-anti-obesity-group.

Australian Government and the Treasury. 2015. 'Response to FOI Requests 1703'. Accessed September 19, 2016. http://www.treasury.gov.au/~/media/Treasury/Access%20to%20Information/Disclosure%20Log/2015/1703/Downloads/PDF/Document_1_1703.ashx.

Australian National Health and Medical Research Council. 2012. 'Freedom of Information'. Accessed September 19, 2016. https://www.nhmrc.gov.au/about/freedom-information.

Banisar, David. 2006. 'Freedom of Information around the World 2006: A Global Survey of Access to Government Information Laws'. Accessed September 19, 2016. http://www.freedominfo.org/documents/global_survey2006.pdf.

Bero, Lisa. 2013. ‘Implications of the Tobacco Industry Documents for Public Health and Policy’. *Annual Review of Public Health* 24(1): 267–88.

Blair, Steven N., Gregory A. Hand and James O. Hill. 2015. ‘Energy Balance: A Crucial Issue for Exercise and Sports Medicine’. *British Journal of Sports Medicine* 49: 970–71.

Brown, Kevin J. 2009. ‘COUNTERBLAST: Freedom of Information as a Research Tool: Realising Its Potential’. *The Howard Journal of Criminal Justice* 48(1): 88–91.

Corderoy, Amy. 2014. ‘Fiona Nash Conflict-of-Interest Documents “Do Not Exist”’. *Sydney Morning Herald*, 20 June. http://www.smh.com.au/federal-politics/fiona-nash-conflictofinterest-documents-do-not-exist-20140620-zsgas.html.

Crotty, James. 2009. ‘Structural Causes of the Global Financial Crisis: A Critical Assessment of the “New Financial Architecture”’. *Cambridge Journal of Economics* 33(4): 563–80.

Cummings, K. Michael, Christopher P. Morley and Andrew Hyland. 2002. ‘Failed Promises of the Cigarette Industry and Its Effect on Consumer Misperceptions about the Health Risks of Smoking’. *Tobacco Control* 11(Supplement 1): i110–17.

Dimopoulos, Georgina, Andrew D. Mitchell and Tania S.L. Voon. 2015. ‘The Tobacco Industry’s Strategic Use of Freedom of Information Laws: A Comparative Analysis’. *Oxford University Comparative Law Forum* (forthcoming). http://ssrn.com/abstract=2725638.

Dorfman, Lori, Andrew Cheyne, Lissy C. Friedman, Asiya Wadud and Mark Gottlieb. 2012. ‘Soda and Tobacco Industry Corporate Social Responsibility Campaigns: How Do They Compare?’ *PLoS Medicine* 9(6): e1001241.

Hamilton, Clive. 2012. ‘The Shadowy Figure of IPA Finances’. *ABC*, 23 February. http://www.abc.net.au/news/2012-02-24/hamilton-the-shadowy-world-of-ipa-finances/3849006.

Hastings, Gerald. 2015. ‘We Got an FOI Request from Big Tobacco – Here’s How It Went’. *The Conversation*. https://theconversation.com/we-got-an-foi-request-from-big-tobacco-heres-how-it-went-46457.

Hurt, Richard D., Jon O. Ebbert, Monique E. Muggli, Nikki J. Lockhart and Channing R. Robertson. 2009. ‘Open Doorway to Truth: Legacy of the Minnesota Tobacco Trial’. *Mayo Clinic Proceedings* 84(5): 446–56.

Mitchell, Andrew D. and Tania S.L. Voon. 2014. ‘Someone to Watch over Me: The Use of FOI Requests by the Tobacco Industry’. *Australian Journal of Administrative Law* 22(2): 18–22.

Monbiot, George. 2012. ‘Freedom of Information: My Monstrous Idea Will Keep Corporate Tyrants at Bay’. *The Guardian*, 7 May. http://www.theguardian.com/commentisfree/2012/may/07/freedom-information-my-monstrous-proposal.

O’Connor, Anahad. 2015. ‘Coca-Cola Funds Scientists Who Shift Blame for Obesity Away from Bad Diets’. *The New York Times*, 9 August. http://well.blogs.nytimes.com/2015/08/09/coca-cola-funds-scientists-who-shift-blame-for-obesity-away-from-bad-diets/.

Peters, Silvy, Helia Costa, David Stuckler, Martin McKee and Anna Gilmore. 2016. ‘The Revision of the 2014 European Tobacco Products Directive: An Analysis of the Tobacco Industry's Attempts to "Break the Health Silo"'. *Tobacco Control* 25(1): 108–17.

Ries, Nola. 2015. 'Tobacco Companies Should Be Free to Use Freedom of Information Laws, Even If We Don't Like It'. *The Conversation*, 20 August. https://theconversation.com/tobacco-companies-should-be-free-to-use-freedom-of-information-laws-even-if-we-dont-like-it-46408.

Sourcewatch. 2009. 'Think Tanks'. Accessed September 19, 2016. http://www.sourcewatch.org/index.php/Think_tanks.

UK Government. 2015. 'The Leveson Inquiry: Culture, Practice and Ethics of the Press'. Accessed September 19, 2016. http://webarchive.nationalarchives.gov.uk/20140122145147/http:/www.levesoninquiry.org.uk/.

Chapter 20

Tracking Down and Using Grey Literature

Marianne Sullivan and Mark Patrick Taylor

This chapter examines the use of 'grey literature' to support research on corporations and global health governance (GHG). *Grey literature* is defined as documentation 'produced on all levels of government, academics, business and industry in print and electronic formats, but which is not controlled by commercial publishers' (New York Academy of Medicine 2016). Such literature includes dissertations and theses; government reports; think tank publications; industry documents; studies by advocacy groups; findings of government inquiries, commissions and panels; and raw data produced by government, industry or consultants. Many of these sources have applicability to research on understanding corporations and GHG, but are often overlooked in academic research because they are not subject to peer review, the 'gold standard' in academic published research.

Since the mid-1980s, library scientists and researchers have been debating the role of grey literature in scientific research and have been developing organisational systems for these informational resources so that they are more readily accessible to researchers (Alberani, De Castro Pietrangeli and Mazza 1990; New York Academy of Medicine 2016). The first international conference on grey literature was held in 1993, and since then there have been concerted attempts to organise grey literature in a variety of fields, including through the development of searchable grey literature repositories (Biagioni et al. 2014).

The impetus for making grey literature more accessible has also come from perceived gaps in commercial publishing. For example, the majority of research abstracts accepted for presentation at biomedical conferences are not subsequently published as journal articles (Von Elm et al. 2003). Grey literature may provide the primary source of data for public policy research (Lawrence et al. 2015). In environmental health, many biomonitoring studies are conducted by local or state governments, or consultants, and cannot be identified or accessed through traditional literature searches.

This chapter provides an overview of how to access and use grey literature. It draws on examples from research on the mining and smelting sectors in order to demonstrate how grey literature has been used effectively to study the adverse health impacts from industrial emissions and the policy controversies involved. However, the issues and approaches identified are applicable to the use of grey literature in other research areas.

TYPES OF RESEARCH QUESTIONS USING GREY LITERATURE

There are many research questions relevant to corporations and GHG that can be informed by grey literature. Studies of local problems or issues, which may not be published in national or international journals, are frequently described in grey literature. These could include local environmental impacts of polluting industries, results of environmental or human testing for a particular site and evaluations of local and state public health policies and programmes. Other local studies may inventory and analyse proposed policy measures (e.g. taxes, labelling) aimed at controlling harmful products (e.g. e-cigarettes, tobacco or sugar-sweetened beverages). Such geographically bounded grey literature may, in turn, contribute to case studies across multiple locales aimed at developing generalisable findings and lessons. Grey literature may also contribute insights for studying policy making at other jurisdictional levels, including the role of corporate actors in GHG.

Grey literature is especially suited to researching internal corporate decision making, governmental and regulatory decision making, analyses of power relationships among stakeholders in GHG, policy implementation and studies examining the cost-effectiveness of public health interventions. As well as filling gaps in knowledge, there is a need to study how grey literature itself plays a role in information pathways informing policy making. For example, MacDonald et al. (2012) argue that efforts to understand the 'processes by which scientific information is incorporated into environmental policy decisions' should include the role and influence of grey literature. Other examples of specific types of questions, relevant to corporations and GHG, which can be addressed using grey literature, are the following:

- What specific activities undertaken by corporations have public health and environmental impact?
- What do existing data reveal about their impact on human and planetary health?

- What are the policy debates within regulatory bodies concerning the industry in questions in relation to public health?
- What are the concerns of community members regarding environmental and public health impacts?
- How have government and industry responded to possible environmental and public health issues?
- Have polluting activities exceeded accepted environmental and human health guidelines and has any action been taken?

Finally, for systematic reviews in clinical research, it is customary to identify grey literature to avoid publication bias. This bias arises because studies with statistically significant or clinically favourable results are more likely to be published (Hopewell et al. 2009).

ACCESSING GREY LITERATURE

Because of its diverse nature, there is no single strategy to identify and access all pertinent grey literature. Researchers need to use multiple approaches depending on the types of materials they seek to identify (Von Hendy 2014). There are, however, organised efforts in some disciplines to make the process more efficient. In the United States, the New York Academy of Medicine has been publishing the Grey Literature Report since 1999 with the purpose to 'fill the gaps in peer-reviewed journal articles and published books in the public health literature' (Aiola 2012). The report indexes grey literature relevant to health research and policy in the United States, and its purview is being expanded to include similar grey literature from low- and middle-income countries (Kaplan, Myohanen and Taylor 2011).

In Europe, the Grey Literature Network Services (GreyNet) is working to systematise and digitalise access to European grey literature. An Open Grey Repository has been developed, which includes over 700,000 grey literature references from numerous fields (OpenGrey 2016). GreyNet also maintains the *Grey Source Index*, which lists grey literature databases in different subject areas, and is developing a data archive (GreyNet International 2016). Similarly, Australian Policy Online is a publicly available database of policy and scholarly reports that includes over '30,000 research resources' from nearly 4,000 organisations, primarily from Australia and New Zealand, including grey literature. Full-text resources are made freely available through this service (Australian Policy Online 2016).

Other strategies for identifying grey literature use Internet search engines such as Google Scholar and Infotopia, which can yield unpublished materials. However, given their vast reach, Internet searches may not be the most efficient approach to finding literature for targeted research questions. Some commonly used research databases, for focused searching for grey literature, include Business Source Premier, CINAHL, Ergo Abstracts, PapersFirst, Proceedings First, Scopus, ProQuest Digital Dissertations and Web of Science (Mahood, Van Eerd and Irvin 2014; Von Hendy 2014). Finally, researchers seeking to identify grey literature can consult librarians, with many university libraries publishing general and specialised grey literature guides. In addition, researchers can consult with research, policy or practice experts in their subject area to identify other pertinent grey literature (Mahood, Van Eerd and Irvin 2014).

USING GREY LITERATURE TO STUDY THE MINING AND SMELTING INDUSTRIES

How grey literature can be used

Non-ferrous (e.g. copper, lead and zinc) metal mining and smelting are highly polluting industrial practices that release significant quantities of toxic heavy metals into the environment. Emissions from mining and smelting are associated with adverse impacts on soil, vegetation, habitat, water quality and wildlife (Galbraith, LeJeune and Lipton 1995; Li et al. 2014), and significant public health concerns due to human exposure to heavy metals (Zhang et al. 2012; Mackay et al. 2013; Taylor et al. 2014).

Primary smelting is the process of extracting metals from mined ore. Residents near mining and smelting sites may be exposed to toxic metals through multiple pathways, including ingestion of toxic metals from soil, house dust, locally grown produce and drinking water, as well as inhaled aerosol particles (Li et al. 2012). Given the potential health harms, including lead poisoning in children, there is often considerable controversy about the extent of emissions, contamination and health problems in mining and smelting communities (Taylor and Schniering 2010; Sullivan 2014; Taylor et al. 2015a).

Interdisciplinary case studies, drawing heavily on grey literature that documents site-specific environmental conditions and public health impacts, are critical for addressing environmental and public health threats in affected communities. Local studies can lay the foundation for documenting the global impact of mining/smelting sites and understanding the most effective ways to regulate and control toxic emissions. Researchers studying environmental contamination near industrial point sources will often start by collecting primary data on current emissions and depositions. However, this approach is time consuming and expensive, providing only a snapshot of cumulative impacts. An alternative strategy is to identify, collect and synthesise existing grey literature on the pollution source and health impacts.

This approach could be applied to studying environmental health problems of all types, where there is a point source or multiple point sources responsible for environmental contamination. If a point source of localised and stationary pollution has operated in a particular place for a significant time period, numerous studies from different disciplinary perspectives, examining different aspects of its pollution, are likely. These sources sometimes allow compilation of a more complete record of emissions and pollution impacts. For example, near the Broken Hill lead mine in New South Wales, Australia, human health concerns relating to lead poisoning date to the late 1800s (Thompson 1893). In the Silver Valley of Idaho, United States, site of the Bunker Hill Mining Superfund Megasite, pollution impacts on streams, rivers, drinking water and agriculture have been documented in lawsuits and research dating to the early twentieth century (Casner 1989). Historical documents, detailing the environment at the start of mining activity, can be critical to challenging claims that contemporary contamination is 'naturally occurring', a common argument used by companies to contest responsibility (Kristensen and Taylor 2016).

Beyond environmental health studies, grey literature has wide application to studying corporations and GHG, including studies of policy development and implementation, corporate behaviour and government and community responses to corporate health threats. For example, tobacco researchers have relied extensively on grey literature such as internal industry documents and unpublished industry studies to understand corporate behaviour and the industry's influence on science and public policy (Proctor 2011). Another example of the diversity of uses of grey literature is a recent policy study examining the implementation of a carbon tax in British Columbia (Bumpus 2015). Collectively these studies reveal the utility of grey literature for understanding health impacts arising from activities or products produced by corporations.

Identifying grey literature on the mining and smelting industries

To identify relevant grey literature, the first step is to search holdings in the local library where the industry is operating. Local libraries may contain government or industry documents, or local histories, about the site, and librarians may be familiar with the industry's history. Pertinent databases can also be searched, such as PapersFirst and ProQuest Digital Dissertations.

The second step is to interview regulators, health professionals, local university scientists, environmental consultants and, if legal action has been taken, lawyers who may be familiar with the site. Interviewees may identify and even provide unpublished materials. Regulators may point to unpublished studies of emissions and environmental media. Health professionals may know whether unpublished human biomonitoring studies (e.g. urinary arsenic, blood lead, heavy metals in hair) have been conducted in the surrounding communities. Local/regional university-based scientists may be able to identify student dissertations and unpublished research reports. Similarly, environmental consultants may have conducted, but not published, assessments. When there has been legal action, plaintiffs' lawyers may have commissioned additional studies, or possess documents turned over by the industry, during legal discovery processes, that may cast light on environmental or public health problems.

The third step is to identify archives and agency record repositories where documentation about the site, environmental test results and other studies may be archived. Each country, and sometimes states and localities, will have different rules and procedures for accessing archived government data or active government records. These records are important for establishing the history of regulatory efforts. In the United States and Australia, many agency reports and documents will be available online and identifiable through Internet searches. Older studies are unlikely to be available in electronic format and may require searches at agency or state libraries in person. For example, the US Environmental Protection Agency (EPA) maintains Superfund sites files that are usually accessible at EPA regional offices. Some government records, documents and studies may require a public records or Freedom of Information (FOI) request (see Chapter 19). Once all possible grey literature is identified, information should be organised chronologically, allowing the primary facts to be collated. This will allow data gaps and research opportunities to be identified.

Examples of research on the mining and smelting industries using grey literature

There are several examples of studies using grey literature on mining and smelting point sources. Taylor and colleagues (Taylor et al. 2014, 2015a) used grey literature (air quality data collected by the smelting company and the state government) to investigate and analyse air emissions near the Port Pirie (South Australia) and the Mount Isa (Queensland) smelter in Australia. The researchers found that, despite regulatory standards, emissions from the smelter are a significant ongoing source of contamination and exposure for the local community (Taylor et al. 2015b). A study examining lead mining emissions and the association with decrements in childhood development and behavioural and school performances on Broken Hill children (New South Wales) relied on a mixture of government, industry and newly collected data (Dong et al. 2015). The study revealed overwhelming evidence of the adverse effect on childhood development and school performance due to arsenic-, cadmium- and lead-contaminated exposures via aerosols, dust and soils benchmarked against standardised national childhood development and school performance metrics.

Glass (2003) produced a 'Credible Evidence Report' which laid out evidence, much of it drawn from grey literature, of the American Smelting and Refining Company's responsibility for soil contamination with arsenic and lead in the Puget Sound Region, Washington State. The report synthesises studies by local, state and federal agencies; consulting firms; and university researchers that examine contamination of air and residential and garden soil, as well as other media. Similarly, Sullivan (2014) uses grey literature to intensively study the environmental and human health impact of three smelters in the United States.

STRENGTHS AND WEAKNESSES OF USING GREY LITERATURE

It is increasingly inadequate in academic research to limit literature reviews, systematic reviews and policy studies to published materials. Identifying and analysing grey literature is a necessary and useful tool for studying a range of research questions. In the context of environmental point sources of pollution, grey literature resources offer an underused but critical starting point for research aimed at quantifying their environmental and public health impacts. The monetary value of such studies may be in the hundreds of thousands of dollars, providing more data points than can typically be accumulated in a single, temporally restricted study. This approach is applicable to a variety of point-source industrial facilities (e.g. dairy and pig farms, chemical production), particularly those with a long history of operations. In certain circumstances, analysis of grey literature may be sufficient to mark an end point of the research.

Researchers may disregard grey literature sources because they may mistakenly consider them inferior to their own field data or peer-reviewed research. This rich source of data can provide historical context, a weight of evidence and, sometimes, critical detail often lacking elsewhere. Regarding decision making by industry and government, grey literature often forms the primary source material for regulatory advice, even if it has not been subject to peer review. Validation procedures of regulatory authorities differ from those of academia, but the criteria are similar: independent analysis and reporting and internal and/or external review by recognised experts. Moreover, analysis of grey literature can be typically less expensive because it is previously collected data. Finally, the inherently multidisciplinary nature of a grey literature review will likely yield a more comprehensive picture of the topic under study.

At the same time, there are limitations to using this data source. Grey literature may be hampered by a lack of availability or data in raw form (often presented in graphs or charts). Data may not be continuously collected, using the same methodology, and/or made available to researchers. Another potential drawback is that details of the quality assurance and quality control (QA/QC), or external review, of data are often absent and cannot be retrospectively acquired or verified. Although many such studies use data collected and processed by accredited laboratories, the QA/QC procedures are often not fully described.

In addition, many countries and states did not collect independent environmental data until the 1970s or later. Therefore, industry data may be one of few pre-1970–1980s' data sources, and it may be difficult or impossible to access industry data unless it has been presented as evidence in court. In developing countries, systems may not yet be in place to routinely collect data on emissions and environmental contamination, and there may be fewer resources for conducting environmental and human health studies.

There may also be actual variability in the quality and rigour of grey literature. Pappas and Williams (2011) stress the importance of carefully evaluating 'the accuracy and validity of the information gleaned'. For historical, community-based environmental studies, there might be changes in measurement, changes in location of sampling or changes in accepted methods that can limit comparability of data over time. Moreover, there may be questions about the objectivity of specific studies or assessments. For example, an industry-funded study conducted for internal consumption may be more objective than an industry-funded study conducted for external consumption. Many of these hurdles can be overcome by weight of evidence, especially where findings among separate studies are consistent.

Finally, a major limitation to using grey literature can be the availability of grey literature in the form needed. It can be time consuming to search for, acquire and assemble data needed, particularly if not readily accessible in electronic form. For some populations or communities, there may simply be limited data available, or it may take time and effort to obtain through FOI requests. Industry may itself collect the most data but not make it publicly available. In some cases, industry records used as evidence in court are sealed by court order, making them unavailable to researchers.

CONCLUSION

Grey literature can play an important role in helping to answer many types of research questions concerning corporations and GHG, especially when few published studies exist in the peer-reviewed literature. This chapter discusses how grey literature has been essential for understanding the historical context of contemporary community-level environmental health problems. A broad range of studies have reached beyond primary data collection, to draw upon these additional data sources to contextual interpretation of results, fill gaps in causal explanation and generate a strong evidence base for decision makers. There is significant potential for a wider application of grey literature to strengthen growing research on corporations and GHG.

FURTHER READING

Lawrence, Amanda, Julian Thomas, John Houghton and Paul Weldon. 2015. 'Collecting the Evidence: Improving Access to Grey Literature and Data for Public Policy and Practice'. *Australian Academic & Research Libraries* 46(4): 229–49.

Taylor, Mark, Peter Davies, Louise Kristensen and Janae Csavina. 2014. 'Licensed to Pollute but Not to Poison: The Ineffectiveness of Regulatory Authorities at Protecting Public Health from Atmospheric Arsenic, Lead and Other Contaminants Resulting from Mining and Smelting Operations'. *Aeolian Research* 14: 35–52.

Von Hendy, Matthew. 2014. 'Fifty Shades of Scientific and Technical Grey Literature'. *Online Searcher* 38(3): 60–65.

REFERENCES

Aiola, Danielle. 2012. 'Why Grey Literature?' New York Academy of Medicine, 24 August. Accessed 25 March 2016. http://nyamcenterforhistory.org/2012/08/24/why-grey-literature/.

Alberani, Vilma, Paola De Castro Pietrangeli and Anna Maria Rossi Mazza. 1990. 'The Use of Grey Literature in Health Sciences: A Preliminary Survey'. *Bulletin of the Medical Library Association* 78(4): 358–63.

Australian Policy Online. 2016. 'About Policy Online'. Accessed September 19, 2016. http://apo.org.au/about.

Biagioni, Stefania, Carlo Carlesi, Joachim Schöpfel, Dominic Farace and Jerry Frantzen. 2014. 'GreyGuide – Guide to Good Practice in Grey Literature: A Community Driven Open Resource Project'. *Grey Journal* 10(1): 51–55.

Bumpus, Adam G. 2015. 'Firm Responses to a Carbon Price: Corporate Decision Making under British Columbia's Carbon Tax'. *Climate Policy* 15(4): 475–93.

Casner, Nicholas. 1989. 'Leaded Waters: A History of Mining Pollution on the Coeur d'Alene River in Idaho 1900–1950'. Master's Thesis, Boise State University.

Dong, Chenyin, Mark Patrick Taylor, Louise Jane Kristensen and Sammy Zahran. 2015. 'Environmental Contamination in an Australian Mining Community and Potential Influences on Early Childhood Health and Behavioural Outcomes'. *Environmental Pollution* 207(December): 345–56.

Galbraith, Hector, Katherine LeJeune and Joshua Lipton. 1995. 'Metal and Arsenic Impacts to Soils, Vegetation Communities and Wildlife Habitat in Southwest Montana Uplands Contaminated by Smelter Emissions: I. Field Evaluation'. *Environmental Toxicology & Chemistry* 14(11): 1895–1903.

Glass, Gregory. 2003. 'Credible Evidence Report: The ASARCO Tacoma Smelter and Regional Soil Contamination in Puget Sound, Final Report'. Prepared for Tacoma-Pierce County Health Department and Washington State Department of Ecology. https://fortress.wa.gov/ecy/gsp/DocViewer.ashx?did=5786.

GreyNet International. 2016. 'Grey Literature Network Service'. Accessed September 19, 2016. http://www.greynet.org/greysourceindex.html.

Hopewell, Sally, Kirsty Loudon, Mike J. Clarke, Andrew D. Oxman and Kay Dickersin. 2009. 'Publication Bias in Clinical Trials Due to Statistical Significance or Direction of Trial Results'. *Cochrane Database of Systematic Reviews* (1): MR000006.

Kaplan, Janie, Lea Myohanen and Elizabeth Taylor. 2011. 'Global Grey Literature in Health: Identification, Preservation, and Sustainability'. *Grey Journal* 7(1): 41–44.

Kristensen, Louise Jane and Mark Patrick Taylor. 2016. 'Unravelling a "Miner's Myth" That Environmental Contamination in Mining Towns Is Naturally Occurring'. *Environmental Geochemistry and Health*: 39(4): 1015–27.

Lawrence, Amanda, Julian Thomas, John Houghton and Paul Weldon. 2015. 'Collecting the Evidence: Improving Access to Grey Literature and Data for Public Policy and Practice'. *Australian Academic & Research Libraries* 46(4): 229–49.

Li, Qian, Hongguang Cheng, Tan Zhou, Chunye Lin and Shu Guo. 2012. 'The Estimated Atmospheric Lead Emissions in China, 1990–2009'. *Atmospheric Environment* 60: 1–8.

Li, Zhiyuan, Zongwei Ma, Tsering Jan van der Kuijp, Zengwei Yuan and Lei Huang. 2014. 'A Review of Soil Heavy Metal Pollution from Mines in China: Pollution and Health Risk Assessment'. *Science of the Total Environment* 468: 843–53.

MacDonald, Elizabeth M. De Santo, Kevin Quigley, Suzuette S. Soomai and Peter Wells. 2012. 'Tracking the Influence of Grey Literature in Public Policy Contexts: The Necessity and Benefit of Interdisciplinary Research'. Dalhousie University. http://greynet.org/images/GL14-S2P,_MacDonald_et_al.pdf.

Mackay, A., Mark Patrick Taylor, N. Munksgaard, K. Hudson-Edwards and L. Burn-Nunes. 2013. 'Identification of Environmental Lead Sources and Pathways in a Mining and Smelting Town: Mount Isa, Australia'. *Environmental Pollution* 180: 304–11.

Mahood, Quenby, Dwayne Van Eerd and Emma Irvin. 2014. 'Searching for Grey Literature for Systematic Reviews: Challenges and Benefits'. *Research Synthesis Methods* 5(3): 221–34.

New York Academy of Medicine. 2016. 'What Is Grey Literature'. Grey Literature Report. http://www.greylit.org/about.

OpenGrey. 2016. 'OpenGrey'. Accessed September 19, 2016. http://www.opengrey.eu/.

Pappas, Cleo and Irene Williams. 2011. 'Grey Literature: Its Emerging Importance'. *Journal of Hospital Librarianship* 11(3): 228–34.

Proctor, Robert. 2011. *Golden Holocaust: Origins of the Cigarette Catastrophe and the Case for Abolition*. Berkeley: University of California Press.

Sullivan, Marianne. 2014. *Tainted Earth: Smelters, Public Health, and the Environment*. New Brunswick, NJ: Rutgers University Press.

Taylor, Mark Patrick, Peter J. Davies, Louise Jane Kristensen and Janae Lynn Csavina. 2014. 'Licenced to Pollute but Not to Poison: The Ineffectiveness of Regulatory Authorities at Protecting Public Health from Atmospheric Arsenic, Lead and Other Contaminants Resulting from Mining and Smelting Operations'. *Aeolian Research* 14: 35–52.

Taylor, Mark Patrick, Louise J. Kristensen, Peter J. Davies, Janae Lynn Csavina, A.K. Mackay, N.C. Munksgaard and K.A. Hudson-Edwards. 2015a. 'Omissions about the Sources of Contaminant Emissions and Depositions – A Reply to Comments on Taylor, MP, Davies, PJ, Kristensen, LJ, Csavina, J., 2014. Licenced to Pollute but Not to Poison: The Ineffectiveness of Regulatory Authorities at Protecting Public Health from Atmospheric Arsenic, Lead and Other Contaminants Resulting from Mining and Smelting Operations. *Aeolian Research*, 14:35–52'. *Aeolian Research* 17: 205–13.

Taylor, Mark Patrick and Carolyn Schniering. 2010. 'The Public Minimization of the Risks Associated with Environmental Lead Exposure and Elevated Blood Lead Levels in Children, Mount Isa, Queensland, Australia'. *Archives of Environmental & Occupational Health* 65(1): 45–48.

Taylor, Mark Patrick, Sammy Zahran, Louise Kristensen and Marek Rouillon. 2015b. 'Evaluating the Efficacy of Playground Washing to Reduce Environmental Metal Exposures'. *Environmental Pollution* 202: 112–19.

Thompson, A.J. 1893. 'Report of Board Appointed to Inquire into the Prevalence and Prevention of Lead Poisoning at the Broken Hill Silver–Lead Mines'. Sydney: NSW Legislative Assembly Government Printer.

Von Elm, Erik, Michael C. Costanza, Bernhard Walder and Martin R. Tramèr. 2003. 'More Insight into the Fate of Biomedical Meeting Abstracts: A Systematic Review'. *BMC Medical Research Methodology* 3: 1–11.

Von Hendy, Matthew. 2014. 'Fifty Shades of Scientific and Technical Grey Literature'. *Online Searcher* 38(3): 60–65.

Zhang, Xiuwu, Linsheng Yang, Yonghua Li, Hairong Li, Wuyi Wang and Bixiong Ye. 2012. 'Impacts of Lead/Zinc Mining and Smelting on the Environment and Human Health in China'. *Environmental Monitoring and Assessment* 184(4): 2261–73.

Chapter 21

Legal and Ethical Considerations

Kelley Lee, Benjamin Hawkins and Diego S. Silva

The conduct of research on corporations – particularly to document their effects on global health and to inform the development of effective governance responses – gives rise to a range of legal and ethical considerations. It is important that researchers are cognisant of these considerations at all stages of the research process, anticipate the potential risks arising from them and manage them in acceptable ways. This chapter sets out the main ethical and legal considerations that arise when conducting research in this area, and considers how researchers might effectively address them. In some cases, there are overlaps between the legal and ethical dimensions of the decisions researchers must take, in designing and executing their research. For the purpose of this chapter, we have sought to maintain an analytical distinction between them, while highlighting relevant examples where overlap occurs.

This chapter should be read as a broad overview of these complex issues and does not constitute an exhaustive guide. At the very least, researchers will need to understand specific policies and ethical guidelines set out by the institution(s) within which their research is located, along with the relevant legal jurisdictions where they are situated and/or the research is undertaken. Moreover, funding bodies may have additional guidelines related to ethical dimensions of a project (e.g. data protection), which will need to be considered (see Chapter 22). Finally, there may also be specific challenges arising for individual research projects, which require specialist advice from legal or ethics experts. We hope, however, that this chapter will help readers to be more fully aware of key considerations and to enable critical reflection on how their research (and that of others) is conducted.

LEGAL ISSUES

Legal obligations by corporations to provide access to data

Access to appropriate data can, in many cases, be a major challenge, and corporations may not share information for a variety of reasons. First, corporations may only be obliged to disclose a limited range of information about their activities. For example, in most jurisdictions there are annual reporting requirements and obligations to publish annual accounts. However, the specific content of reports may be imprecisely defined, allowing corporations to present information in ways that are opaque. State-owned enterprises, in whole or part, can be subject to fuller public disclosure requirements such as freedom of information (FOI) (see Chapter 19). Corporations in the private sector, however, are not bound by FOI and other transparency requirements. Some corporations may also be privately owned companies and, hence, not subject to regulatory requirements to disclose financial and other information applicable to publicly traded companies (shares publicly traded in equity markets). In general, the latter must report on assets and operations, management structure and finances as certified by independent accountants (see Chapter 18). Another reason for nondisclosure is the need to keep certain information, known as trade secrets, away from competitors. This includes confidential business information that provides a competitive edge to the firm (e.g. manufacturing processes, ingredients, particular organisational features). Corporations are also permitted to keep undisclosed, and private, information about its personnel or clientele, and interactions with legal counsel (termed *attorney–client privilege*).

Beyond the reporting requirements and protections set out under company law, corporations may be reluctant to provide access to information that may be unfavourable to the firm or specific individuals. In some cases, a company may even claim legal privilege as a pretext. The tobacco industry, for example, has been shown to inappropriately assert privilege and protected status over some internal documents (Ciresi, Walburn and Sutton 1999; LeGresley and Lee 2016). In other instances, a firm may simply not provide information unless it is compelled to do so by law. This information may include financial contributions to charities, think tanks, consultants, scholars and other third parties, which may be relevant to corporate efforts to shape the informational and regulatory environments in which they are active. There may also be a reluctance to participate in key informant interviews, with researchers perceived to be potentially critical of the corporation's activities (see Chapter 11).

Intellectual property rights

Data legally obtained by researchers may be subject to protection under intellectual property rights (IPRs) – copyright, patent and trademark – which restrict their subsequent use. Researchers seeking to study corporate activities may wish to use as data artefacts protected by IPRs, such as marketing and advertising campaigns, print and broadcast media and speech acts. However, corporations may wish to protect the use of such data. For example, research on media coverage of the European Union in British newspapers wanted to reproduce articles and cartoons which appeared in certain publications to illustrate their findings (Anderson and Weymouth 1999). While the material is freely available in the public domain, and easily accessible by the researchers, permission to reproduce them directly was denied by the media corporations. Instead, the researchers gave detailed descriptions of the content in question but were unable to reproduce the images and articles as originally published.

Confidentiality agreements

Corporate employees routinely have access to proprietary information in the normal course of their daily work. This information may include internal correspondence, client lists, business strategies and plans, financial data and market research. A corporation may require an employee to sign a confidentiality or nondisclosure agreement, as part of its terms of employment, to prevent access by external parties. Such agreements require the employee to abide by company rules regarding privacy and confidentiality of proprietary information, including the unauthorised use and provision of such information to third parties, including researchers. Such agreements can extend beyond the period of employment for a specified period, which may extend to several years. Employees who violate such agreements can be subject to legal action by the corporation.

Use of unauthorised data

Data may be obtained from corporations in a number of unauthorised ways, and the decision to use such data for research purposes requires careful legal and ethical consideration. Obtaining data through practices such as wire-tapping, hacking, eavesdropping or bugging devices is strictly illegal and unethical, and should not be used by researchers (Soghoian 2008).

Another potential data source is 'whistle-blowers', or corporate insiders, who might disclose information about corporate activities, including internal company documents, without formal consent. Notwithstanding confidentiality agreements, whistle-blowers act out of concern for illegal, immoral or otherwise illegitimate practices engaged in by their employers. Their intent is to disclose information to individuals or organisations that may be able to address such practices. In many countries, whistle-blowers are protected under law where they act to protect the public interest. The United States adopted the Whistleblower Protection Act (1989) and Whistleblower Protection Enhancement Act (2012) to protect federal government employees who report agency misconduct.

In the private sector, there are few protections available to whistle-blowers. In 1996, Jeffrey Wigand, the former vice-president of research and development for Brown & Williamson (B&W, British American Tobacco's US subsidiary), appeared on US television, stating that the company intentionally manipulated its tobacco blend to increase the amount of nicotine and, therefore the addictiveness, of its cigarettes. Wigand subsequently endured extensive legal and personal pressures to disclose or keep confidential company activities (as portrayed in the film *The Insider*).

Given the limited protection to whistle-blowers, the anonymous leaking of information has become increasingly common. In 1995 another B&W employee, working under the pseudonym Mr. Butts, sent 4,000 pages of incriminating documents to Professor Stanton Glantz and various media outlets. The documents were subsequently used in litigation against the tobacco industry, scholarly papers and the book *The Cigarette Papers* (Glantz et al. 1998). Electronic data storage and communication has also made leaks more possible. Drafts of the Transatlantic Trade and Investment Partnership, currently under negotiation between the United States and the European Union, were leaked to and published by Greenpeace. The documents revealed unprecedented powers to be granted to corporations to challenge policies, including public health and safety regulations, which they deem counter to their interests (Hilary 2016). In 2016, another anonymous source leaked 11.5 million records of offshore and shell companies facilitated by a Panamanian law firm Mossack Fonseca, to the International Consortium of Investigative Journalists (ICIJ 2016). The creation of Wikileaks in 2006 has prompted fierce debate on the legality and ethics of such data, and its potential use for research purposes (Michael 2015, 194). In some instances, there may be obligations to return documents to their legal owners. Some political science journals and scholars decline to publish papers making use of such sources, while other fields have availed themselves readily of their contents. Researchers considering using this type of data are advised to proceed with caution and seek guidance from ethics boards, funding bodies and potentially legal counsel.

Academic freedom

The principle of academic freedom lies at the very heart of the research process. According to the American Association of University Professors (AAUP 1940):

> Institutions of higher education are conducted for the common good and not to further the interest of either the individual teacher or the institution as a whole. The common good depends upon the free search for truth and its free exposition.. . . Freedom in research is fundamental to the advancement of truth.

For researchers abiding by recognised legal and ethical requirements, institutional support is essential to academic freedom. Researchers should clarify what support their institutions will provide them if, for example, a legal challenge is mounted by a disgruntled company or a researcher receives personal threats.

Pressure may be exerted on researchers via their funding sources. Some funding agencies are mandated not to support political activism. In 2014, Stanton Glantz's research on the links between the Tea Party and tobacco industry, funded by the National Cancer Institute (Fallin, Grana and Glantz 2013), was criticised as 'political lobbying paid for by the taxpayer' (Frezza 2013). This led to unsuccessful calls for his funding to be rescinded by vested interests seeking to stifle research critical of their activities (Intemann and de Melo-Martin 2007). The line between political analysis and advocacy concerning research on corporations can be unclear to funders more familiar with basic science and public health interventions.

Similarly, there is evidence that FOI laws (see Chapter 19) are increasingly being used to harass and intimidate researchers and hinder the progress of work (Halpern 2015). The purpose may be to deter them from investigating issues deemed by corporations to be harmful to their interests. With growing awareness of this problem, there are recommendations for universities to clarify their policies on such requests and legislators to review FOI exemptions to protect academic freedoms.

Avoiding defamation

Defamation concerns any intentional and untrue statement, communicated in either physical (libel) or oral (slander) form, which damages a person's standing, reputation or respect. The negative impact may include public ridicule, contempt or other injurious effects on a person in his or her professional or business capacity. Defamation laws are intended to protect persons against such statements or compensate them through awarded damages. For researchers studying corporations, what one is permitted to say or not say, for fear of defamation, varies across national jurisdictions (Falconer 2014). The consequent risk of legal action and associated costs may also have a 'chilling effect' on researchers (Cressey 2013). In some cases, defamation laws 'can be used by people with enough money to pay for expensive legal services as a means of intimidating researchers who have a legitimate interest in matters of public concern' (Ellis 2014, 50). Researchers can reduce the risk of defamation by rigorous attention to the quality of data sources, validation of interpretations, careful recordkeeping and conscious use of language and meaning. Scholars may usefully draw on guides on defamation developed by journalists (see Further Reading).

In an interesting twist, public health researchers in New Zealand announced legal action against an online blogger for using his website to make personal attacks against them and their work (Dudding 2016). The action followed revelations that the blogger, Cameron Slater, had close connections with lobbyists and consultants working for the tobacco industry. It is alleged he published material written by consultants under his own byline (Hager 2014). The legal action is intended to reveal how lobbyists use blogs and other web-based media, which have lower levels of editorial oversight, as a political tactic. Claims and accusations are made on the Internet regardless of their evidence base which, once in the public domain, can be widely repeated and assumed by some to be true. As such, online material can be effectively deployed by corporate lobbyists to discredit legitimate researchers whose work runs counter to their interests. If successful, the legal action seeks to deter or temper similar practices in future, and encourage online readers to critically assess such material. It is notable that this case is also noteworthy, in the context of this chapter, given that the revelations about Slater emerged from emails hacked from his computer (see below).

Undergoing legal review

When a paper under peer review raises potential sensitive legal matters, such as claims of corporate misconduct, an editor may refer the paper for legal review. The review will not only check the efficacy of assertions but also ensure that the burden of proof meets legal requirements to avoid defamation. The latter will require the production of data to the reviewer, which will need to be taken into account when seeking ethical approval. As well as slowing down peer review, the cost of legal review can be prohibitive.

ETHICAL ISSUES

Most discussions of research in the field of corporate actors' research mainly concern the involvement of human subjects in corporate settings. For researchers seeking to study the activities of corporations, where human subjects are involved, there are few ethical guidelines. For example, guidelines by the US Department of Health and Human Services (2009), Council for International Organizations of Medical Sciences (CIOMS 2002) and World Health Organization (WHO) do not cover corporations. Nor does the academic or grey literature address this subject directly. The Canadian Tri-Council Policy Statement: Ethical Conduct for Research Involving Humans (TCPS2 2014) provides some guidance that informs the following sections.

Recognised ethical principles governing human subject research establish a duty of care towards research subjects by protecting them from harm, and securing and respecting their rights and interests through procedures such as informed consent (CIOMS 2002). These principles must be abided by, when involving human subjects, such as when interviewing employees or surveying stakeholders affected by corporate activity. In such cases, the research must undergo evaluation and approval by the relevant ethics review board (ERB) before commencing. In the first instance, this is likely to be in the researcher's home institution, but ERBs in other institutions may also be necessary (e.g. fieldwork location). Appropriate time, funding and expertise to secure ethics approval need to be planned in advance to prevent delays in the research process. While it is beyond the scope of this chapter to address the full range of ethical issues related to research on corporations, the challenges concerning informed consent, and privacy, confidentiality and disclosure are worthy of careful attention.

Informed consent

Informed consent is an ethical and legal requirement for research involving human subjects. This means that the subject must be informed of all aspects of a study so that a decision can be made by the subject whether to participate. To secure consent, the subject should be told about his or her rights; study purpose; procedures to be undertaken; potential risks of and benefits from participating (including risk to reputation, stigma or employment); study duration; how data will be analysed, stored, used and disposed of; who will have access to the data; and what degree of anonymity will be provided (Nijhawan et al. 2013). Options for attribution (e.g. subject's name, company, position, sector), and data collection and use, are included in these terms. Study information should be provided as a summary document to subjects prior to their participation, and subjects should be allowed sufficient time to read and understand the information. Subjects are often requested to complete and sign a consent form confirming their willingness to voluntarily participate in the study, and the terms by which they agree to do so. The WHO's Consent Form Template web page (WHO 2016) provides links to informed consent templates for a number of different types of study designs, and these templates are a useful resource for researchers to draw on in developing their own study consent forms. Importantly, consent is an ongoing process and is thus not merely signing an informed consent form. Study information sheets should provide subjects with the option to withdraw from a study at any point if they so wish.

Informed consent has been strictly applied in the biomedical and health sciences (e.g. clinical trials). For social science researchers, however, the direct transfer of informed consent procedures from biomedical research is not always straightforward and can influence data generated. Telling interview respondents, for example, about the exact purpose of the study can potentially bias their responses. The informed consent process can change how key informants express their positions to researchers or way inadvertently cue them to focus on certain aspects of their experiences over others.

There are instances when participant observation could be undertaken without informed consent. For example, researchers may use participant observation to gather information on corporate behaviour in selected public settings such as industry conferences and meetings. The validity of this method is dependent on the researcher not disrupting or influencing the normal activity of those observed. As such, gaining informed consent (discussed later) can be problematic. Where public presentations by corporate actors are being observed, this can usually be treated as public domain, and thus, informed consent is generally not needed. However, where the researcher poses questions to an individual, such as during a question and answer session, or afterwards in a social setting, the method becomes closer to an interview. The researcher should normally disclose his or her identity and purpose in such cases, and may need to seek informed consent.

It may also not be possible to set out all the potential risks to a subject from participating in a study. While this may be possible in a tightly controlled, clinical trial setting, research on corporations takes place in diverse social contexts where many factors lay beyond the control of the researcher. This makes it difficult to set out all possible risks, and doing so can be off-putting to the subject. Moreover, researchers may be studying illegal activities involving subjects who may themselves be subject to prosecution. In such cases, informed consent is critical to protect corporate employees who may also face retribution for speaking to researchers. Potential subjects should be informed of the risks of participation (e.g. if there is a data breach) and that the corporation in question has not approved the study. A participant must be assured that he or she may withdraw from the study at any point without any penalties or repercussions. Finally, upholding privacy and confidentiality in such instances is critical (see the following section).

Corporations do not need to give their consent to research about them. Indeed, research that might be critical of corporations serves public interest. According to the TCPS2 (2014, 34):

> Where social sciences or humanities researchers seek knowledge that critiques or challenges the policies and practices of institutions, governments, interest groups or corporations, researchers do not need to seek the organization's permission to proceed with the proposed research. If institutional approval were required, it is unlikely that research could be conducted effectively on such matters as institutional sexual abuse or a government's silencing of dissident scientists. Important knowledge and insights from research would be forgone.

This means that the social value of research, that is providing knowledge to serve the public interest, is ultimately what justifies not needing to obtain consent from an organisation, including corporations. This justification extends to research of illegal or potentially illegal activities.

Finally, researchers may decide to seek informed consent from corporate representatives for their study in the hope that data access will be more forthcoming. This may lead to potential collaborations with corporations in undertaking the research. However, collaborating with corporations generally raises concerns about potential conflicts of interest. Based on the tobacco industry's long and extensive history of interference in research and policy, for example, most academic researchers now avoid contact with that industry. However, similar conflicts arise from collaborations with other industries whose interests pertain to the research in question. Despite this, some researchers continue to collaborate with corporations or accept research funding from them, although the dangers of this, as with the tobacco industry, are being increasingly highlighted (Hawkins et al. 2016). Many funding bodies now require detailed conflict of interest declarations to ensure an appropriate arms-length relationship is maintained. A corporation may also seek to prevent publication of findings if harmful to its interests. Where the researcher has been funded by the corporation, or has a close relationship, this can be within its rights. In such cases, the researcher should agree a data sharing or ownership agreement prior to engagement, which protects academic freedom including the dissemination of findings.

Privacy, confidentiality and disclosure

Maintaining the confidentiality of subjects throughout the research process is critical when researching corporations, including when the activities of a corporation are potentially morally or legally illicit. As Palys and Lowman (2000, 163) write, 'Pledging and maintaining strict confidentiality provides the foundation of trust and rapport that allows researchers to gather valid data to promote understanding of the human condition, and provide the basis for rational social policy.' A detailed data management plan (see Chapter 22) forms the basis of this protection, and informed consent should explain the steps researchers will take to protect confidentiality of subjects and data. Finally, since informed consent is a process and not necessarily a signed consent form, it is acceptable to forgo a signed consent form if doing so limits the possibility of disclosure of private information. In such instances, careful dialogue before, during and after research ethics submission with ERBs is critical and should be welcomed.

It is also important, however, for the researcher to be honest about any institutional or personal limitations. While journalists, in many countries, have a legal right to the protection of sources, equivalent rights might not be afforded to researchers. This becomes particularly problematic where mandatory reporting laws create a duty to report by researchers (e.g. subject at risk of physical harm, public security). The scope of such duty varies across jurisdictions, and informing subjects of this duty can have a chilling effect. A researcher should consider beforehand whether the study will collect information of this kind and, if so, the extent to which the researcher is legally permitted and ethically willing to maintain confidentiality. How the study will handle such data must be disclosed to a subject as part of the informed consent process.

CONCLUSION

Research on corporations is an evolving endeavour that requires consideration of a broad range of legal and ethical issues. There is also a need to appreciate variation across disciplines on how to address these considerations. Overall, the challenge is to balance the goals of complying with legal obligations, minimising harm to subjects and producing valid research that serves the public interest. This chapter should be seen as a first step for researchers engaging with these issues in the field of corporations and GHG. Careful attention will need to be paid to these issues, and additional sources drawn upon, to ensure compliance with relevant standards and procedures.

FURTHER READING

Halpern, Michael. 2015. *Freedom to Bully: How Laws Intended to Free Information Are Used to Harass Researchers*. Centre for Science and Democracy, Union of Concerned Scientists. Accessed September 19, 2016. http://www.ucsusa.org/center-science-and-democracy/protecting-scientists-harassment/freedom-bully-how-laws#.V-BqcUf_paQ.

Michael, Gabriel. 2015. 'Who's Afraid of Wikileaks? Missed Opportunities in Political Science Research'. *Review of Policy Research* 32(2): 175–99.

Palys, Ted and John Lowman. 2000. 'Protecting Research Confidentiality: Towards a Research Participant Shield Law'. *Canadian Journal of Law and Society* 21(1): 163–85.

REFERENCES

AAUP. 1940. 'Statement of Principles on Academic Freedom and Tenure, with 1970 Interpretive Comments'. Accessed September 19, 2016. https://www.aaup.org/file/1940%20Statement.pdf.

Anderson, Peter & Tony Weymouth. 1999. Insulting the Public? British Press and the European Union. New York: Routledge.

Canadian Institutes of Health Research, Natural Sciences and Engineering Research Council of Canada, and Social Sciences and Humanities Research Council of Canada. 2014. 'Tri-Council Policy Statement: Ethical Conduct for Research Involving Humans'. Accessed Septmeber 19, 2016. http://www.pre.ethics.gc.ca/pdf/eng/tcps2-2014/TCPS_2_FINAL_Web.pdf.

CIOMS/WHO. 2002. *International Ethical Guidelines for Biomedical Research Involving Human Subjects*. Geneva: Council for International Organizations of Medical Sciences.

Ciresi Michael V., Roberta B. Walburn and Tara D. Sutton. 1999. 'Decades of Deceit: Document Discovery in the Minnesota Tobacco Litigation'. *William Mitchell Law Review* 25(2): 477–510.

Cressey, Daniel. 2013. 'England's Libel Laws Reformed in a Victory for Science Campaigners'. *Nature*, 24 April. http://www.nature.com/news/england-s-libel-laws-reformed-in-a-victory-for-science-campaigners-1.12874.

Dudding, Adam. 2016. 'Public Health Researchers Fighting Back against Lobbyists'. http://www.stuff.co.nz/national/politics/81194202/Public-health-researchers-fighting-back-against-lobbyists.

Ellis, Stephen. 2014. 'Face to Face with England's Libel Laws'. *Socio* 3: 49–62.

Falconer, Sam. 2014. 'Defamation Act 2013: What Scientists Need to Know'. *Times Higher Education Supplement*, 16 January. https://www.timeshighereducation.com/comment/opinion/defamation-act-2013-what-scientists-need-to-know/2010434.article.

Fallin, Amanda, Rachel Grana and Stanton Glantz. 2013. ' "To Quarterback behind the Scenes, Third-Party Efforts": The Tobacco Industry and the Tea Party'. *Tobacco Control* 23(4): 322–31.

Frezza, Bill. 2013. 'National Cancer Institute Funds Tea Party Witch Hunt'. *Huffington Post*, 19 February. http://www.huffingtonpost.com/bill-frezza/national-cancer-institute_1_b_2703072.html.

Glantz, Stanton, John Slade, Lisa Bero, Peter Hanauer and Deborah Barnes. 1998. *The Cigarette Papers*. Berkeley: University of California Press.

Hager, Nicky. 2014. *Dirty Politics: How Attack Politics Is Poisoning New Zealand's Political Environment*. Nelson, New Zealand: Craig Potton Publishing.

Halpern, Michael. 2015. *Freedom to Bully: How Laws Intended to Free Information Are Used to Harass Researchers*. Center for Science and Democracy, Union of Concerned Scientists. Accessed September 19, 2016. http://www.ucsusa.org/center-science-and-democracy/protecting-scientists-harassment/freedom-bully-how-laws#.V-BqcUf_paQ.

Hawkins, Benjamin, Chris Holden, Jappe Eckhardt & Kelley Lee. 2016. 'Reassessing policy paradigms: A comparison of the global tobacco and alcohol industries.' Global Public Health (epub).

Hilary, John. 2016. 'After the Leaks Showed What It Stands For, Could This Be the End for TTIP?' *Independent*, 2 May. http://www.independent.co.uk/voices/ttip-leaks-shocking-what-are-they-eu-us-deal-a7010121.html.

ICIJ. 2016. 'ICIJ Releases Database Revealing Thousands of Secret Offshore Companies'. Washington, DC: International Consortium of Investigative Journalists. https://panamapapers.icij.org/blog/20160509-offshore-database-release.html.

Intemann, Kristen and Immaculada de Melo-Martin. 2007. 'Regulating Scientific Research: Should Scientists Be Left Alone?' *The FASEB Journal* 22(3): 654–58.

LeGresley, Eric and Kelley Lee. 2016. 'Analysis of British American Tobacco's Questionable Use of Privilege and Protected Document Claims at the Guildford Depository'. *Tobacco Control* (epub). doi:10.1136/tobaccocontrol-2016-052955.

Michael, Gabriel. 2015. 'Who's Afraid of Wikileaks? Missed Opportunities in Political Science Research'. *Review of Policy Research* 32(2): 175–99.

Nijhawan, Lokesh P., Manthan D. Janodia, B.S. Muddukrishna, K.M. Bhat, K.L. Bairy, N. Udupa and Prashant B. Musmade. 2013. 'Informed Consent: Issues and Challenges'. *Journal of Advanced Pharmaceutical Technology and Research* 4(3): 134–40.

Palys, Ted and John Lowman. 2000. 'Protecting Research Confidentiality: Towards a Research Participant Shield Law'. *Canadian Journal of Law and Society* 21(1): 163–85.

Soghoian, Chris. 2008. 'Researchers Could Face Legal Risks for Network Snooping'. *CNET*, 24 July. http://www.cnet.com/news/researchers-could-face-legal-risks-for-network-snooping/.

US Department of Health and Human Services. 2009. 'Code of Federal Regulations – Title 45 Public Welfare CFR 46'. Accessed September 19, 2016. http://www.hhs.gov/ohrp/regulations-and-policy/regulations/45-cfr-46/index.html.

WHO (World Health Organization). 2016. 'Informed Consent Form Templates'. Accessed September 19, 2016. http://www.who.int/rpc/research_ethics/informed_consent/en/.

Chapter 22

Developing a Data Management Plan

Natalia Carrillo Botero and Jennifer Fang

Ensuring appropriate management and secure storage of data, through the development of a data management plan (DMP), is important for any research project, but this is especially the case when conducting research involving sensitive information. What is considered 'sensitive' varies by project and should be defined by the researchers at the outset. Typically, this relates to issues of privacy and ethical considerations associated with human subjects' participation in the research. Sensitive items could include, but are not limited to, participant information such as names and other identifying data, interview content (i.e. recordings and transcripts) and preliminary research results in which participants and their responses are identified. There are well-established processes and mechanism for data management and security relating to the involvement of human subjects in the clinical and biomedical sciences. However, these issues are fast becoming a concern for a growing range of social science research, including the study of corporations and global health. Where research on corporations and global health governance (GHG) involves the collection and analysis of sensitive information, developing a plan to ensure appropriate data management and security is critical.

A growing number of funding bodies also encourage grantees to archive and share data to maximise utility to the research community and reduce the duplications of data collection. As a relatively new requirement in many fields, however, the guidance provided by funders on how to comply with their requirements in this area varies from comprehensive guidelines to broad principles of best practice to leaving researchers to develop their own mechanisms. Research teams unfamiliar with data curation practices or digital archiving technologies may find themselves unsure what to do, and whether the structures put in place are adequate. While there are resources and guidance online, the vast majority are focused on biomedical settings and may not be applicable for research projects such as those on corporations and which occur outside the laboratory environment where often qualitative data is collected. Biomedical guidelines may not be helpful or appropriate in dealing with the data management challenges arising in this type of research, or facilitate the specific ways in which researchers in this field engage with their data sets. This chapter aims to serve as a basic guide for developing a DMP for research on corporations and GHG.

WHAT IS DATA MANAGEMENT?

Data management is 'the process of controlling the information generated during a research project' (PennState University Libraries n.d.). This information includes, but is not limited to, the personal information of human subjects, sources of data, raw data collected through fieldwork or desk research and analysis and results. The requirement to control this information, in the context of research, spans the entire duration of the project: from the initial design of the project prior to its formal start to a specified period after the formal end of the project. Many research projects specify during the ethical approval process that they will retain data generated, such as interview recordings and transcripts, for a specific period of time, which may be several years. DMPs, and project budgets, will need to cover this entire period.

It is also important to consider any funding body requirements for data management when planning the data life cycle. For example, the researcher may decide that saving all information on a flash drive in a locked office drawer is sufficiently secure. However, the funding agency may require data to be stored in a secure location with special security protocols. The latter would thus need to be included as part of the DMP, even if the researchers themselves deem it unnecessary.

THE DATA LIFE CYCLE

The first step in designing a DMP is to understand how the relevant information in the project will be produced and used in the project, which is often termed the *data life cycle* (Figure 22.1).

The life cycle of data begins with data collection (creating data). During this phase, it is necessary to consider project methodology and the types of data generated, considering the following:

- What data will be collected: media analysis, document analysis or interview data?

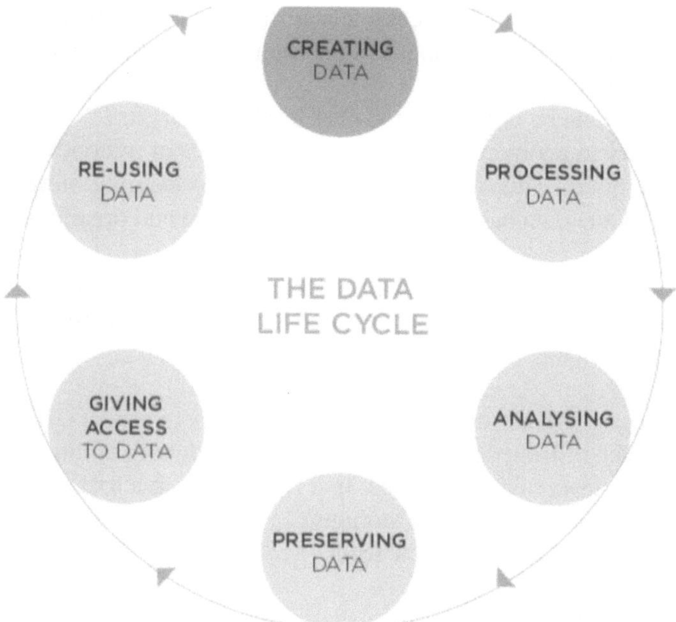

Figure 22.1. Research data life cycle
Source: UK Data Service (2015a).
Reused with permission from UK Data Services.

- Will there be interviews or focus groups? Who are the interviewees (industry informants, government representatives, etc.)?
- How will the data be recorded: as questionnaires, audio recordings, videos, photographs, spreadsheets?
- How will the data be stored: on flash drives, CDs, personal computers and so on?
- How will the data be organised? Creating an organisation system with clear descriptors is the first step in creating metadata (data about data), as it will not only help organise and categorise raw data but also ensure usability by other team members and researchers.

The second step is to consider how to transfer the data from the collection site to the storage site where it will be processed. Details to consider here include the following:

- How will interview audio files or other raw data be transferred: email, flash drive or third-party platform?

- How will the raw data be processed: will the audio files be transcribed? By whom? Who will enter and digitise data from questionnaires into an electronic format?
- How will the data be organised and classified for analysis?
- Is it necessary to anonymise the data, such as names of interviewees? How will this be done? This adds descriptive details to existing metadata, describing how the data has been processed, classified and organised for use.

From here, the life cycle continues into data analysis, where the team starts working on the clean, organised and systematised data. Key aspects to consider are the following:

- Level of access: do all team members need access to all data, or does access need to be restricted for certain data (e.g. the identity of interviewees)?
- How will electronic data be stored: in a flash drive in a locked cabinet in an office or using secure virtual storage?
- How will data be accessed by the team?

With current technology, virtual data sharing mechanisms are readily available from anywhere with an Internet connection. At the same time, these technologies have created new data security risks such as hacking or accidentally making data available to third parties (e.g. by not logging out of a shared server on a public computer). Consequently, there is a need to put in place additional measures to ensure data security when using virtual data sharing mechanisms.

The next stage, preserving data, is of critical importance in the life cycle, as this directly impacts the legacy of the project (Pollard, Mencoiffe and O'Brien 2011). Researchers need to consider which formats are the most suitable to store the type of data generated and where it is going to be stored. The reliability of the data storage site is critical to quality and security of data, and provisions need to be made for storage sites other than personal computers or laptops used by researchers, which can be easily lost or damaged. For this purpose, data should be replicated and/or stored on a separate, secure server that is continuously backed up. The latter also allows easier data sharing than information stored on individual computers.

The next step, giving access to data, is optional and relevant only if it is intended for data to be shared with other researchers. This may be more relevant to the natural sciences, where data sets are more commonly shared. For example, data sets generated by biologists studying a particular characteristic of a species may be shared with and used by another project studying a different aspect of the same species. In clinical research, data can also be shared between teams, but previous consent from human subjects is required.

However, data obtained for social sciences projects can also potentially be shared: if a team studying tobacco industry tactics to influence public policy and promote its products has created a database of key marketing strategies used in the United States in the 1960s, the same material could be valuable to other research teams working on related aspects of tobacco industry activity, such as cigarettes marketing aimed at particular demographics such as children or women. The application of this data could even be extended to other industries, such as the food and alcohol industries (see e.g. Bond, Daube and Chikritzhs 2009, 2010).

The final stage, reusing data, illustrates the importance of maintaining detailed metadata, which is 'data about data', or a brief description of each category of raw data collected. This is critical to ensure reusability of data, especially if the raw data is to be shared with individuals not familiar with the original project and the context of data production. Other uses of metadata include subsequent phases of the project, corroborating findings, comparing with new data or teaching purposes. Reusing data will also be much easier if all previous steps have been followed (see New York University Health Sciences Library 2015). Data sharing is increasingly being recognised as a way to improve efficiency and create better value for money, with some major funders, such as the US National Institutes of Health, introducing mandates to facilitate data sharing with the purpose of 'open scientific inquiry' (NIH 2012).

Table 22.1 summarises the key activities that need to be undertaken at each stage of the data management process.

Table 22.1. Activities for data life cycle steps

Creating data	• Design research • Plan data management (formats, storage, etc.) • Plan consent for sharing • Locate existing data • Collect data (experiment, observe, measure, simulate) • Capture and create metadata
Processing data	• Enter data, digitise, transcribe and translate • Check, validate and clean data • Anonymise data where necessary • Describe data • Manage and store data
Analysing data	• Interpret data • Derive data • Produce research outputs • Author publications • Prepare data for preservation

(Continued)

Table 22.1. Continued

Preserving data	• Migrate data to best format • Migrate data to suitable medium • Back up and store data • Create metadata and documentation • Archive data
Giving access to data	• Distribute data • Share data • Control access • Establish copyright • Promote data
Reusing data	• Follow-up research • New research • Undertake research reviews • Scrutinise findings • Teach and learn

Source: UK Data Service (2015b).

PLANNING A DATA MANAGEMENT STRATEGY

Data management should be addressed at the project planning and grant application stages to allow for the appropriate allocation of resources depending on project needs, institutional support and infrastructure available and funding agency requirements. It is recommended that 5–10% of a project's budget be set aside for data management needs (Pollard, Mencoiffe and O'Brien 2011), such as physical and virtual storage, software and equipment. Early planning is especially important for collaborative projects spread across different geographical settings, involving the sharing of data, or where added measures need to be developed to ensure the anonymity and confidentiality of study participants.

Where the funder has more stringent data management requirements than the project's host institution, the infrastructure and associated resources needed for compliance with the funder's requirement will have to be identified from external sources. For example, compliance with funder requirements to ensure data security requires the use of encrypted secure channels for data transfer, but the service is not available through the researchers' institution. In this case, an external service provider will need to be engaged. The lack of institutional support and infrastructure for data management may be used as the basis to negotiate possible changes in the funder's data protection requirements. While institutions are typically familiar with strict requirements for biological/biomedical research involving patient data or substances which could represent a biohazard (waste or samples of microorganism, virus or toxin), support for social research is often lacking, as the data it generates is often not quantitative and may be considered as a lesser source of hazard. However, library and archival services can often provide suggestions on data storage and analysis. Researchers not affiliated with a higher education institution will need to develop their own organisational guidelines and procedures. Public libraries and online guidelines (see further readings) can support this endeavour.

DEVELOPING A DMP

Once the data management life cycle has been considered, it is necessary to develop a DMP. This is a practical, project-specific tool for systematising, documenting and disseminating data management guidelines. It is important to emphasise that the DMP is a living document systematising best practices at each step of the data's life cycle.

The DMP should cover each stage of the data life cycle set out earlier. It should stipulate very clearly the *what*, the *how* and the *when* at each stage in the project and be agreed upon by all the research teams. While considering the data life cycle helps to identify *what* needs to be done and *how* these measures can be put in place, a plan will create a clear, written strategy to establish this in more detail and set out precisely *when* these actions need to be taken.

A useful exercise prior to developing a DMP is to conduct a risk assessment exercise to identify high-risk areas or weak points in the life cycle of the data. This exercise will encourage researchers to think about the security levels required by different types of data at each stage of the data life cycle. Different models of risk assessments can be found in project management texts (see Watt 2014; Wells and Kloppenborg 2015). Once the types of data and stages of data life cycle have been evaluated, the security requirements can be estimated for different types of data sets by classifying the level of sensitivity of each type of information at each stage. High-risk areas could then be targeted with stronger measures in the corresponding section of the DMP, and researchers can be advised to be especially vigilant in this context. This can be done, for example, by using the Harvard Data Classification Table, part of the Harvard Research Data Security Policy, to more accurately estimate security needs (see Figure 22.2). It should be noted that the higher the risk levels and security protection needs, the greater the need for early resource planning.

Since the DMP is based on the project's data life cycle, its key components are strongly related to the stages of the life cycle. Table 22.2 lists the stages of the data life cycle, key DMP components and sample text (see ICPSR 2012 for full list).

Level	Data Classification and Examples (abridged version)
5	***Information that would cause severe harm to individuals or the University if disclosed.***
Examples	• Research information classified as Level 5 by an IRB or otherwise required to be stored or processed in a high security environment and on a computer not connected to the Harvard data networks • Certain individually identifiable medical records and genetic information, categorized as extremely sensitive
4	***Information that would likely cause serious harm to individuals or the University if disclosed.***
Examples	• High Risk Confidential Information (HRCI) and research information classified as Level 4 by an IRB • Personally identifiable financial or medical information • Information commonly used to establish identity that is protected by state, federal, or foreign privacy laws and regulations • Individually identifiable genetic information that is not Level 5 • National security information (subject to specific government requirements) • Passwords and Harvard PINs that can be used to access confidential information
3	***Information that could cause risk of material harm to individuals or the University if disclosed.***
Examples	• Research information classified as Level 3 by an IRB • Information protected by the Family Educational Rights and Privacy Act (FERPA) to the extent it is not covered under Level 4 including non-directory student information and directory information about students who have requested a FERPA block • HUIDs associated with names or any other information that could identify individuals • Harvard personnel records (employees may discuss terms and conditions of employment with each other and third parties) • Institutional financial records • Individual donor information • Personal information protected under most other state, federal and foreign privacy laws not classified as Level 4 or 5
2	***Information the disclosure of which would not cause material harm, but which the University has chosen to keep confidential.***
Examples	• Unpublished research work and intellectual property not in Level 3 or 4 • Research information classified as Level 2 by an IRB • Patent applications and work papers, drafts of research papers • Building plans and information about the University physical plant
1	***Public information.***
Examples	• Research data that has been de-identified in accordance with applicable rules • Published research • Published information about the University • Course catalogs • Directory information about students who have not requested a FERPA block • Faculty and staff directory information

Need more detailed information? See the expanded Data Classification Table.
Need to talk to an expert? Contact rdsap@harvard.edu for research data and data use agreement questions and ithelp@harvard.edu for all other security questions. Report any data breach to your Help Desk. *Eff. 7.16.13*

Figure 22.2. Data classification

Source: Harvard Information Security (n.d.). Reused with permission from Harvard University.

Apart from the components in Table 22.2, there are some aspects that are applicable across all stages of the data life cycle. It is important to clearly identify roles and responsibilities for each team member, including a central contact person for any data management and security-related questions. For large multi-centre projects, it is recommended that a 'data scientist' be designated, who will have the sole responsibility of managing data (Pollard, Mencoiffe and O'Brien 2011). Second, it is also important to consider ongoing data security, which is especially applicable in long-term projects in order to keep up with technological advancements.

The DMP cannot be 'one size fits all' and needs to be tailored according to the data management needs of specific individual projects. It is advised that each component of the data life cycle is evaluated for applicability and its ability to meet the specific needs of the project. There are two further points to consider when writing a DMP, which apply to all sections of the plan. First, it is essential to *be precise*. Do not write 'data collected will be stored on a hard drive in an office'; instead, write 'data collected will be stored on a password-protected computer and uploaded to a secure database, whose server is located at location X'. Do not write 'data will be collected by research team members', but do write 'data will be collected by Drs X, Y, Z, and supported by a, b, c' (Glenn 2011). Second, be flexible*:* the DMP needs to be flexible in order to be able to respond to the changing needs of the project team. For example, the DMP may require all interviews to be transcribed by a designated transcription agency, but there are some interviews conducted in a language other than those spoken by the agency's transcribers, or with accents that are difficult for transcribers in that location to understand. If the plan does not specify what to do in this case, the designated responsible person (i.e. *data scientist*) needs to evaluate the situation, assess the alternatives available to the project team and expand it to include these situations. Interviews in another language may then be sent to another agency, or be transcribed by a team member/third party, who will be required to comply with data protection measures. Furthermore, as a DMP should be drafted and agreed upon prior to data collection, there may be inherent differences between theory and practice which emerge only during the conduct of the project, so flexibility is needed to adapt procedures and guidelines if they prove to be impossible to follow or insufficient once in the field.

Finally, a DMP itself cannot ensure data security, and only its ongoing and effective implementation by all team members will. All the relevant procedures can be in place, and the resources available to follow the plan, but non-compliance with even one step in the life cycle could compromise data security. If a researcher fails to ensure data is protected on the USB flash drive before transferring it to the central server and the memory is

Table 22.2. Stages and corresponding key components of a DMP

Stage of data life cycle	*Key component of DMP*
Creating data	**Data description** • Nature, scope and scale of data to be generated • Format of data • Designation of sensitive and non-sensitive information Sample text: The project will generate various data from key informant interviews with subjects from industry, governments and advocacy organisations. It will also generate information on key informant identities, primary analysis of raw material and scientific paper drafts. Formats will include audio files, Word files and handwritten notes. All files will be stored on the most appropriate format for Microsoft and Apple users. All files marked 'confidential' are considered 'sensitive data'. *Note*: It is recommended that text data, such as interview records or transcripts, be converted formats used for long-term preservations. At the time of writing,. txt and. rtc are recommended instead of Microsoft Word, and audio recordings are recommended to be stored as. mp3 or. mp4 formats, and. wav or. flac for high-quality recordings. **Metadata** • 'Data about data' • Content and context of data files • Organisation and classification of information to facilitate storage, usage and information cross-reference Sample text: All interviews will be logged into a database with information on date, location, interviewer and interviewee. **Ethics and privacy** • How informed consent will be handled • How privacy will be protected through the life cycle (see Chapter 21) Sample text: The informed consent forms approved by the Ethics Committee will be made available to each informant beforehand. The interviewer should discuss any questions/issues with the informant before proceeding. Audio recording will require formal approval as confirmed by signature by the informant in the consent form. For each interview, the recorded data will have all identifying information removed and will be relabelled with project code numbers. A database which links project codes to consent forms and identifying information will be stored separately from transcriptions and audio files on a secure central data repository.
Processing and analysing data	**Data storage policies** • Where and how to temporarily store data such as during fieldwork • Where and how to store data throughout and beyond project duration

Processing and analysing data	• Who will process the data Sample text: All data will be transferred to, and stored on, a secure central repository hosted by the home institution, which will be regularly backed up. Audio files from interviews will be stored on a password-protected USB flash drive until the researcher can upload it to the central repository. Handwritten notes will be scanned or typed, and then uploaded to the server. Originals will be kept in a locked cabinet accessible only by the researcher. An original file will be deleted from the recording device once the data manager confirms reception of the file. Use of email communication to transfer files will be strictly forbidden. All audio files from interviews will be transcribed by an appointed transcribing agency, which will sign a confidentiality agreement and guarantee secure transfer of files via a safe server. *Note*: You may consider encryption of USB flash drives if the data is extra-sensitive (e.g. data on informant's identity that if disclosed could jeopardise his or her employment situation or put him or her in any danger). If the researcher is not affiliated with an institution that can provide safe storage, private storage providers should be considered. When using a private provider, a careful checking of server locations (as it will determine the legislation that will apply in case of litigation) and the company's level of access to data is needed. Ensure the provider is compliant with privacy legislation and standards in your country/region. The use of free cloud storage is not recommended as these storage options are not secure.
Processing/ analysing data	**Data transfer** • How and where to transfer data to ensure maximum security • Where the weak links potentially might be when uploading to a central repository Sample text: All researchers will have access to the central repository and will ensure login details are kept confidential. Safe Internet connections will be used, and the use of public computers to upload/download data will not be permitted. All personal laptops and computers, where information is to be downloaded or saved for uploading, will be password protected, along with USB flash drives to transport data.
Analysing data	**Data access** • Who will have access to data • How data access will be controlled • Whether a 'gatekeeper' will need to be designated • If access is to be granted on a case-by-case basis, what time period access will be provided Sample text: The project coordinator will be responsible for granting access to data if relevant. Non-sensitive data will be accessible by all team members, but access to sensitive data such as identities of informants will be granted only on a need-to-know basis.
Preserving data	**Data ownership** • If data is stored at a central repository, who the ultimate owner of data will be • What sharing of data ownership there will be with the institution, funder(s), research collaborators, practitioners or service providers of secure storage Sample text: The main grantee will maintain full ownership of all data. Collaborating institutions shall transfer all the data stored by their research teams no later than six months after the end of the project.

Source: Inter-university Consortium for Political and Social Research (ICPSR) (n.d.).

lost, or if personal computers and laptops are not password protected and data is accessed by unauthorised persons, then the whole chain of security is broken.

CRITICAL REFLECTIONS ON THE USEFULNESS OF THIS METHOD IN THESE DISCIPLINES

Research involving corporations and GHG may be particularly sensitive as data generated can contain information about powerful agents – individuals, companies, organisations or institutions. As discussed in this volume, studying these actors implies dealing with spheres of economic and political power and 'digging up' information that does not necessarily support their public persona or that reveals less desirable impacts of their practices. Appropriate management and protection of data within this context is thus vital for the success of the project.

Corporate actors have a history of attempting to discredit scientific evidence to counter results that demonstrate the harmfulness of their practices. Researchers have revealed such practices among the tobacco, alcohol and food industries among others (see e.g. Nestle 2002; Bero 2005; MacCambridge, Hawkins and Holden 2013; Kenworthy, MacKenzie and Lee 2016). Safe storage and effective data management practices can decrease the chances of research results being leaked prior to publication, and the risks of being accused of slander/libel and facing litigation from powerful corporate actors.

In terms of data sharing within the context of GHG research, non-confidential information such as data sets containing public internal industry document analysis, systematic press research data on marketing practices of the food industry, for example, can be used by other research teams or analysed from a different perspective, such as to compare strategies with other industries (Suzuki and Moon 2016). Even within the same industry, data collected for one specific country could be reused in later stages, such as to compare with other countries (MacKenzie and Lee 2016). It could also provide a methodological model of analysis to apply to other industries, organisations, institutions and global governance dynamics not studied before. This can constitute a valuable asset for current and future researchers and knowledge users interested in the field. It could also provide a methodological model of analysis to apply to other industries, organisations, institutions and global governance dynamics not studied before. This can constitute a valuable asset for current and future researchers and knowledge users interested in the field. Permissions and procedures to share (if any), as well as restrictions, must be included in the DMP.

CONCLUSION

Technological advancements are making it increasingly easier to collect, transfer, analyse, store and share data; however, this also exposes researchers to added security risks. Multi-centre research teams can be especially vulnerable due to geographical spread, and GHG researchers are particularly at risk when pitted against powerful corporate actors, or when their research has the potential to damage corporate interests. DMPs are a practical tool that few social scientists are familiar with, and it is suggested as a best practice to manage, identify and address security risks at each stage from data collection to archiving.

FURTHER READING

Corti, Louise, Veerle Van den Eynden, Libby Bishop and Matthew Woollard. 2014. *Managing and Sharing Research Data: A Guide to Good Practice*. Sage. Companion website to the book, UK Data Service: Accessed September 19, 2016. http://ukdataservice.ac.uk/manage-data/handbook.

Inter-university Consortium for Political and Social Research (ICPSR). 2012. *Guide to Social Science Data Preparation and Archiving: Best Practice throughout the Data Life Cycle*, 5th edition. Ann Arbor, MI. Accessed September 19, 2016. http://www.icpsr.umich.edu/files/deposit/dataprep.pdf.

University of California Curation Centre, California Digital Library. n.d. 'DMPTool'. Accessed September 19, 2016. https://dmptool.org/community_resources.

REFERENCES

Bero, Lisa A. 2005. 'Tobacco Industry Manipulation of Research'. *Public Health Chronicles* 120: 200–208.

Bond, Laura, Mike Daube and Tanya Chikritzhs. 2009. 'Access to Confidential Alcohol Industry Documents: From "Big Tobacco" to "Big Booze"'. *Australasian Medical Journal* 1(3): 1–26.

Bond, Laura, Mike Daube and Tanya Chikritzhs. 2010. 'Selling Addictions: Similarities in Approaches between Big Tobacco and Big Booze'. *Australasian Medical Journal* 3(6): 325–32.

Glenn, Jacob. 2011. 'NSP ENG Data Management Plan Template for the University of Michigan College of Engineering'. Accessed September 19, 2016. https://deepblue.lib.umich.edu/bitstream/handle/2027.42/86586/CoE_DMP_template_v1.pdf?sequence=1&isAllowed=y.

Harvard Information Security. n.d. 'Data Classification Table'. Accessed September 19, 2016. http://security.harvard.edu/dct.

Inter-University Consortium for Political and Social Research (ICPSR). 2012. *Guide to Social Science Data Preparation and Archiving: Best Practice throughout the Data Life Cycle*, 5th edition. Ann Arbor, MI. Accessed September 19, 2016. http://www.icpsr.umich.edu/files/deposit/dataprep.pdf.

Inter-University Consortium for Political and Social Research (ICPSR). n.d. 'Guidelines for Effective Data Management Plans'. Accessed September 19, 2016. http://www.icpsr.umich.edu/icpsrweb/content/datamanagement/dmp/.

Kenworthy, Nora, Ross MacKenzie and Kelley Lee, eds. 2016. *Case Studies on Corporations and Global Health Governance: Impacts, Influence and Accountability*. London: Rowman & Littlefield International.

MacCambridge, Jim, Benjamin Hawkins and Chris Holden. 2013. 'Industry Use of Evidence to Influence Alcohol Policy: A Case Study of Submissions to the 2008 Scottish Government'. *PLoS Medicine* 10(4): e1001431.

MacKenzie, Ross and Kelley Lee. 2016. 'Tobacco Industry Strategies to Influence Global Governance in Three Asian Countries'. In *Case Studies on Corporations and Global Health Governance: Impacts, Influence and Accountability*. pp. 159–174, edited by Nora Kenworthy, Ross MacKenzie and Kelley Lee. London: Rowman & Littlefield International.

National Institutes of Health (NIH). 2012. 'NIH Data Sharing Policy and Implementation Guidance'. Accessed September 19, 2016. http://grants.nih.gov/grants/policy/data_sharing/data_sharing_guidance.htm.

Nestle, Marion. 2002. *Food Politics: How the Food Industry Influences Nutrition and Health*. Los Angeles: University of California Press.

New York University Health Sciences Library. 2015. 'Data Sharing and Management Snafu in 3 Short Acts'. Accessed September 19, 2016. http://hslguides.med.nyu.edu/data_management.

PennState University Libraries. n.d. 'What Is Data Management?' Accessed July 13, 2016. https://www.libraries.psu.edu/psul/pubcur/what_is_dm.html.

Pollard, Raymond T., Gwen Mencoiffe and Todd D. O'Brien. 2011. 'The IMBER Data Management Cookbook. A Project Guide to Good Data Practices'. Integrated Marine Biogeochemistry and Ecosystem Research-IMBER Report No. 3, IPO Secretariat, Plouzané, France. http://www.imber.info/index.php/Science/Working-Groups/Data-Management/Cookbook.

Suzuki, Elina and Suerie Moon. 2016. 'Informal Channels of Corporate Influence on Global Health Policymaking: A Mapping of Strategies across Four Industries'. In *Case Studies on Corporations and Global Health Governance: Impacts, Influence and Accountability*. pp. 73–88, edited by Nora Kenworthy, Ross MacKenzie and Kelley Lee. London: Rowman & Littlefield International.

UK Data Service. 2015a. 'Research Data Lifecycle'. Accessed September 19, 2016. https://www.ukdataservice.ac.uk/manage-data/lifecycle.

UK Data Service. 2015b. 'Create and Manage Data'. Accessed September 19, 2016. http://www.data-archive.ac.uk/create-manage/life-cycle.

Watt, Adrienne. 2014. *Project Management*. Victoria, BC: BCcampus, BC Open Textbook Project.

Wells, Kathryn and Timothy Kloppenborg. 2015. *Project Management Essentials*. New York: Business Expert Press.

Index

About the Contributors

CO-EDITORS

Kelley Lee

Kelley Lee is Tier 1 Canada Research Chair in Global Health Governance in the Faculty of Health Sciences, Simon Fraser University. She is a fellow of the UK Faculty of Public Health and Canadian Academy of Health Sciences. Her research focuses on the need for collective action to address the public health impacts of globalisation. Her most recent books include *Global Health and International Relations* (2012 with Colin McInnes), *Transformations in Global Health Governance* (2014 with Colin McInees and others) and *Case Studies on Corporations and Global Health Governance* (2016 with Nora Kenworthy and Ross McKenzie).

Benjamin Hawkins

Benjamin Hawkins is lecturer in global health policy at the London School of Hygiene and Tropical Medicine. His current research concerns the role of research evidence and corporate actors in health policy making at the national and global levels in particular, focusing on the global alcohol and tobacco industries. Prior to entering academia he worked in sales and marketing for the alcohol producer Diageo.

CONTRIBUTORS

Michelle Carnegie

Michelle Carnegie is a research fellow in the School of Environmental and Rural Science at the University of New England, in Armidale, Australia. She is a human geographer who conducts research on rural livelihoods and development in Southeast Asia and the Pacific. Previous to her current position, Michelle held lecturing appointments at Macquarie University and the Australian Catholic University in Sydney, where she taught undergraduate development studies.

Natalia Carrillo Botero

Natalia Carrillo Botero holds a degree in anthropology from the University of the Andes in Colombia and sociology from the Post-Graduate Institute of Latin American Studies (IHEAL), University of Paris III, in France. Her research interests have been largely in rural development and social movements in Latin America, but have expanded to global health through work in in France, the United Kingdom and now Canada. She is currently a member of the Global Tobacco Control Research Programme based at Simon Fraser University, Canada.

Rebecca Cassidy

Rebecca Cassidy is professor of anthropology at Goldsmiths, University of London. She has written on kinship, class and thoroughbred breeding in the horseracing industries of Newmarket and Kentucky. She has conducted fieldwork in the United Kingdom with gamblers and members of the gambling industries since 1996. Her recent work, supported by the European Research Council, focuses on the production and circulation of knowledge about gambling.

Brandon Barclay Derman

Brandon Barclay Derman is assistant professor of environmental studies, University of Illinois at Springfield. He researches and teaches in the areas of environmental and natural resource policy and politics, political ecology, socio-legal studies and geographic information systems/science. His recent work has appeared in the *Annual Review of Law and Social Science*, *Climate Policy* and the *South African Journal on Human Rights*.

Jappe Eckhardt

Jappe Eckhardt is lecturer in politics and international relations at the University of York. His research and teaching interests are in the fields of international political economy, international organisations, global governance and economic regionalism. His research to date has focused on trade politics, the role and influence of non-state actors in (economic) policy making and the political economy of global value chains. His works have been published in *Global Public Health*; *Journal of Common Market Studies*; *Journal of European Public Policy*; *Journal of International Constitutional Law*; *Journal of World Trade* and *World Trade Review*. He is also the author of the book *Business Lobbying and Trade Governance: The Case of EU-China Relations* (2015).

Jennifer Fang

Jennifer Fang has a degree in nutritional science from the University of British Columbia and is currently pursuing a master of public health at the University of Liverpool. She is a part of the Global Tobacco Control Research Programme at Simon Fraser University, Canada. Prior to joining SFU, Jennifer worked in the field of China–Africa health cooperation in Beijing, China. She is co-author of *A Historical Dictionary of the World Health Organization* (2012).

Kevin Farnsworth

Kevin Farnsworth is reader in comparative and global social policy, University of York. He is founder and co-editor of the *Journal of International and Comparative Social Policy*, and has published widely on corporate power, corporate welfare and social policy. His most recent books include *Social versus Corporate Welfare* (2012), *Social Policy in Challenging Times* (edited with Zoe Irving) and *Social Policy in Times of Austerity* (edited with Zoe Irving).

Becky Freeman

Becky Freeman is an NHMRC early career research fellow at the School of Public Health, University of Sydney. Her primary research interests include tobacco control, obesity prevention and how online and social media influence public health. Prior to pursuing her research interests in Australia, Becky worked for both government and not-for-profit organisations in Canada and New Zealand.

Chris Holden

Chris Holden is reader in international social policy at the University of York, United Kingdom. He has published widely on the relationships between the global economy, transnational corporations and health and social policy. He has been a member of the editorial board of the *Journal of Social Policy* and of the international advisory board of the journal *Global Social Policy*. He co-edited *The Global Social Policy Reader* (2009) and *Social Policy Review* (2009–2011).

Nora J. Kenworthy

Nora J. Kenworthy is assistant professor in the School of Nursing and Health Studies at the University of Washington Bothell. Her research focuses on global health governance, corporate social responsibility and the politics of HIV treatment in southern Africa. She is author of the forthcoming book *Mistreated: The Political Consequences of the Fight against AIDS in Lesotho* and co-editor, with Richard Parker, of *HIV Scale-Up and the Politics of Global Health* (2014).

Stephen Kline

Stephen Kline is professor at the School of Communication, Simon Fraser University, Canada. His research interests include advertising, children's media and culture, audience research, public health campaigns and non-broadcast video designs and uses. His published work includes numerous journal articles, book chapters and books including *Globesity, Food Marketing and Family Lifestyles.*

Alexandra Mack

After earning her BA, cum laude in English from Carleton College, Alex spent 15 years in the private sector working in the food industry. While in these jobs she became interested in food as a social justice issue and moved her focus from profits to social change. She earned Master degrees in public health (MPH) and urban planning (MPL) from the University of Southern California in 2016.

Ross MacKenzie

Ross MacKenzie is lecturer in the Department of Psychology at Macquarie University in Sydney, Australia. His research interests include the implications of global expansion of the tobacco industry, global health governance and medicalisation of smoking cessation. He has previously worked at the Centre for Global Change and Health at the London School of Hygiene &

Tropical Medicine where he received his PhD; School of Public Health, University of Sydney; and Action on Smoking and Health (ASH) Thailand.

Raymond Michalowski

Raymond Michalowski is a sociologist and Arizona Regent's Professor in Criminology and Criminal Justice at Northern Arizona University. He is the author of *Order, Law and Crime*, *Run for the Wall: Remembering Vietnam on a Motorcycle Pilgrimage*, *State-Corporate Crime: Wrongdoing at the Intersection of Business and Politics* and over 50 articles and chapters on the political economy of crime and justice. His current research projects explore the evolving political economy of corporate power under neoliberalism, the cultural foundations of contemporary conflicts over immigration and the future of human rights in a changing geopolitical environment.

Richard G. Parker

Richard G. Parker is a medical anthropologist. His research focuses on the social and cultural construction of gender and sexuality; the social and political aspects of HIV/AIDS; and the relationship between social inequality, stigma, discrimination and the social determinants of health. He is especially well known for his work on the politics of global health and on the role of social movements and community mobilisation in responding to public health challenges. Dr. Parker has conducted long-term research in Brazil since the early 1980s, as well as comparative studies in Asia, Africa, North America and other parts of Latin America and the Caribbean. He is the author of more than 200 publications, and his recent books include *Sexuality, Health and Human Rights*, *The Routledge Handbook on Global Public Health* and *Structural Approaches in Public Health.*

Diego S. Silva

Diego Silva is assistant professor at the Faculty of Health Sciences, Simon Fraser University, specialising in bioethics and public health ethics. His main research project currently focuses on ethical and political challenges related to tuberculosis, including new technologies. He also works with the World Health Organization on broader topics related to health ethics. Former projects focus on global health ethics and governance issues related to transnational research.

Michael Stevenson

Michael Stevenson is lecturer at the University of Waterloo and a research fellow at the Balsillie School of International Affairs. His research relates to governance innovation focused on meeting the health needs of marginalised populations and the implications of the rise of private authority in domains long associated exclusively with state stewardship.

Marianne Sullivan

Marianne Sullivan received her doctorate in public health from the Department of Sociomedical Sciences, Mailman School of Public Health at Columbia University. She is currently associate professor of public health at William Paterson University of New Jersey. Her book *Tainted Earth: Smelters, Public Health and the Environment* was published in 2014. She has also published numerous papers on occupational and environmental health and community-based research.

Mark Taylor

Mark Taylor is professor of environmental science at Macquarie University, Sydney, Australia. His main research, teaching and consulting interests are in environmental health. His research programme investigates environmental pollution and risks to human health from aerosols, dust, sediments, soil and water. He has published more than 200 research papers and research reports. He provides expert evidence and advice to government, industry, lawyers and community on a range of environmental matters, particularly environmental pollution. In October 2015, he was appointed by the environment minister of New South Wales to review NSW EPA's management of contaminated sites.

William H. Wiist

William H. Wiist holds a Courtesy Faculty appointment in International Health at Oregon State University. Prior to retirement, he was professor and senior scientist at Northern Arizona University. He edited and co-authored *The Bottom Line or Public Health* (2010). He conducted community-based research on the prevention of heart disease, cancer and violence in African-American, Latino and Native American communities. His course teaching included corporations and health, and economic globalisation and health. His recent policy publications focus on public health's role in the prevention of war.

Heather Wipfli

Heather Wipfli is assistant professor in the Department of Preventative Medicine at the Keck School of Medicine at the University of Southern California (USC) and associate director for the USC Institute for Global Health. Her research focuses on international cooperation and governance approaches to improve health, specifically in regard to global chronic disease control, including tobacco use, obesity and exposure to air pollution. Dr. Wipfli previously directed research and training for the Institute for Global Tobacco Control at the Johns Hopkins Bloomberg School of Public Health and worked on the development of the Framework Convention on Tobacco Control as technical officer at the World Health Organization, Geneva. She has published work on global tobacco control, globalisation and health, capacity building in low- and middle-income countries and health security. Dr. Wipfli's book *The Global War on Tobacco* was published in 2015.

www.ingramcontent.com/pod-product-compliance
Ingram Content Group UK Ltd.
Pitfield, Milton Keynes, MK11 3LW, UK
UKHW012036150926
475560UK00001B/31

9 781783 483594